UroGynecology Simplified

UroGynecology Simplified

Editors

Nandita Palshetkar
MD FCPS FICOG FRCOG (UK)
Scientific Director, Bloom IVF, Mumbai
Professor
Department of Obstetrics and Gynecology
Dr DY Patil Medical College,
Hospital and Research Centre
Navi Mumbai, Maharashtra, India
President, FOGSI (2019–20)
President, AMOGS (2018–20)
President, IAGE (2017–18)
Chairperson, MSR (2017–18)

Shakir Tabrez Z
MS (General Surgery) MCh (Urology)
FICS FIAGES Dip in MAS (Urology)
Dip in Robotic Surgery (Lorraine University, France)
Senior Consultant – Urology, Uro-Oncology,
Andrology, Kidney Transplant and
Robotic Surgery
Fortis Hospitals
Bengaluru, Karnataka, India

Co-Editors

Rubina Shanawaz Z
MS (Obs & Gyn) FICS CU DRM (Germany)
Consultant – Urogynecology, Gynec Endoscopy,
and Robotic Surgery
Fortis Hospitals
Bengaluru, Karnataka, India

Selvapriya Saravanan
MD (Obs & Gyn) FICOG DRM (Kiel)
Fellow in Fetal Medicine (MGR Univ)
Director
SPring Fertility Fetocare Fetogene Centre
Kanyakumari, Tamil Nadu, India

Forewords
S Shantha Kumari
Hrishikesh D Pai

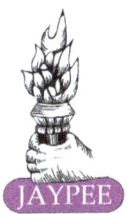

JAYPEE BROTHERS MEDICAL PUBLISHERS
The Health Sciences Publisher
New Delhi | London

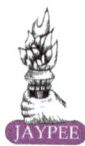 **Jaypee Brothers Medical Publishers (P) Ltd**

Headquarters
Jaypee Brothers Medical Publishers (P) Ltd
EMCA House, 23/23-B
Ansari Road, Daryaganj
New Delhi 110 002, India
Landline: +91-11-23272143, +91-11-23272703
+91-11-23282021, +91-11-23245672
Email: jaypee@jaypeebrothers.com

Corporate Office
Jaypee Brothers Medical Publishers (P) Ltd
4838/24, Ansari Road, Daryaganj
New Delhi 110 002, India
Phone: +91-11-43574357
Fax: +91-11-43574314
Email: jaypee@jaypeebrothers.com

Overseas Office
JP Medical Ltd
83 Victoria Street, London
SW1H 0HW (UK)
Phone: +44 20 3170 8910
Fax: +44 (0)20 3008 6180
Email: info@jpmedpub.com

Website: www.jaypeebrothers.com
Website: www.jaypeedigital.com

© 2022, Jaypee Brothers Medical Publishers

The views and opinions expressed in this book are solely those of the original contributor(s)/author(s) and do not necessarily represent those of editor(s) of the book.

All rights reserved. No part of this publication may be reproduced, stored or transmitted in any form or by any means, electronic, mechanical, photocopying, recording or otherwise, without the prior permission in writing of the publishers.

All brand names and product names used in this book are trade names, service marks, trademarks or registered trademarks of their respective owners. The publisher is not associated with any product or vendor mentioned in this book.

Medical knowledge and practice change constantly. This book is designed to provide accurate, authoritative information about the subject matter in question. However, readers are advised to check the most current information available on procedures included and check information from the manufacturer of each product to be administered, to verify the recommended dose, formula, method and duration of administration, adverse effects and contraindications. It is the responsibility of the practitioner to take all appropriate safety precautions. Neither the publisher nor the author(s)/editor(s) assume any liability for any injury and/or damage to persons or property arising from or related to use of material in this book.

This book is sold on the understanding that the publisher is not engaged in providing professional medical services. If such advice or services are required, the services of a competent medical professional should be sought.

Every effort has been made where necessary to contact holders of copyright to obtain permission to reproduce copyright material. If any have been inadvertently overlooked, the publisher will be pleased to make the necessary arrangements at the first opportunity. The **CD/DVD-ROM** (if any) provided in the sealed envelope with this book is complimentary and free of cost. **Not meant for sale.**

Inquiries for bulk sales may be solicited at: jaypee@jaypeebrothers.com

UroGynecology Simplified

First Edition: **2022**

ISBN: 978-93-5465-205-9

Dedicated to

*Our parents and teachers for guiding and
encouraging us to keep learning and growing*

Our patients for their unshakeable trust and faith in us

Contributors

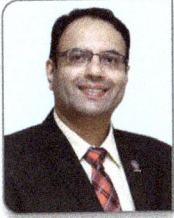

Ameya C Purandare MD DNB FCPS DGO DFP MNAMS FICMCH FICOG
Fellowship in Gyn Endoscopy (Germany)
Consultant (Obstetrics and Gynecology)
Purandare Hospital, KJ Somaiya Medical College and Research Centre,
Sir HN Reliance Foundation Hospital and Research Centre, Bhatia Hospital,
Masina Hospital, Mumbai Police Hospital
Mumbai, Maharashtra, India
2nd Vice President Elect, AMOGS (2022–24)
Joint Secretary, FOGSI (2019)
Peer Reviewer, Journal of Obstetrics and Gynaecology of India

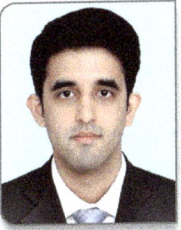

Anuj Thakre MBBS
Consultant
Welcare Speciality Hospital
Ahmedabad, Gujarat, India

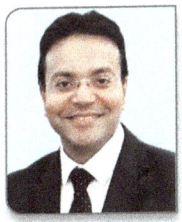

Ashish Kale MD DNB MNAMS FICOG FICMCH
IVF Consultant and Laparoscopic Surgeon
Director
Ashakiran Hospitals and Asha IVF Centers
Pune, Maharashtra, India

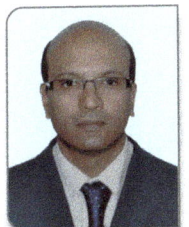

Ashwin Shetty MD (Obs & Gyn) MRCOG FRCOG CCST
Consultant – Obstetrics, Gynecology and Urogynecology
Sir HN Reliance Foundation Hospital and Research Centre
Mumbai, Maharashtra, India

Contributors

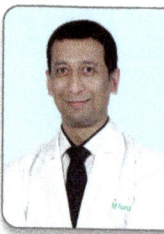

Basavaraj Neelagar MBBS MS (General Surgery) DNB (Urology)
Consultant – Urology, Uro-Oncology, Andrology, Renal Transplant and Robotic Surgery
Fortis Hospitals
Bengaluru, Karnataka, India
Visiting Specialist
Aster Al Raffah Hospital, Ghubra
Muscat, Oman

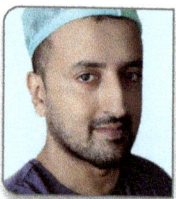

Bimal M John MS FMIGS (France)
Senior Laparoscopic Surgeon and IVF Specialist
Credence Hospital
Thiruvananthapuram, Kerala, India

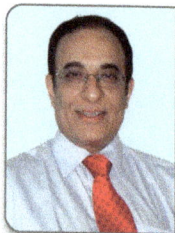

Chander P Lulla MD DMRD
Consultant, Sonologist and Fetal Medicine Specialist
Head, Department of Ultrasound
Jaslok Hospital, Mumbai
Consultant, Department of Ultrasound
Sir HN Reliance Foundation Hospital and Research Centre, Mumbai
Consultant, Ria Clinic
Mumbai, Maharashtra, India

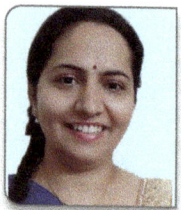

Deepa Chaudhary MBBS MS (Obs & Gyn) FMAS (Hysteroscopic and Laparoscopy) Dip Urogyne (GERMANY) FARM (IVF)
Associate Professor
Department of Obstetrics and Gynecology
SMS Medical College
Jaipur, Rajasthan, India

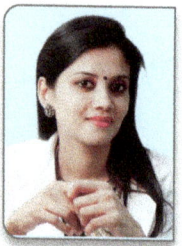

Deepa Ganesh MBBS MS FMAS DMAS FICRS FIMA Dip in MIS (Germany) Dip in ALS (France) Dip in ACG (USA) FIMSA Fellowship in Robotics (USA)
Gynecologist, Advanced Laparoscopic and Robotic Surgeon,
Cosmetic Gynecologist, and Vaginal Laser Surgery Specialist
Founder and Director, Laser Vaginal Rejuvenation Institute of India (LVRII)
DG Laser and Cosmetic Gynecology Clinic
Chennai, Tamil Nadu, India

Contributors ix

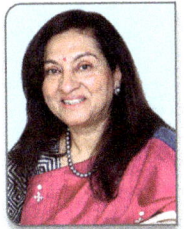

Jaideep Malhotra MD FICMCH FICOG FICS FMAS FIAJAGO FRCOG FRCPI
Managing Director (ART)
Rainbow IVF Hospital, Agra, Uttar Pradesh, India
Professor, Dubrovnik International University, Croatia
Imm Past President, IMS
President Elect, SAFOMS (2019–2021); President Elect, ISPAT
Editor-in-Chief, SAFOMS and SAFOG Journal
Member, FIGO, Reproductive Endocrinology and Infertility
Member, FIGO, RDEH
Regional Director of South Asia Ian Donald School of Ultrasound
Vice President, ISARM

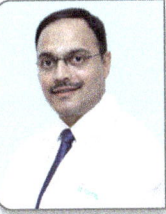

Karthik Rao MBBS MS MCh (Urology) DNB (Genitourinary Surgery)
Consultant – Urology, Uro-Oncology, Andrology and Renal
Transplant Surgery
Fortis Hospitals
Bengaluru, Karnataka, India

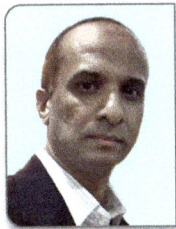

Kiran Ashok MS (Obs & Gyn) Fellowship in Urogynecology
Consultant – Gynecology and Urogynecology
ESIC Hospital, Peenya
Bengaluru, Karnataka, India

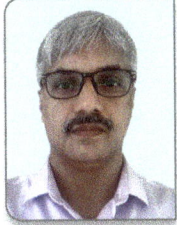

Madhusudhan Naidu MBBS DGO MRCOG CCST (Urogynecology, London)
Director and Consultant – Urogynecology
Gynaaecare
Bengaluru, Karnataka, India

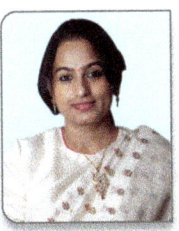

Mala Raj MBBS DGO FICOG Dip in Advanced Endoscopic Surgery (Germany, France, Taiwan)
Dip in Reproductive Medicine (Germany) Fellowship in Aesthetic Gynecology (USA)
Managing Director
Firm Hospitals
Chennai, Tamil Nadu, India

Contributors

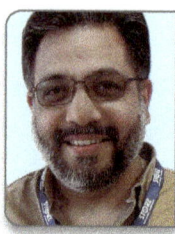

Manish Machave MD DNB MNAMS LLB Dip in Endoscopy (Germany)
Adv Dip in Gyn Endoscopy (France) ISSA (Italy)
Director and Consultant
Machave Hospital—Center for High Risk Pregnancy and Advanced Endoscopy, Pune
Consultant Endoscopist and Postgraduate Teacher
Ruby Hall Clinic, Kamla Nehru Hospital
Pune, Maharashtra, India

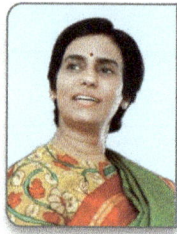

Manjula Anagani MD FICOG
Padmashree Awardee
Clinical Director and Head
Department of Obstetrics and Gynecology
Care Hospitals
Hyderabad, Telangana, India

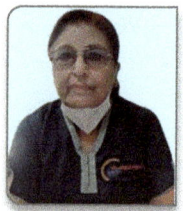

Manpreet Sharma MBBS MS (Obs & Gyn)
Consultant
Department of Obstetrics and Gynecology
Rainbow Hospital
Agra, Uttar Pradesh, India

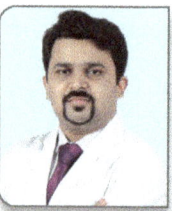

Mohan Balaiah Aswathaiya MBBS MS DNB (Urology)
Consultant – Urology, Andrology and Kidney Transplant Surgery
Fortis Hospitals
Bengaluru, Karnataka, India

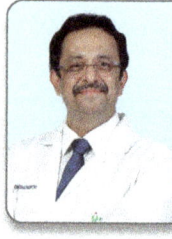

Mohan Keshavamurthy MBBS MS MCh (Urology) FRCS(C) FASTS FICS Fellowship in Trans Surg (Canada) Fellowship in Urogyn Onc (TMH, Mumbai) Dip in Robotic Surgery (France)
Director – Urology, Uro-Oncology, Urogynecology, Andrology, Transplantation and Robotic Surgery
Fortis Hospitals, Bengaluru, Karnataka, India
Visiting Consultant – Urology
Aster Al Raffah Hospital, Oman
Norvik Hospital, Uganda

Contributors xi

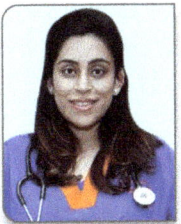

Molina Patel MD Dip RM MRCOG
Consultant
Akanksha Hospital and Research Institute, Anand
Assistant Professor, Shree Krishna Hospital and Medical Research Center
Anand, Gujarat, India
Fellow in Aesthetic Gynecology, IAAGSW, London School of Medicine

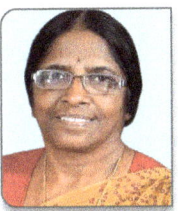

N Rajamaheswari MD DGO MCh (Urology)
Director, Urogynecology Research Center, Chennai
Consultant, Department of Urogynecology
Chennai Urology and Robotics Institute
Chennai, Tamil Nadu, India
President, Urogynecology and Reconstructive Pelvic Surgery Society of India (URPSSI)

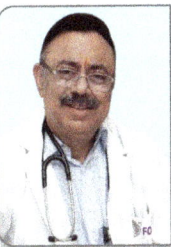

Narendra Malhotra MD FICOG FICS FRCOG FMAS FIAP FICMCH
Managing Director
Global Rainbow Health Care and MNMH (P) Ltd, Agra, Uttar Pradesh, India
Professor, Sarajevo School of Science and Technology, Croatia
President, INSARG
Past President, FOGSI/IFUMB/ISPAT/ISAR
Vice President, WAPM/SAFOG

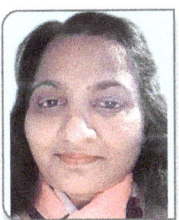

Neeta Mishra MBBS MD (Obs & Gyn)
Consultant
Department of Obstetrics and Gynecology
Director
Nitya Maternity and Nursing Home
Ahmedabad, Gujarat, India

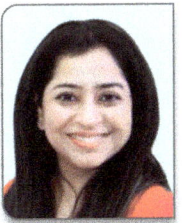

Neharika Malhotra MD (Obs & Gyn) DRM (Germany) ICOG
Fellowship in Reproductive Medicine and Ultrasound
Infertility Consultant
Rainbow IVF
Agra, Uttar Pradesh, India

Contributors

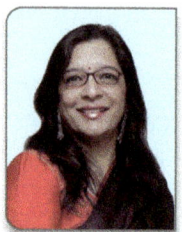

Nita Thakre MD
Gynecologist, Obstetrician and Urogynecologist
Director, Welcare Speciality Hospital, Ahmedabad
Senior Consultant, KD Hospital
Ahmedabad, Gujarat, India
Hon Joint Secretary, AOGS (2021-22)
West Zone Coordinator, FOGSI (2020-21)
Chairperson, FOGSI Urogynaecology Committee (2017-19)

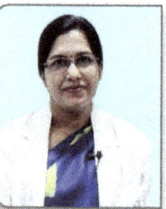

Prabha Agrawal MD FICOG FMAS
Senior Consultant
Department of Obstetrics and Gynecology
Care Hospitals
Hyderabad, Telangana, India

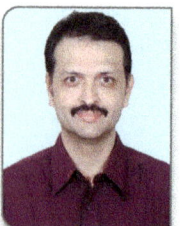

Prashanth K Adiga MD
Professor
Department of Obstetrics and Gynecology
Kasturba Medical College (KMC), Manipal
Manipal Academy of Higher Education (MAHE) University
Manipal, Karnataka, India

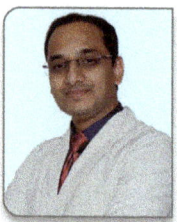

Premkumar Krishnappa MS (General Surgery) DNB (Genitourinary Surgery)
Consultant
Urologist, Urogynecologist, Andrologist, Uro-Oncologist,
Robotic and Renal Transplant Surgeon
Fortis Hospitals
Bengaluru, Karnataka, India

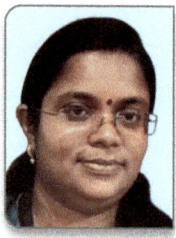

Raji S MS DNB DGO
Consultant Gynecologist
Credence Hospital
Thiruvananthapuram, Kerala, India

Contributors xiii

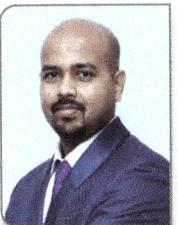

Ramesh Hanumegowda MS MCh (Urology)
Consultant – Urology, Andrology and Renal Transplant Surgery
Fortis Hospitals
Bengaluru, Karnataka, India

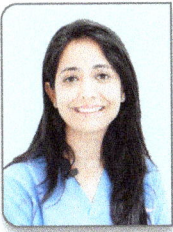

Ritu Hinduja MD MRM (UK) DRM (Germany) FICOG Fellowship in Reproductive Medicine (India, Spain, Israel) Certificate in Genetic Counseling
Senior Consultant
Fertility Specialist
Nova IVF Fertility Center
Mumbai, Maharashtra, India

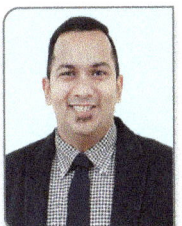

Rohan Palshetkar MS (Obs & Gyn) FRM DRME (Germany) ADRM (Germany)
ART Consultant and Endoscopic Surgeon
Associate Professor, DY Patil Medical College, Hospital and Research Centre
Unit Head, DY Patil Bloom IVF, Navi Mumbai
Consultant, Department of Obstetrics and Gynecology
Surya Hospitals, Breach Candy Hospital Trust
Palshetkar Patil Nursing Home
Mumbai, Maharashtra, India

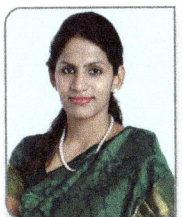

Rubina Shanawaz Z MS (Obs & Gyn) FICS CU DRM (Germany)
Consultant – Urogynecology, Gynec Endoscopy and
Robotic Surgery
Fortis Hospitals
Bengaluru, Karnataka, India

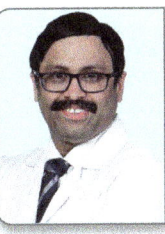

Santosh Kumar Subudhi MBBS MS DNB (Urology)
Consultant – Urology, Uro-Oncology, Andrology, Urogynecology and
Kidney Transplant Surgery
Fortis Hospitals, Bengaluru
Visiting Consultant, Jayashree Multispeciality Hospital, Bengaluru, Karnataka
Teja Nursing Home, Hindupur, Andhra Pradesh
Chirayu Hospital, Gulbarga, Karnataka, India

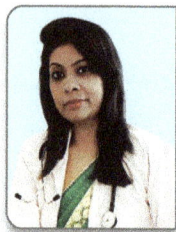
Selvapriya Saravanan MD OG FICOG DRM (Kiel) Fellow in Fetal Medicine (MGR Univ)
Director
SPring Fertility Fetocare Fetogene Centre
Kanyakumari, Tamil Nadu, India

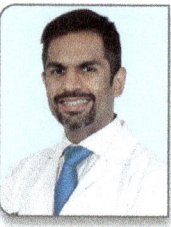
Shakir Tabrez Z MS (General Surgery) MCh (Urology) FICS FIAGES Dip in MAS (Urology)
Dip in Robotic Surgery (Lorraine University, France)
Senior Consultant – Urology, Uro-Oncology, Andrology,
Kidney Transplant and Robotic Surgery
Fortis Hospitals
Bengaluru, Karnataka, India

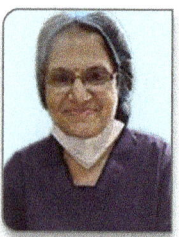
Shemi Bansal MBBS DIPGO
Consultant
Department of Obstetrics and Gynecology
Rainbow Hospital
Agra, Uttar Pradesh, India

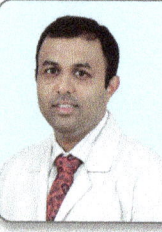
Shreyas Nagaraj MBBS MS DNB (Urology)
Consultant
Department of Urology
Fortis Hospitals
Bengaluru, Karnataka, India

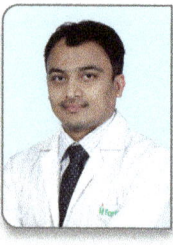
Sreeharsha Harinatha MS (General Surgery) MCh (Urology) Dip in Robotic Surgery (France)
Dip in Urogynecology (Germany)
Consultant – Urology, Uro-Oncology, Urogynecology, Andrology,
Transplant and Robotic Surgery
Fortis Hospitals
Bengaluru, Karnataka, India

Contributors

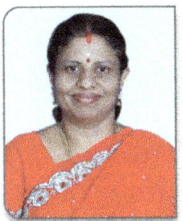

T Srikala Prasad MD (Obs & Gyn) DGO MCh (Urology)
Professor and Head, Department of Urology
Chengalpattu Medical College
Chengalpattu, Tamil Nadu, India
Past Secretary, OGSSI
Secretary, Tamil Nadu Chapter of SOVSI (Society of Vaginal Surgeons of India)
Nominated Indian Member of the Urogynecology Committee of AOFOG

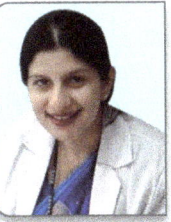

Urvashi Neelagar MBBS MS (Obs & Gyn) Fellowship in Fetal Medicine
Assistant Professor
Department of Obstetrics and Gynecology
Ramaiah Medical college,
Bengaluru, Karnataka, India

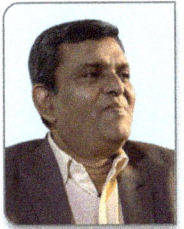

Vineet Mishra MD (Obs & Gyn)
President
SAFUG (South Asian Federation of Urogynecology)
Professor Director
Institute of Kidney Diseases and Research Centre, Medicity, Asarwa
Ahmedabad, Gujarat, India

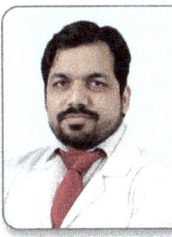

Vishal MBBS MS MCh (Urology)
Consultant – Urology, Uro-Oncology, Urogynecology and Andrology
Fortis Hospitals
Bengaluru, Karnataka, India

Foreword

UroGynecology Simplified is a novel attempt to enhance the knowledge of gynecologists with regard to female urological clinical dilemmas. The editors have aimed to include the most important topics which present in day-to-day clinical practice. The authors, each being doyens in their field, have presented their approach benefitting the reader with both their knowledge and perspective of the subject.

This book is a necessary addition to every aspiring pelvic surgeon, be it gynecologist or urologist or urogynecologist as it covers the most pertinent aspects right from basics to clinical approach to surgeries up to the latest advances.

Wishing the book all success.

S Shantha Kumari
MD DNB FICOG FRCPI (IRELAND) FRCOG (UK)
President, FOGSI (2021–22)
Senior Consultant, Department of Obstetrics and Gynecology
Laparoscopic Surgeon, Yashoda Hospitals
Hyderabad, Telangana, India
Chairperson, ICOG (2018–19)
Secretary, ICOG (2015–17)
Member, FIGO Working Group on Violence against Women (2015–18)
ICOG Governing Council Member (2012–15)
IAGE Managing Committee Member (2012–18)
National Corresponding Editor for JOGI (2011–13)

Foreword

Having been a part of various societies and panels over the past few decades, I have always noticed the lacunae when it comes to the specialty of urogynecology and the apprehensions by many fellow gynecologists in treating the conditions such as pelvic organ prolapse or genitourinary fistulae and many more. This compilation of chapters painstakingly put together, incorporates a wealth of information starting from the relevant clinical anatomy and physiology to the multifarious investigations available and including the various treatment modalities available to treat these conditions. It is an exhaustive body of work clearly elucidating comprehensively yet succinctly the otherwise complex world of Urogynecology and also aptly titled *UroGynecology Simplified*!

I congratulate the authors, renowned specialists from across the nation, for their earnest efforts in penning down these chapters and to the editors for having compiled this book, through this trying pandemic. I wish the authors and editors all the very best and hope it will serve to enlighten many in our fraternity, and enable them to not just counsel their patients appropriately but also treat them with absolute confidence and trust.

Hrishikesh D Pai
MD FCPS FICOG MSc (USA) FRCOG
President Elect, FOGSI (2022)
Gynecologist and Head of IVF Unit
Lilavati Hospital
Mumbai, Maharashtra, India
Scientific Director, Bloom IVF
Chief Administrator, FOGSI Manyata Project
Director, Corporate Affairs, IFFS
Secretary General, FOGSI (2015–17)

Preface

Ever so often, we have so many of our gynecologist colleagues approaching us with various concerns ranging from urinary incontinence to pelvic organ prolapse to urinary calculi to bladder or ureteric injuries amongst others.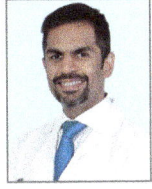

This book is our honest endeavor to reach out to all our gynecologist colleagues and general surgeons performing pelvic surgery and take that element of apprehension or anxiety out of this sometimes intricate field and allow them not just to understand it better but manage all these conditions and any possible complications on their own.

I would like to express our immense gratitude to the stellar group of contributors, all of whom are superstars in their chosen fields from across the nation who have taken the time and effort to put together this impressive tome.

The endeavor has been to cover the entire palette of topics which cover urogynecology, and present them in a format which would make an interesting read and also serve as a ready reckoner at any point for reference and application during everyday clinical practice.

Though COVID-19 and its various manifestations did delay our work significantly, with contributions pouring in from the length and breadth of our wonderful nation, we have had the pleasure of editing and compiling this one of a kind work, which we hope will reach and enlighten a wide section of gynecologists, and not just introduce them but give them a wholesome picture of the hitherto enigmatic field of urology and urogynecology.

Shakir Tabrez Z

From the Editor's Desk

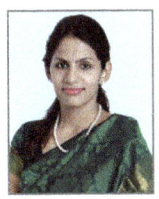

Greetings on behalf of the editorial board on which I am privileged to be a part of, along with Dr Nandita Palshetkar, Dr Selvapriya Saravanan and Dr Shakir Tabrez Z.

With the ongoing pandemic, it has been a Herculean task to bring to reality our brainchild of collaborating Gynecologists, Urologists and Urogynecologists to share their knowledge in a single book.

The idea behind this book is to simplify the concepts of urogynecology for the Gynec practitioners and enable better quality-of-care delivered to the patient. We felt this comprehensive amalgamation of allied specialties is essential in this present day of subspecialization and rapidly evolving technology.

We are proud of the fact that ours is the first such venture in India where experts from the allied specialties have come together to share their knowledge in a single book. We hope every reader of this book is benefited and empowered with the right approach to various diagnostic dilemmas in urogynecology.

Rubina Shanawaz Z

Acknowledgments

We are grateful to Dr S Shantha Kumari and Dr Hrishikesh D Pai for taking time out to review our book and giving us a heartening feedback. We thank M/s Jaypee Brothers Medical Publishers (P) Ltd, New Delhi, India, for patiently working with us through the COVID-19 upheaval and making our efforts see the light of day. Our heartfelt gratitude goes out to each and every author for their well-researched and earnestly articulated chapters. We are indebted to the authors of the reference articles that we have used for paving the way for us and making our task smoother. None of this would have been possible, if not for the support of our spouses and families who have been our pillars of support and encouragement.

Thank you readers for trusting your time with us and we assure you, it will be worth it.

Contents

1. **Pelvic Ureter and Its Applied Anatomy** 1
   Rubina Shanawaz Z

2. **Pelvic Floor: Anatomy and Significance in Urogynecology** 5
   Kiran Ashok

3. **Retroperitoneum: What to Expect?** 14
   Santosh Kumar Subudhi

4. **Important Renal Physiological and Biochemical Parameters** 20
   Ritu Hinduja, Rohan Palshetkar

5. **History and Clinical Assessment of Lower Urinary Tract Symptoms** 26
   Shreyas Nagaraj

6. **Imaging in Urogynecology** 33
   Chander P Lulla, Selvapriya Saravanan

7. **Basics of Urodynamics** 42
   Premkumar Krishnappa

8. **Stress Urinary Incontinence: Assessment and Management** 53
   Nita Thakre, Anuj Thakre

9. **Tension-free Vaginal Tape** 67
   Shakir Tabrez Z

10. **Tension-free Transobturator Tape Insertion** 70
    Ashish Kale

11. **Autologous Rectus Fascia Sling** 72
    T Srikala Prasad

12. **Urge Urinary Incontinence: Management Options** 82
    Urvashi Neelagar, Basavaraj Neelagar

13. **Assessment and Management of Patient with Obstructive Lower Urinary Tract Symptoms** 88
    Vishal

14. **Current Trends in the Management of Recurrent Urinary Tract Infections** 97
    Karthik Rao

15. **Urinary Tract Calculi in Pregnancy** 101
    Mohan Balaiah Aswathaiya

16. **Basics of Cystoscopy** 107
    Ramesh Hanumegowda

17. **Urinary Tract Injuries in Difficult Gynecologic Surgeries: Tips and Tricks to Anticipate and Avoid** 114
    Manjula Anagani, Prabha Agrawal

18. **Identification and Management of Ureteric Injuries in Gynecological Surgeries** 122
    Sreeharsha Harinatha

19. **Urinary Bladder Injuries during Cesarean Section** 129
    Mala Raj, Prashanth K Adiga

20. **Postpartum Urinary Issues and Management** 135
    Ameya C Purandare, Ashwin Shetty

21. **Identification and Management of Genitourinary Fistulae** 140
    Madhusudhan Naidu

22. **Genital Prolapse** 150
    Manish Machave

23. **Vaginal Apical Suspension Procedures** 165
    T Srikala Prasad

24. **High Uterosacral Ligament Suspension for Apical Prolapse** 175
    N Rajamaheswari

25. **Abdominal Apical Suspension Procedures for Pelvic Organ Prolapse** 185
    Bimal M John, Raji S

26. **Advances in Pelvic Repair and Reconstructive Surgeries** 194
    Vineet Mishra, Neeta Mishra, Deepa Chaudhary

27. **Robotics in Urogynecology** 204
    Mohan Keshavamurthy

28. **Female Genital Cosmetic Surgery** 209
    Deepa Ganesh

29. **Her Unspoken Problems** 217
    Narendra Malhotra, Molina Patel, Neharika Malhotra, Jaideep Malhotra, Manpreet Sharma, Shemi Bansal

Index 225

Contents

1. **Pelvic Ureter and Its Applied Anatomy** 1
   Rubina Shanawaz Z

2. **Pelvic Floor: Anatomy and Significance in Urogynecology** 5
   Kiran Ashok

3. **Retroperitoneum: What to Expect?** 14
   Santosh Kumar Subudhi

4. **Important Renal Physiological and Biochemical Parameters** 20
   Ritu Hinduja, Rohan Palshetkar

5. **History and Clinical Assessment of Lower Urinary Tract Symptoms** 26
   Shreyas Nagaraj

6. **Imaging in Urogynecology** 33
   Chander P Lulla, Selvapriya Saravanan

7. **Basics of Urodynamics** 42
   Premkumar Krishnappa

8. **Stress Urinary Incontinence: Assessment and Management** 53
   Nita Thakre, Anuj Thakre

9. **Tension-free Vaginal Tape** 67
   Shakir Tabrez Z

10. **Tension-free Transobturator Tape Insertion** 70
    Ashish Kale

11. **Autologous Rectus Fascia Sling** 72
    T Srikala Prasad

12. **Urge Urinary Incontinence: Management Options** 82
    Urvashi Neelagar, Basavaraj Neelagar

13. **Assessment and Management of Patient with Obstructive Lower Urinary Tract Symptoms** 88
    Vishal

14. **Current Trends in the Management of Recurrent Urinary Tract Infections** 97
    Karthik Rao

15. **Urinary Tract Calculi in Pregnancy** 101
    Mohan Balaiah Aswathaiya

16. **Basics of Cystoscopy** 107
    Ramesh Hanumegowda

17. **Urinary Tract Injuries in Difficult Gynecologic Surgeries: Tips and Tricks to Anticipate and Avoid** 114
    Manjula Anagani, Prabha Agrawal

18. **Identification and Management of Ureteric Injuries in Gynecological Surgeries** 122
    Sreeharsha Harinatha

19. **Urinary Bladder Injuries during Cesarean Section** 129
    Mala Raj, Prashanth K Adiga

20. **Postpartum Urinary Issues and Management** 135
    Ameya C Purandare, Ashwin Shetty

21. **Identification and Management of Genitourinary Fistulae** 140
    Madhusudhan Naidu

22. **Genital Prolapse** 150
    Manish Machave

23. **Vaginal Apical Suspension Procedures** 165
    T Srikala Prasad

24. **High Uterosacral Ligament Suspension for Apical Prolapse** 175
    N Rajamaheswari

25. **Abdominal Apical Suspension Procedures for Pelvic Organ Prolapse** 185
    Bimal M John, Raji S

26. **Advances in Pelvic Repair and Reconstructive Surgeries** 194
    Vineet Mishra, Neeta Mishra, Deepa Chaudhary

27. **Robotics in Urogynecology** 204
    Mohan Keshavamurthy

28. **Female Genital Cosmetic Surgery** 209
    Deepa Ganesh

29. **Her Unspoken Problems** 217
    Narendra Malhotra, Molina Patel, Neharika Malhotra, Jaideep Malhotra, Manpreet Sharma, Shemi Bansal

Index 225

Pelvic Ureter and Its Applied Anatomy

Rubina Shanawaz Z

INTRODUCTION

Iatrogenic injury to the urinary tract can be caused by any surgeon operating in or around the pelvis and the retroperitoneal abdominal space, with a general incidence of 0.3–1.5%.[1]

Of the urinary tract, the ureter is the most vulnerable to injury as it can be encountered at any level in the retroperitoneum and upper pelvis. This along with the occasional unexpected congenital anomaly makes the ureter especially vulnerable to injury.

COURSE OF PELVIC URETER WITH OPERATIVE SIGNIFICANCE (FIG. 1)

The ureter is 25–30 cm long in adults and courses down the retroperitoneum in an S curve. It consists of the abdominal, the pelvic, and the intramural segment.

The ureter begins at the level of the renal artery and vein posterior to these structures. This ureteropelvic junction usually coincides with the second lumbar vertebra on the left, with the right being marginally lower.

The ureter then continues anteriorly on the psoas major muscle, crossing under the gonadal vein at the level of the inferior pole of the kidney. The ureters course medial to the sacroiliac joint and then curve laterally in the pelvis. The colon and its mesentery are associated anterior to the ureters. Specifically, the cecum, appendix, and ascending colon lie over the right ureter, and the descending and sigmoid colon lie over the left ureter.

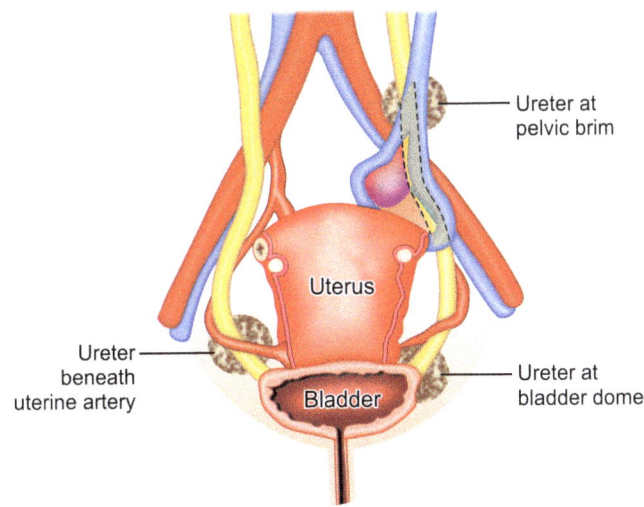

Fig. 1: Course of pelvic ureter with operative significance.
Source: Adapted from Reference 2.

The ureter enters the pelvis at the pelvic brim at the base of the infundibulopelvic ligament, crossing the external iliac vessels from lateral to medial. This is one of the most common areas of ureteric injury during oophorectomy which can be avoided by two simple surgical principles: stay as close to the ovary as possible and if no adhesions, always lift and ligate.

The ureter then traverses down the lateral pelvic wall anterior and medial to the internal iliac artery.

It then crosses under the uterine artery (water under the bridge) at 1–1.5 cm away from the vaginal fornices on its way to the bladder insertion (**Fig. 2**).[3]

This is another vulnerable area of injury when ligating the uterosacral pedicle and also when suturing the vault which can be avoided by staying as close as possible to the uterus.

An important anatomical fact to note is that the left ureter has a more close relation to the anterior wall of vagina than the right,[4] which explains why it is the left ureter close to the ureterovesical junction, which gets most commonly injured during hysterectomies.

The ureter has three physiologic narrowings: (1) the ureteropelvic junction, (2) the crossing over the iliac vessels, and (3) the ureterovesical junction. This is crucial in the manifestations of calculus disease. These narrowings may result in ureteral stones becoming trapped and obstructing at these specific levels. These narrowings may also limit retrograde instrumentation performed for diagnostic or therapeutic purposes.

SURGICAL SIGNIFICANCE OF URETERIC BLOOD SUPPLY

The nutrient arteries generally approach the ureteric wall from one direction which needs to be kept in mind by the surgeon to avoid devascularizing the ureter. Above the pelvic brim, the nutrient arteries approach from the

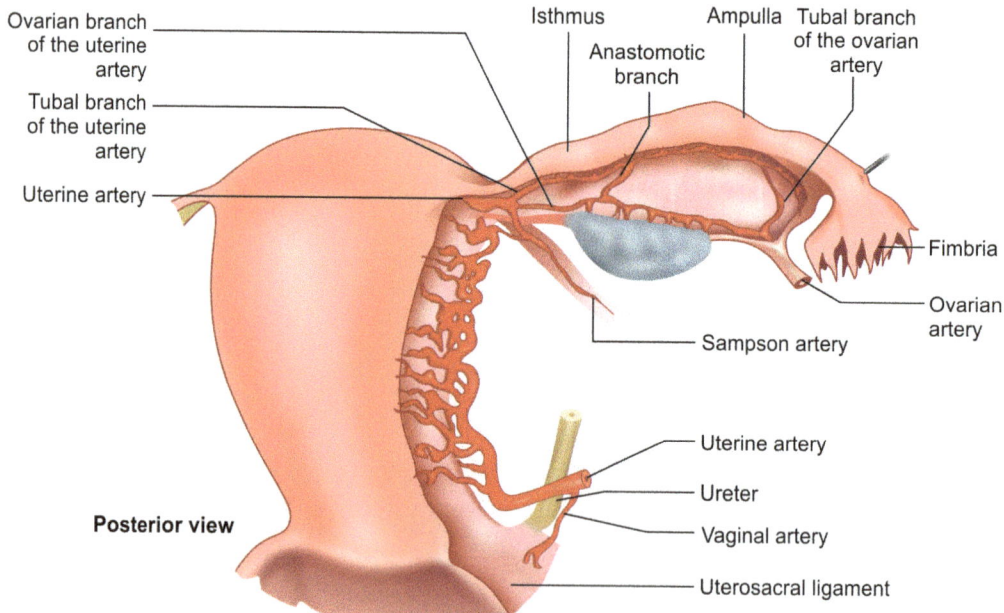

Fig. 2: Pelvic ureter crossing uterine artery.
Source: Adapted from Reference 3.

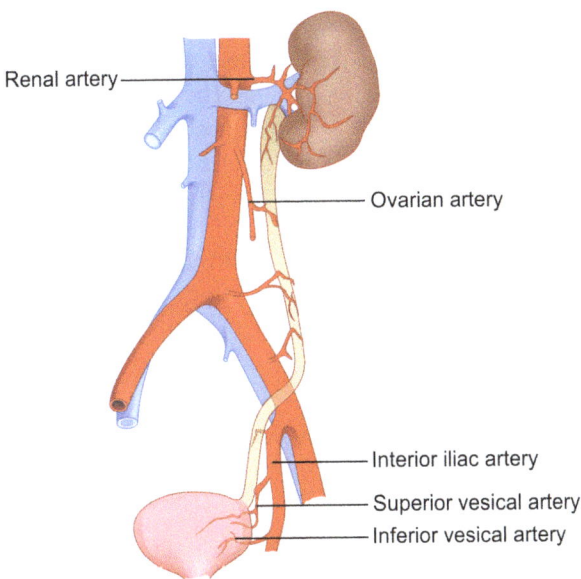

Fig. 3: Surgical significance of ureteric blood supply.

medial side and below the pelvic brim from the lateral side of the ureter.[2]

The supplying arteries and veins run through a layer of loose connective tissue to the adventitial vascular plexus called the mesoureter. This means that even if an arterial inflow is ligated, there will not be necrosis of the ureter because of its rich collateral anastomoses within the adventitial vascular plexus. But, unnecessary and excessive mobilization can devascularize the ureter and increase the risk of postoperative ureteric stricture **(Fig. 3)**.

SURGICAL SIGNIFICANCE OF URETERIC NERVE SUPPLY

The sympathetic nerves supplying the ureter originate from the aortic plexus and its continuation, the superior hypogastric plexus, the paired hypogastric nerve, and the subsequent inferior hypogastric (pelvic) plexus. The nerves accompany the nutrient branches of the neighboring arteries and form circumarterial plexuses or run free in the connective tissue.

The parasympathetic pelvic splanchnic nerves usually arising from the second, third, and fourth sacral root traverse the inferior hypogastric plexus before its partition in its specific plexuses for the pelvic viscera.

In female, the branches of the uterovaginal plexus are themselves positioned a little lower than the uterine artery and the ureter. The branches of the vesical plexus run inferior to the terminal ureter and extend to the trigone of the bladder.

Note: In an antireflux procedure there is a high risk of injury to the nervous structures if dissection is performed dorsally to the trigone and dorsocaudally to the vesicoureteric junction. Careful dissection close to the terminal ureter (within the layer of mesoureter) avoids intraoperative injury to the pelvic autonomic nerves.

Mucosal irritation and luminal distention stimulate nociceptors whose afferents travel with sympathetic nerves and confer the visceral-type referred pain that results in the manifestations of ureteral colic. Pain or hyperesthesia may be sensed from the region of the ipsilateral ribs down to the labia.

MALFORMATIONS OF THE URETER

The ureter can be duplicated completely or incompletely, unilaterally or bilaterally.

Duplications of the ureter are of practical importance; the incidence of a ureteric duplication is 1:100. "Ureter duplex" denotes complete duplication of the ureter on one or both sides. The ureter arising from the cranial part of the renal sinus usually opens into the bladder more caudally than normal, while the ureter arising from the lower part of the renal sinus enters the bladder higher than the dystopic ureter (Weigert-Meyer law). Duplex ureter is due to the presence of two ureteric buds on one or both sides during embryogenesis.

Note: In cases of duplicated ureter, there is a common vascular supply within the ureteric sheath, so that resection of one of the ureters can endanger the blood supply of the remaining ureter and may lead to its necrosis.

The other ureteric anomalies include ureterocele, ectopic ureteral orifice, megaureter, ureteral atresia, ureteral diverticula, or a retrocaval ureter.

REFERENCES

1. Rosemarie F. Surgical Anatomy of the Ureter. Surgery Illustrated; 2007. Available from https://bjui-journals.onlinelibrary.wiley.com/doi/pdf/10.1111/j.1464-410X.2007.07207.x [Last accessed on April, 2021].
2. Sankpal RS, Karoshi M, Keith LG (Eds). Textbook of Simplified Laparoscopic Hysterectomy: Practical, Safe and Economic Methodology. New Delhi: Jaypee Brothers Medical Publishers; 2018. Also available from glowm.com [Last accessed on April, 2021].
3. American Association for the Surgery of Trauma. [online] Available from: http://www.aast.org/injury/t15-20.html#ureter [Last accessed on March, 2019].
4. Bartsch G, Poisel S (Eds). Operative Zugangswege in der Urologie. Stuttgart New York Thieme; 1994.

2. Pelvic Floor: Anatomy and Significance in Urogynecology

Kiran Ashok

INTRODUCTION

Pelvic floor is the region between perineal skin and the caudal peritoneal cavity. This region contains muscles, connective tissues, anorectum, urethra, bladder, vagina, uterus, vessels, and nerves. Muscles and connective tissues anchor the visceral organs to the pelvic bone.

The sacrum, the coccyx and the two innominate hip bones containing pubis, ischium and ileum make up the pelvic bone. The pelvic bones are connected by ligaments which help in providing stability and mobility. The bony pelvis and ligaments also act as anchoring points for pelvic floor muscles and connective tissue which in turn support the viscera of the pelvis. The sacrospinous ligament **(Fig. 1)** runs from the lateral aspect of the sacrum to the ischial spine, and is an excellent supporting structure for fixing the vaginal apex following hysterectomy for prolapse uterus or during vaginal vault prolapse repair. Near the ischial spine, the pudendal neurovascular bundle curves around the sacrospinous ligament posteriorly and enters the pudendal canal. Approximately at the middle of the sacrospinous ligament, inferior gluteal artery runs posterior to the sacrospinous ligament **(Fig. 1)**. Hence caution should be exercised while taking a suture on the sacrospinous ligament—not to go near the ischial spine and should not be very deep. Iliopectineal (Cooper's) ligament is a thickening of the periosteum that overlays the pectineal line of the pubis which is reinforced by fibers that extend from the inguinal ligament and the

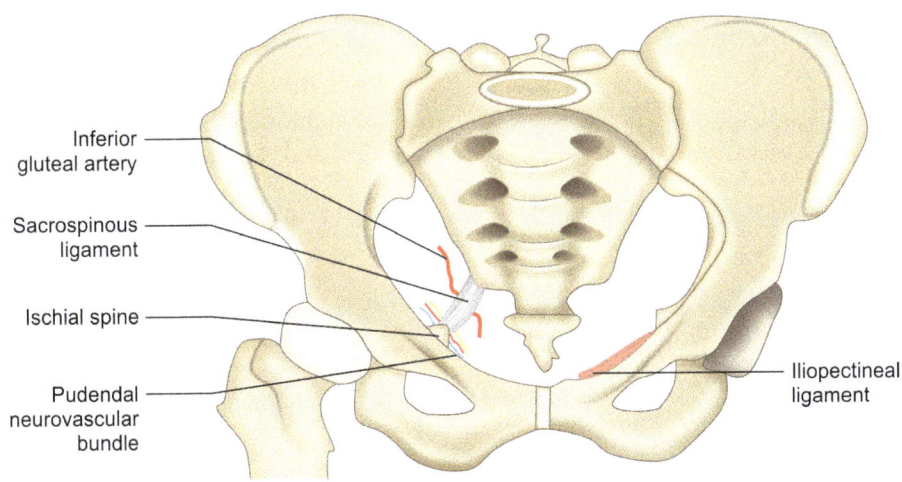

Fig. 1: Bony pelvis with sacrospinous and iliopectineal ligament.

lacunar ligament. Burch colposuspension involves suspending the paraurethral fascia to the Cooper's ligament to treat stress urinary incontinence (SUI).

MUSCLES FORMING THE PELVIC FLOOR

Obturator internus along with its fascia forms the lateral boundary of the pelvic cavity and lines the inner surface of the ischium, ilium and pubic bones **(Fig. 2)**. Obturator internus along with its fascia provides attachment to the major portion of the levator ani muscle. Obturator internus fascia also provides attachment to the pubocervical and rectovaginal fasciae at the arcus tendineus fascia pelvis (ATFP) and arcus tendineus fascia rectovaginalis, respectively. These fasciae will be described later.

The most important muscle that forms and provides support to the pelvic floor is the levator ani. Levator ani is muscle is arbitrarily divided into puborectalis, pubococcygeus, iliococcygeus and coccygeus muscle groups **(Fig. 3)**. The puborectalis and pubococcygeus portion arise from the posterior aspect of symphysis pubis on either side, run along the direction of ATFP and fuse in the midline forming median raphe. Between the right and the left puborectalis muscles lies the genital hiatus, through which the urethra, the vagina and the anorectal canal exit the pelvic cavity. The puborectalis and pubococcygeus muscles pass posteriorly around the rectum, and contraction (and constant tone) of these muscles pull the rectum anteriorly toward symphysis, creating anorectal angle (approximately 90°) and closes the anorectal junction and the vagina **(Fig. 4)**. Even when there is external anal sphincter injury, the puborectalis mechanism can maintain continence to some degree.[1]

The portion of the levator ani muscle raphe which lies between the anorectal junction and the coccyx is called the levator plate and it supports the upper vagina, uterus and the rectum.

Pelvic floor dysfunction results from the lack of support provided by the pelvic floor muscles and fascia, especially the levator

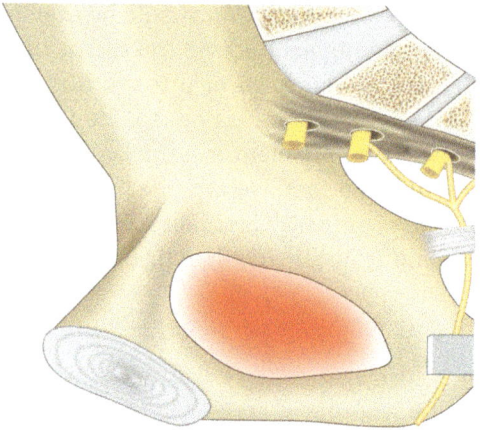

Fig. 2: Obturator internus (red shade) covering lateral pelvic wall.

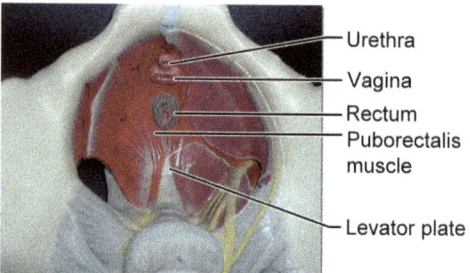

Fig. 3: Levator ani muscle.

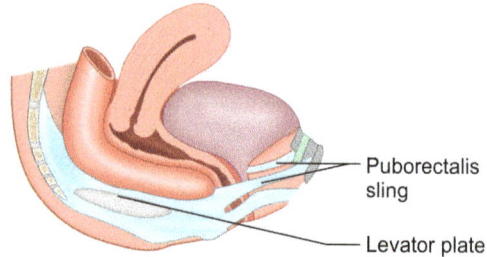

Fig. 4: Puborectalis sling and levator plate on which proximal vagina and rectum lie.

ani muscle complex.² During the process of vaginal delivery, the passage of the fetal head causes significant deformations in the pelvic floor. The puborectalis muscle fibers and the medial portion of the pubococcygeus muscle stretch 3.26 more times than other pelvic muscles during the expulsion of the fetus, albeit without any traumas during an uneventful vaginal delivery.³ However, in certain traumatic deliveries, the puborectalis portion of the levator ani can get avulsed from its attachment to the pubic bone.

Levator detachment (noted in 20% of women who deliver vaginally)⁴ appears as loss of vaginal lateral sulcus on axial MRI or 3D ultrasound **(Figs. 5 and 6)**.

Compared with spontaneous vaginal birth, forceps assisted vaginal delivery has been associated with three times increased risk of levator damage. Levator avulsion leads to increase in the size of genital hiatus with loss of anorectal angle. This predisposes to development of pelvic organ prolapse, especially when the levator hiatal area is greater than 25 cm².⁶

Levator defects are always accompanied by concomitant injury to the endopelvic fascia and the pelvic nerves especially the pudendal nerve when the fetal head engages during labor. This is found in 38–42% of vaginal deliveries.⁸

Most nerve lesions regenerate spontaneously within a year. However, pudendal nerve damage may actually be more pronounced as time lapses.

Women operative vaginal birth has been associated with SUI. The odds of surgical intervention for SUI are three times higher for women who delivered vaginally and 20 times higher for those who have experienced forceps assisted delivery compared with women who gave birth exclusively via cesarean delivery.⁹

With regards to external anal sphincter injury, women with third and fourth degree perineal lacerations have a higher rate of flatus and fecal incontinence.¹⁰

The above findings are not to say that cesarean delivery offers complete protection against pelvic floor injury. Pregnancy itself has been shown to increase postpartum muscle weakness independent of the mode of delivery.¹¹

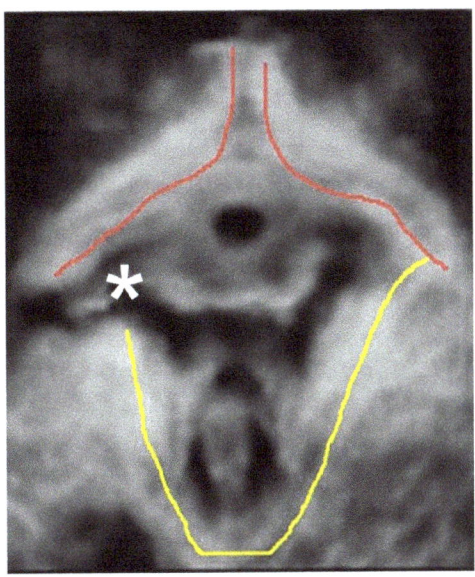

Fig. 6: Unilateral puborectalis detachment. Red lines outline pubic bone and rami. Yellow line outlines puborectalis. Asterisk is the area of puborectalis detachment from pubic bone.

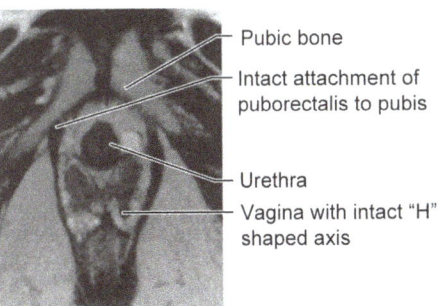

Fig. 5: Normal attachments of puborectalis to pubic bone.

Pelvic Fascia

Kovac has demonstrated the following findings about endopelvic fascia in cadaveric dissections. Endopelvic fascia is a dense connective tissue that overlies the pelvic floor and extends to the pelvic sidewalls and the perineum. This connective tissue extends throughout the pelvic floor and attaches the muscles and pelvic viscera to the bony pelvis. This connective tissue sheath is thickest at two regions: (1) uterosacral ligaments and (2) ATFP.[1]

The upper vagina and the cervix are supported by condensed connective tissue structures which are termed cardinal-uterosacral complex. These constitute Level 1 supports in DeLancey's classification. This connective tissue condensation stretches from the upper vagina and cervix to the level of the anterior aspect of the sacrum. Discrete breaks in the cardinal uterosacral complex can lead to prolapse of the uterus or vaginal vault. In such circumstances, the vaginal vault has to be suspended to some stable structure such as sacrospinous ligament or to the sacral promontory, as the uterosacral ligaments are already compromised.

DeLancey's Level 2 support is constituted by the pubocervical and rectovaginal fascia and their attachment to the lateral pelvic wall **(Fig. 7)**. Level 3 supports involve the distal vagina and it is provided by the perineal body, perineal membrane, and pubourethral ligaments. It provides support to the urethra also.

Anterior Compartment of Vagina

The anterior vaginal wall and the bladder are supported by a trapezoid sheet of endopelvic fascia termed pubocervical fascia (PCF).

The PCF is attached proximally to the pericervical ring and uterosacral ligaments, distally to the pubic bone, and laterally on either side to the ATFP **(Figs. 8 and 9)**. ATFP is a linear condensation of the endopelvic fascia on the obturator internus muscle and it extends from ischial spine to the pubic bone on the lateral pelvic wall.

During vaginal delivery, along with levator muscle, endopelvic fascia can also be damaged and torn. As the fetal head descends in the birth canal it stretches the pericervical ring and during descent it can cause detachment

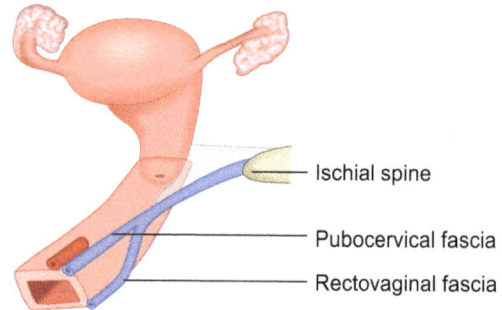

Fig. 7: Pubocervical and rectovaginal fascia in relation to vagina.

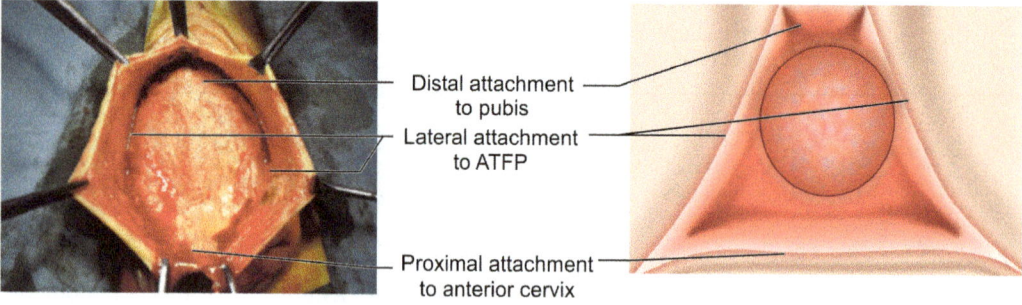

Fig. 8: Pubocervical fascia and its attachments.

of PCF from the pericervical ring due to the downward shearing forces **(Fig. 10)**. This results in proximal or transverse detachment of pubocervical fascia and therefore the bladder can herniate (and thus form cystocele) in the defect between the pericervical ring and the detached proximal edge of the PCF **(Fig. 11)**. As the fetal head descends and undergoes internal rotation, the rotating shearing forces can cause detachment of PCF from the ATFP resulting in a paravaginal defect **(Fig. 12)**. Apical (proximal or transverse) detachment results in a larger cystocele than paravaginal impairment.[12,13] Using functional MRI studies, it has been shown that paravaginal defects are highly correlated with apical descent.[14] This correlation implies that during cystocele repair, apical suspension of vaginal vault is a must to correct the defects and to prevent recurrence.

Posterior Compartment of Vagina

The posterior vaginal wall is supported by the rectovaginal fascia (RVF). RVF is a sheath of connective tissue that extends posteriorly from the posterolateral vaginal sulci, traverses around the rectum, and attaches the vagina

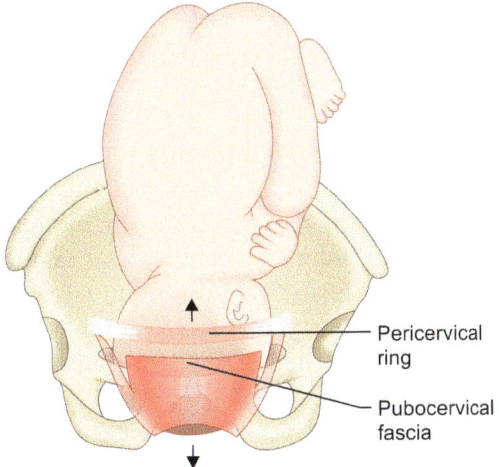

Fig. 10: Detachment of pubocervical fascia (PCF) from pericervical ring during descent of fetal head.
Source: Kovac R, Zimmerman C. Advances in Reconstructive vaginal surgery, 2nd edition. Philadelphia: Lippincott Williams and Wilkins; 2012.
Courtesy: Dr Shivaranjini.

Fig. 9: Pubocervical fascia—view after dissection of anterior vaginal wall.

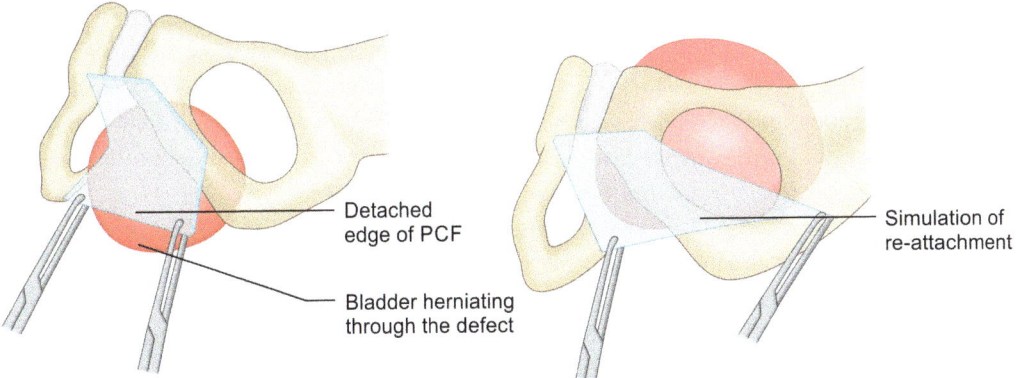

Fig. 11: Pubocervical fascia (PCF)—transverse detachment leading to cystocele formation.
Courtesy: Dr Shivaranjini.

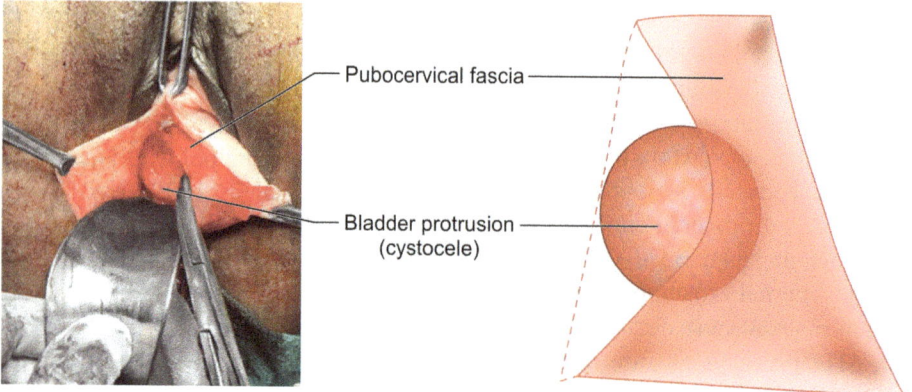

Fig. 12: Paravaginal defect. Detachment of pubocervical fascia (PCF) from right lateral pelvic wall/arcus tendineus fascia pelvis (ATFP).

to the pelvic floor. Inferiorly these fibers blend with the perineal body. The RVF does not have many attachments in the midline, rather it anchors the posterolateral vaginal sulci to the ipsilateral levator ani fascia at arcus-tendineus rectovaginalis. Superiorly the RVF is attached to the pericervical ring and the uterosacral ligaments (**Fig. 13**). The pathology of rectocele is more complicated than cystocele. In general, detachment of RVF from the perineal body and from the uterosacral ligaments has been observed. Therefore, the technique of rectocele repair involves reattachment of RVF superiorly to the uterosacral ligaments, inferiorly to the perineal body and midline plication of RVF.

IMPORTANCE OF PELVIC NERVES AND PLEXUSES IN UROGYNECOLOGY

Peripheral nervous system in relation to bladder can be studied under three categories: (1) sacral parasympathetic, (2) lumbar sympathetic, and (3) somatic pudendal nerves. Formation of superior and inferior hypogastric plexuses is shown in **Figure 14**.

Sacral parasympathetic pathway arises from preganglionic neurons in the intermediolateral horn of S2, S3, S4. These travel through the pelvic nerves to connect with postganglionic

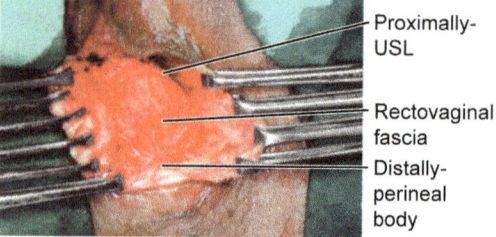

Fig. 13: Posterior vaginal wall dissected to show the rectovaginal fascia.

neurons in the pelvic plexus, bladder wall, and urethra. This parasympathetic system causes contraction of the bladder wall (by cholinergic action through M2 and M3 receptors) and relaxation of the urethral sphincter by release of nitrous oxide.

Thoracolumbar sympathetic pathways: sympathetic pathways to the lower urinary tract originate in the lumbosacral sympathetic chain ganglia and send axons via hypogastric nerve to the bladder and the urethra.

Sympathetic effects on LUT are:
1. Inhibition of detrusor muscle via beta-adrenergic receptors,
2. Excitation of bladder base and urethra via alpha-1 adrenergic receptors, and
3. Inhibition of bladder parasympathetic ganglia via alpha-2 receptors (this helps to modulate bladder storage function).

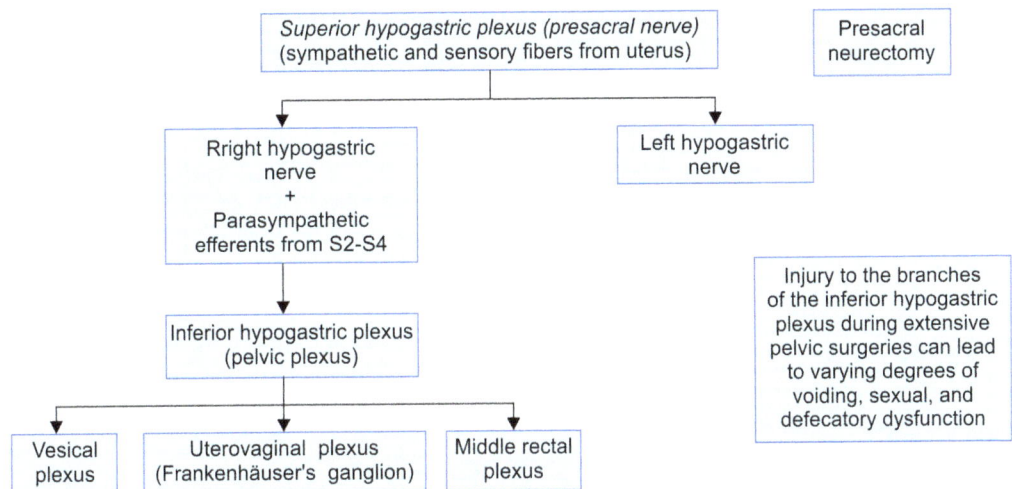

Fig. 14: Formation of pelvic hypogastric plexus.

Somatic efferent pathway: This pathway originates in the motor neurons located in the lateral ventral horn of the sacral spinal cord (the region is termed "Onuf's nucleus"). These motor neurons send axons via pudendal nerve to the striated sphincter muscle of the urethra where they excite the urethral muscle by release of acetylcholine.

Afferent pathways of LUT: The most important afferent neurons of the LUT are those passing in the pelvic nerve to the sacral spinal cord. These neurons are of two types: (1) myelinated A-delta and (2) unmyelinated C-fibers. A-delta fibers respond to gradual distension of bladder and their threshold is between pressures of 5 and 15 cmH$_2$O which correspond to normal sensation of bladder filling. The C-fibers have very high thresholds and generally do not respond to high intravesical pressures. However, activity in C-fibers can be stimulated by chemical irritation or inflammation of bladder mucosa. C-fiber afferents are sensitive to neurotoxins, capsaicin, resiniferatoxin and many other chemical irritants. These substances can modulate afferent nerve excitability and change the response of afferents to mechanical stimulation. Thus, pathological activation of C-fibers may play a role in the pathogenesis of overactive bladder.[15]

ANATOMICAL FACTORS IN STRESS URINARY INCONTINENCE

The female urethra is the seat of continence mechanism which involves the urethral supports and urethral sphincters. The urethra has an intramural smooth muscle sphincter which is a continuation of detrusor muscle. Surrounding the urethra, near its middle part (between the external urethral meatus and the bladder neck) is the striated muscle external urethral sphincter. This striated external urethral sphincter has a horseshoe configuration, surrounding the urethra anteriorly and laterally, but deficient posteriorly **(Fig. 15)**. On the posterior aspect, urethra is supported by the connective tissue of the anterior vaginal wall. During increases in the intra-abdominal pressure (which tends to push the urine out of the bladder) the striated sphincter contracts and compresses the urethra against the underlying fascia, effectively preventing urine leak. This is the mechanism of continence during increases in intra-abdominal pressures.

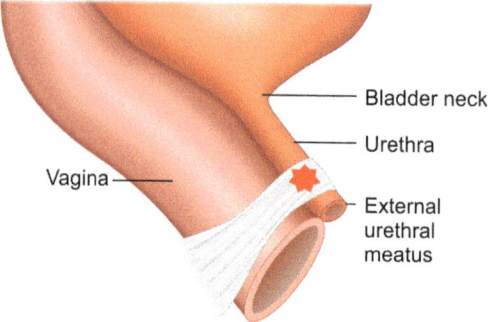

Fig. 15: Configuration of external urethral sphincter (red star).

Two pathophysiological mechanisms have been proposed for the occurrence of SUI (defined as leak of urine through the urethra whenever there is an increase in intra-abdominal pressure such as during coughing, straining, sneezing, etc.). It is easy to understand that weakness of the striated external urethral sphincter can lead to incomplete compression of the urethra during increases in intra-abdominal pressure and, consequently, leak of urine. This phenomenon, termed, intrinsic-sphincter deficiency, can be caused by damage to the sphincter itself or to the nerves supplying it as in spinal cord or nerve root lesions (lumbar disk prolapse), diabetic neuropathy, spinal cord tumors, multiple sclerosis, and extensive pelvic surgery. Any periurethral surgery such as anti-incontinence surgery and urethral diverticulectomy can lead to damage to the sphincter muscle or to the delicate nerves supplying it and can result in intrinsic sphincter deficiency.

Another common theory proposed for the occurrence of SUI is the DeLancey's theory of continence mechanism. Normally, with rise in intra-abdominal pressure, the urethra gets compressed against the supporting structures and prevents loss of urine. So here, it is the stability of this support rather than the position of the urethra that determines stress incontinence. The supporting layer is the fascia underlying the urethra, against which the urethra is compressed and closed (by the external urethral sphincter) during increases in intra-abdominal pressure. Hammock of endopelvic fascia acts as a backboard for the urethra to be compressed against when there are increases in abdominal pressure. If the fascial hammock is deficient or weak, then the urethral compression and closure may not be very effective and hence urine leaks leading to SUI.[16]

REFERENCES

1. Kovac R, Zimmerman C. Advances in Reconstructive Vaginal Surgery, 2nd edition. Philadelphia: Lippincott Williams and Wilkins; 2012.
2. Kearney R, Miller JM, Ashton-Miller JA, DeLancey JO. Obstetric factors associated with levator ani muscle injury after vaginal birth. Obstet Gynecol. 2006;107(1):144-9.
3. Krofta L, Havelkova L, Urbankoba I, Krčmář M, Hynčík L, Feyereisl J. Finite element model focused on stress distribution in the levator ani muscle during vaginal delivery. Int Urogynecol J. 2017;28(2):275-84
4. Rizk DE. Minimizing the risk of childbirth-induced pelvic floor dysfunctions in the developing world: "preventive" urogynecology. Int Urogynecol J. 2009;20(6):615-7.
5. Dietz HP, Lanzarone V. Levator trauma after vaginal delivery. Obstet Gynecol. 2005;106(4):707-12.
6. Dietz HP, Shek C, De Leon J, Steensma AB. Ballooning of the levator hiatus. Ultrasound Obstet Gynecol. 2008;31(6):676-80
7. Dietz HP, Simpson JM. Levator trauma is associated with pelvic organ prolapse. BJOG. 2008;115(8):979-84.
8. Fitzpatrick M, O'brien C, O'connell PR, O'herlihy C. Patterns of abnormal pudendal nerve function that are associated with postpartum fecal incontinence. Am J Obstet Gynecol. 2003;189(3):730-5.
9. Leijonhufvud A, Lundholm C, Cnattingius S, Granath F, Andolf E, Altman D. Risks of stress urinary incontinence and pelvic organ prolapse surgery in relation to mode of childbirth. Am J Obstet Gynecol. 2011;204(1):70.e1-7.

10. Eason E, Labrecque M, Marcoux S, Mondor M. Anal incontinence after childbirth. J Can Med Assoc. 2002;166(3):326-30.
11. Koc O, Duran B, Ozdemirci S, Bakar Y, Ozengin N. Is cesarean section a real panacea to prevent pelvic organ disorders? Int Urogynecol J. 2011;22(9):1135-41.
12. Chen L, Ashton-Miller JA, Hsu Y, DeLency JO. Interaction among apical support, levator ani impairment, and anterior vaginal wall prolapse. Obstet Gynecol. 2006;108(2):324-32.
13. Chen L, Ashton-Miller JA, DeLancey JO. A 3D finite element model of anterior vaginal wall support to evaluate mechanisms underlying cystocele formation. J Biomech. 2009;42(10):1371-7.
14. Larson KA, Luo J, Guire KE, Chen L, Ashton-Miller JA, DeLancey JO. 3D analysis of cystoceles using magnetic resonance imaging assessing midline, paravaginal, and apical defects. Int Urogynecol J. 2012;23(3):285-93.
15. de Groat WC. Integrative control of the lower urinary tract: preclinical perspective. Br J Pharmacol. 2006;147(Suppl 2):S25-40.
16. Delancey JOL. Why do women have stress urinary incontinence? Neurourol Urodyn. 2010;29(Suppl 1):S13-7.

CHAPTER 3

Retroperitoneum: What to Expect?

Santosh Kumar Subudhi

INTRODUCTION

The retroperitoneum can be described as the entirety of the structures contained anteriorly by the posterior reflection of the peritoneum, posteriorly by the posterior abdominal wall with its muscle layers, cranially by the diaphragm and caudally by the extraperitoneal pelvic structures. The retroperitoneum is different from extraperitoneal space which includes the retroperitoneum and the space that circumferentially surrounds the abdominal cavity (**Fig. 1**).

STRUCTURE

The retroperitoneum relevant to the urogynecologists is the pelvic retroperitoneum, which lies between the parietal peritoneum and the parietal pelvic fascia behind the pelvic structures in the pelvis of females (**Fig. 2**).

The pelvic retroperitoneum is a connective tissue space crossed by pelvic ureter, visceral vessels, and nerves.

This space is organized in three functional structures:
1. Visceral ligaments
2. Acollaged visceral surfaces
3. Visceral pelvic fascia

This has great surgical and functional importance in urogynecology, endometriosis and in oncology.

The posterior aspect of the pelvis contains the sacrum and the pelvic girdle formed by ilium, ischium and pubic bones. These bones are lined by the iliacus, psoas major and sometimes psoas minor muscles (**Fig. 3**).

The *visceral ligaments* are connective support of vessels which lie along sagittal-vesicopubic, vesicouterine (pillar bladder), uterosacral laterallateral sacral, parametric and paracervical, lateral rectal (**Fig. 4**).

The *acollaged visceral surfaces* are: septumsvesicouterine, vesicovaginal and rectovaginal; pelvic spaces—paravesical, pararectal, retropubic space of Retzius, retrorectal and presacral.

The *visceral pelvic fascia* lines the pelvic viscera.

The open or the laparoscopic anatomy can be divided into:
- *Sagittal spaces and septums—from posterior to anterior:*
  - Promontory
  - Rectovaginal septum

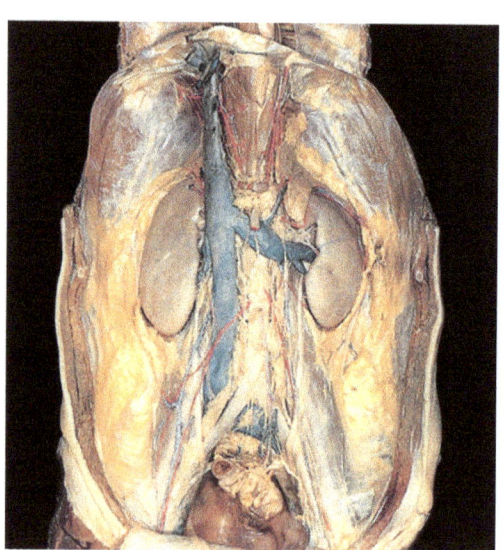

Fig. 1: Dissected retroperitoneum.

Retroperitoneum: What to Expect?

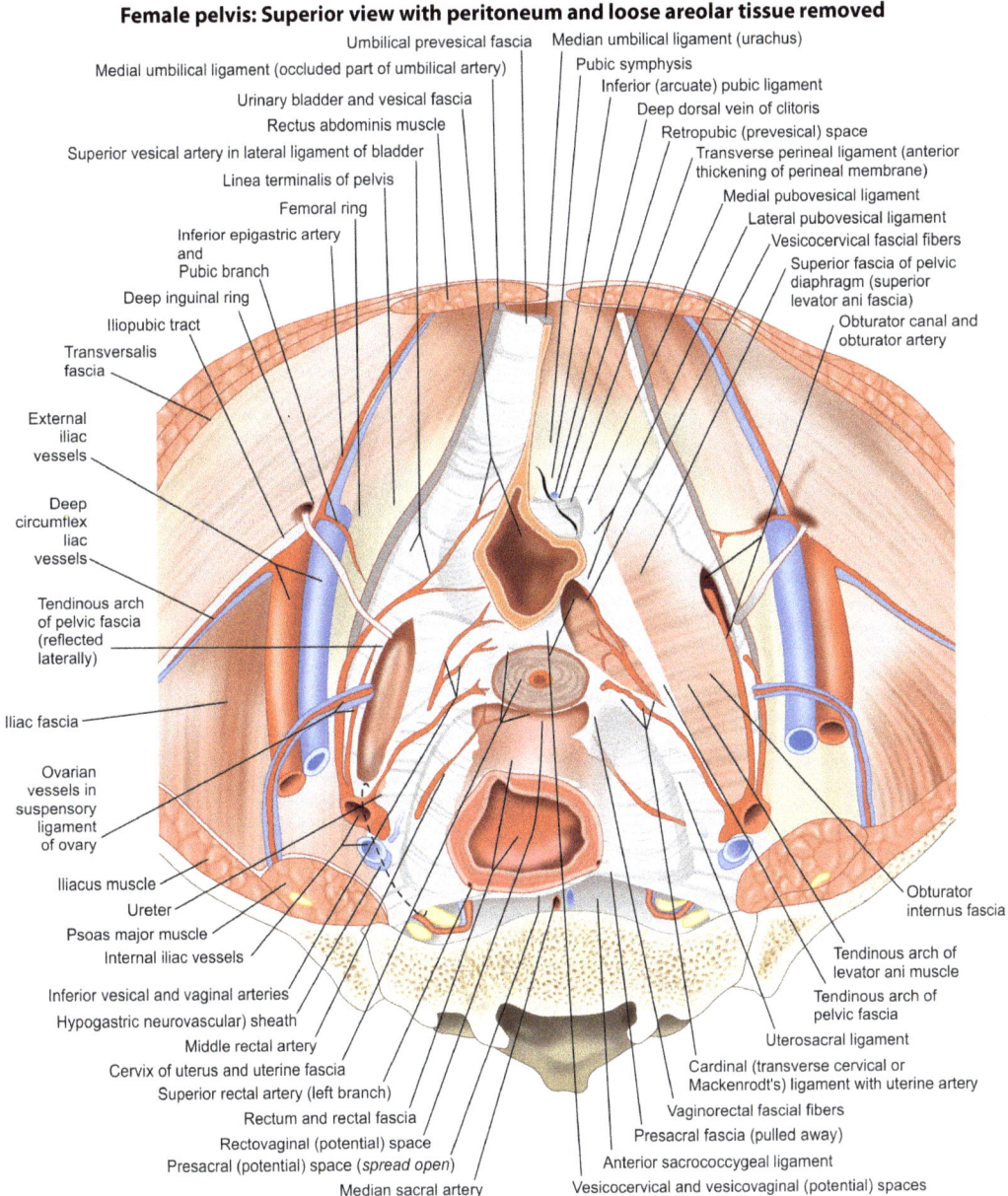

Fig. 2: Pelvic viscera and retroperitoneum.

- Vesicovaginal septum
- Retropubic space of Retzius
■ Lateral spaces:
  - Paravesical and pararectal spaces
  - Parametrium and paracervix
  - Pelvic ureter

Promontory

This is the projection of the first sacral vertebrae into the retroperitoneum and the peritoneal cavity. It constitutes a portion of the margin of the pelvic inlet. It joins at an angle of 30° to the vertebral column and is called the sacrovertebral angle **(Figs. 5A and B)**.

This landmark is important during sacral colpopexy for fixation of mesh in vault prolapse.

Rectovaginal Septum

The rectovaginal septum or the rectovaginal fascia also called fascia of Otto. It is a thin structure separating the vagina from the rectum. Inferiorly and laterally, it is bound by the perineal body **(Fig. 6)**.

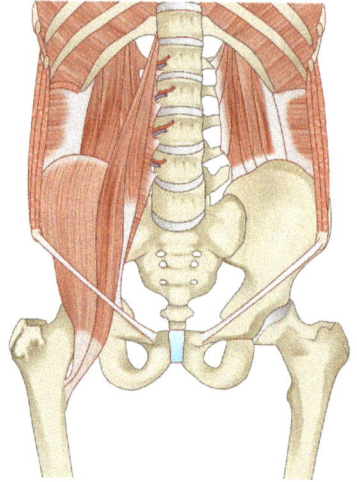

Fig. 3: Muscles of the posterior abdominal wall.

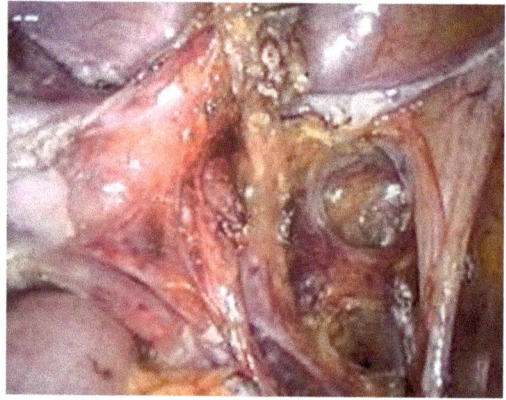

Fig. 4: Visceral ligaments.

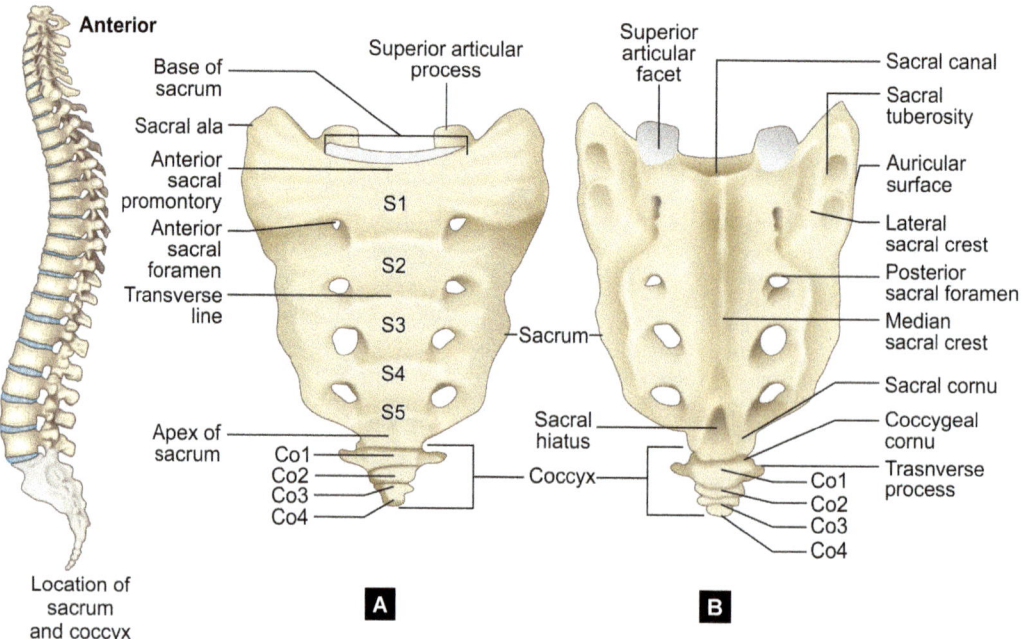

Figs. 5A and B: Structure of the sacrum: (A) Anterior view and (B) Posterior view.

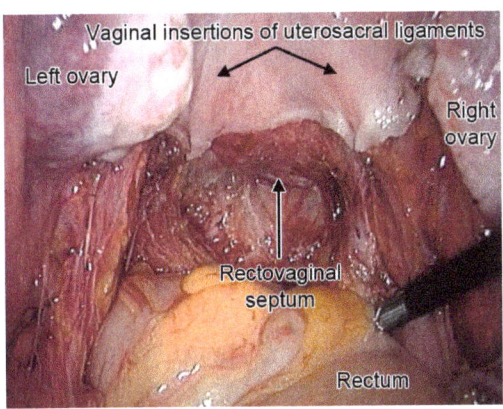

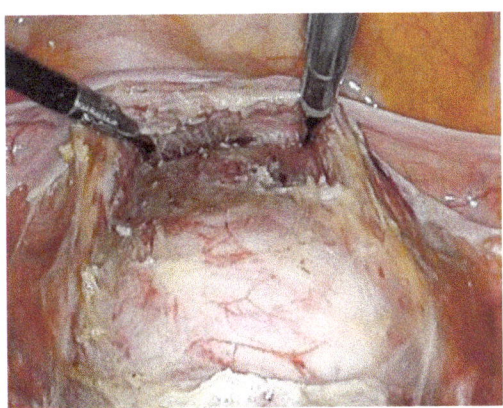

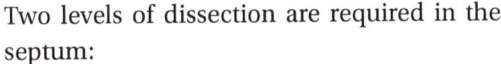
Fig. 6: Rectovaginal septum.

Fig. 7: Vesicovaginal dissection during promontofixation.

Two levels of dissection are required in the septum:
1. *For promontofixation*: Vagina/rectum and the levator ani muscles
2. *For radical hysterectomy or deep endometriosis*: Vagina/rectum/uterosacral ligaments.

Vesicovaginal Septum

The vesicovaginal space is the commonly dissected space by gynecologists. It is a potential avascular space except its lateral boundaries formed by the vesicocervical ligament or bladder pillars (**Fig. 7**). It is demarcated anteriorly by the urinary bladder and posteriorly by the cervix and uterus.

Retropubic Space of Retzius

Retropubic space is a potential extraperitoneal avascular space with vascular borders between the pubic symphysis and the urinary bladder (**Fig. 8**). The retropubic space is a preperitoneal space, behind the transversalis fascia and in front of the peritoneum.

The floor of this space is formed by the paraurethral ligaments and the urethrovesical junction (bladder neck).

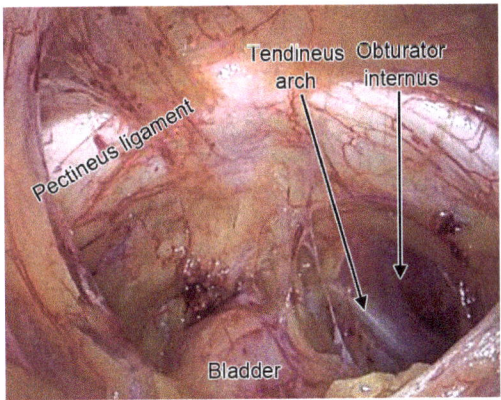
Fig. 8: Retropubic space.

Paravesical Spaces

The paravesical spaces are paired avascular spaces of the pelvis. The paravesical spaces generally contain fat, but can become filled with ascites, blood or pus.

Boundaries

- *Superior*: Lateral umbilical folds
- *Inferior*: Pubocervical fascia as it inserts into the tendinous portion of the levator ani muscle
- *Anterior*: Arcuate rim of the ileum

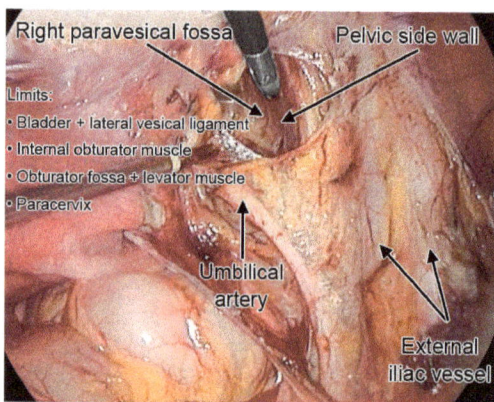

Fig. 9: Paravesical spaces.

- *Posterior*: Cardinal ligament dividing the paravesical spaces from the pararectal spaces
- *Medial*: Bladder pillars
- *Lateral*: Pelvic walls, obturator internus and levator ani muscles

Relations

- Continuous with the retropubic space (space of Retzius), which lies medially
- Continuous with the infrarenal space, which lies superiorly

In approximately 40% of patients, this space is traversed by accessory obturator arteries and veins which originate from the inferior epigastric vessels and drape across the pectineal (Cooper's) ligament on their way to anastomose with the obturator vessels in the obturator canal **(Fig. 9)**. The surgeon must always look for them especially when performing retropubic colposuspension.

Pararectal Space

The pararectal spaces are paired, triangular-shaped spaces in the posterior pelvis.

Boundaries

- *Anterior*: Base of cardinal ligament
- *Medial*: Rectal pillars
- *Lateral*: Levator ani muscle, internal iliac arteries
- *Posterior*: Sacrum

Contents

- Fat
- Connective tissue

Relations

- Separated from the *paravesical spaces* by the cardinal ligament
- Separated from the *presacral (retrorectal) space* by the rectal septa

This space can be easily developed by bluntly dissection lateral to the ureter and posterior to the origin of the uterine artery.

Parametrium and Paracervix

The parametrium is the fibrous and fatty connective tissue that surrounds the uterus.[1] This tissue separates the supravaginal portion of the cervix from the bladder. The parametrium (called cervical stroma in some texts) lies in front of the cervix and extends laterally between the layers of the broad ligaments. It connects the uterus to other tissues in the pelvis.

Contents: Uterine artery and ovarian ligament.

An associated form of pelvic inflammatory disease is inflammation of the parametrium known as parametritis.

THE PELVIC URETER

Out of all the structures mentioned, the ureter is the most feared structure in the retroperitoneum as it is likely to be injured and missed intraoperatively **(Fig. 10)**. The course is important but its recognition by its peristalsis and the crisscrossing vessels on

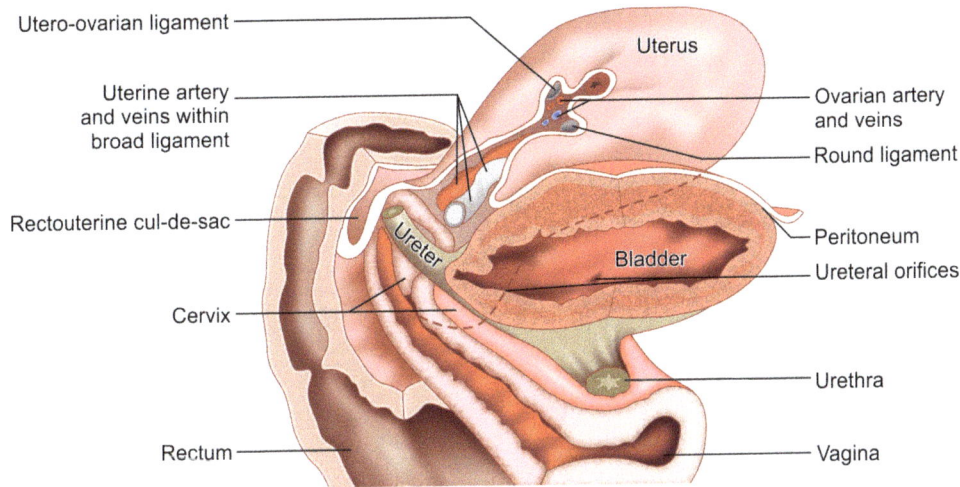

Fig. 10: Pelvic ureter.

the surface would avoid injury in situations where the anatomy is altered due to pathology.

CONCLUSION

The knowledge of this retroperitoneal anatomy would make the surgeon confident doing the surgeries and avoid untoward complication.

REFERENCE

1. Laparoscopy Blog. Intraoperative images from www.laparoscopy.blogs.com.

4 | Important Renal Physiological and Biochemical Parameters

CHAPTER

Ritu Hinduja, Rohan Palshetkar

INTRODUCTION

Kidneys play an important role in the excretion of waste products and toxins such as urea, creatinine and uric acid from the body in urine. They also have a vital role in regulation of extracellular fluid volume, electrolyte concentration and serum osmolality. Kidneys not only play an important role in excretion but also in regulating hormones such as erythropoietin and 1,25-dihydroxyvitamin D and renin. Nephron is the functional unit of the kidney and consists of the glomerulus, proximal and distal tubules, and the collecting ducts.

Assessment of renal function is important in the management of patients with kidney disease or pathologies affecting renal function. Tests of renal function have utility in identifying the presence of renal disease, monitoring the response of kidneys to treatment, and determining the progression of renal disease.[1-4]

COMPOSITION OF URINE

Urine is made up of water and solids. Solids in the urine are made up of organic and inorganic substances **(Fig. 1)**.

RENAL FUNCTION TESTS

Renal function tests are a battery of tests that are performed to assess the functioning of the kidneys.

There are three types of renal function tests:
1. Examination of urine

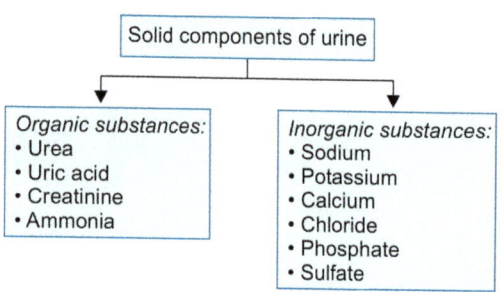

Fig. 1: Solid components of urine.

2. Examination of blood
3. Examination of blood and urine

Examination of Urine: Urinalysis

Urinalysis is performed under the following headings:
- Physical examination
- Microscopic examination
- Chemical analysis

Physical Examination

The interpretation of physical examination of urine are given in **Table 1**.

Microscopic Examination

Microscopic examination is when the urine is centrifuged and then the sediments are examined under a microscope **(Table 2)**. It helps to diagnose renal disease.

Chemical Analysis

Chemical analysis helps to determine the presence of abnormal constituents of urine or presence of normal constituents in abnormal quantities **(Table 3)**.

TABLE 1: Interpretation of physical examination of urine.

Parameter	Normal range	Differential diagnosis
Volume	1,000–1,500 mL/day	Increases due to an increase in protein catabolism and can be due to: • Chronic renal failure • Diabetes insipidus • Glycosuria
Color	Straw color	Abnormal coloration can be due to: • Jaundice • Hematuria • Hemoglobinuria • Medications • Excess urobilinogen • Ingestion of beetroot • Color added to food
Appearance	Clear	Physiological conditions causing turbidity: • Precipitation of crystals • Presence of mucus or vaginal discharge Pathological causes of turbidity: • Presence of blood cells • Bacteria or yeast
Specific gravity	1.010–1.025	• Low—diabetes insipidus • High—diabetes mellitus, acute renal failure and excess medications
Osmolarity	1,200 mOsm/L	Decreased in diabetes insipidus
pH and reaction	pH of 4.5–6 /Slightly acidic	• pH decreases in renal diseases • Slightly alkaline in vegetarians • Acidic in non-vegetarians

TABLE 2: Results of microscopic examination of urine.

Centrifuged sediments	Indicates
Red blood cells	Glomerular disease such as glomerulonephritis
White blood cells	• Acute glomerulonephritis • Infection of urinary tract, vagina or cervix
Epithelial cells	• Nephrotic syndrome • Tubular necrosis
Casts	Glomerulonephritis/tubular necrosis
Crystals	• *Normal crystals*: Calcium oxalate, calcium phosphate, uric acid and triple phosphate (calcium, ammonium and magnesium) • *Abnormal crystals*: Cysteine and tyrosine • Seen in liver disease
Bacteria	$\geq 10^5$ colony-forming units in a midstream urine specimen are diagnostic of an infection (bacteriuria) (Kass et al., 2002)

EXAMINATION OF BLOOD

Estimation of Plasma Proteins

Normal values of plasma proteins:

- *Total proteins*: 7.3 g/dL (6.4–8.3 g/dL)
- *Serum albumin*: 4.7 g/dL
- *Serum globulin*: 2.3 g/dL
- *Fibrinogen*: 0.3 g/dL

Renal failure may alter the above mentioned levels.

TABLE 3: Results of chemical analysis of urine.

Constituent in urine	Normal level	Pathology/Significance in case of presence
Glucose	180 mg/dL	• Glycosuria (>180 mg/dL) • Diabetes mellitus
Protein	30 mg/day	• Proteinuria/albuminuria (>30 mg/day) • Glomerulonephritis • Fever • Severe exercise
Ketone bodies	Nil	Pregnancy, fever, diabetes mellitus, prolonged starvation and glycogen storage diseases
Bilirubin	Nil	• Bilirubinuria • Hepatic and posthepatic jaundice
Urobilinogen	1–3.5 mg/day	*Excess of urobilinogen*: Hemolytic jaundice
Bile salts	Nil	Jaundice
Blood	Nil	• Hematuria • Glomerulonephritis, renal stones, infection or malignancy of urinary tract
Hemoglobin	Nil	• Hemoglobinuria • Excess hemolysis
Nitrite	Nil	Indicates presence of bacteria

Albuminuria and Proteinuria[5]

- Albuminuria refers to the presence of albumin in urine to the magnitude of 30–300 mg/day.
- Albuminuria is used as a marker for incipient nephropathy in diabetics.
- Albuminuria is an independent marker for cardiovascular disease.
- Urine albumin can be measured in 24-hour urine collections or early morning or random specimens to calculate the albumin/creatinine ratio.
- Albuminuria on two separate occasions while excluding urinary infection points towards a glomerular dysfunction.
- Three or more months of albuminuria is indicative of chronic kidney disease.
- More than 300 mg/day of protein loss in the urine is termed as Frank proteinuria. Level of normal protein detected in the urine should be up to 150 mg/day.

Urine protein again can be measured by either resorting to a 24-hour urine collection or random sample urine protein:creatinine ratio (early morning sample preferred).

The KDIGO classification defines three stages of albuminuria:

1. *A1*: Less than 30 mg/g creatinine
2. *A2*: 30–300 mg/g creatinine
3. *A3*: Greater than 300 mg/g creatinine

If protein excreted in the urine exceeds 3.5 g/day it is indicative of nephrotic Syndrome which can manifest with edema, hypoalbuminemia and hypercholesterolemia.

Serum Electrolytes[6,7]

The standard values of serum electrolytes along with conditions caused by electrolyte imbalances are given in **Table 4**.

Renal Function Tests[6,7]

The standard values of the renal function parameters along with the possible differential diagnoses in case of abnormalities are listed in **Table 5**.

TABLE 4: Serum electrolyte values and their interpretation.

Electrolyte	Standard value	Causes
Sodium	135–145 mmol/L	*Hyponatremia:* • *Hypervolemic hyponatremia:* Hypothyroidism, inappropriate antidiuretic hormone secretion, paraneoplastic, chronic lung disease, trauma, postoperative situations, heart failure, liver cirrhosis, nephrotic syndrome, kidney failure • *Hypovolemic hyponatremia:* Diuretic therapy, adrenocortical insufficiency (Addison's disease), salt restriction in chronic kidney disease, chronic diarrhea or vomiting, ileus, burns *Hypernatremia:* • *Hypovolemic hypernatremia:* Profuse sweating, thirst, diarrhea, burns • *Hypervolemic or euvolemic hypernatremia:* Iatrogenic, medication, fever, Cushing syndrome, hyperaldosteronism, diabetes insipidus
Potassium	3.5–5 mmol/L	*Hypokalemia:* • Severe hypokalemia (<2.5 mmol/L) • *Insufficient intake:* Starvation • *Renal loss:* Chronic interstitial nephritis, tubulopathies, polyuria after acute renal failure, diuretics, primary or secondary hyperaldosteronism, Cushing's syndrome, steroid therapy • *Enteral loss:* Chronic diarrhea, chronic vomiting, nasogastric tube, laxative abuse, treatment with cation exchangers • *Potassium shift from extracellular to intracellular space:* Metabolic alkalosis, treatment of pernicious anemia with vitamin B_{12}, familial hypokalemic paroxysmal paralysis *Hyperkalemia:* • Severe hyperkalemia (>6.5 mmol/L) • *Iatrogenic:* Overdose of potassium medication, treatment with penicillin, potassium-sparing diuretics, spironolactone or transfusions • *Insufficient renal elimination:* Acute renal insufficiency with oligo/anuria, terminal renal insufficiency, adrenal insufficiency • *Potassium shift from intracellular to extracellular space:* Acidosis, severe hemolysis, crush syndrome, chemotherapy (tumor lysis syndrome)
Chloride	95–110 mmol/L	• *Hypochloremia:* Diuretics, Cushing's syndrome, hyperaldosteronism, vomiting, respiratory acidosis • *Hyperchloremia:* Chronic renal insufficiency, acid intake, carbonic anhydrase inhibitor, primary hyperparathyroidism, respiratory alkalosis, hyperchloremic metabolic acidosis
Calcium	*Total calcium:* 2.1–2.6 mmol/L *Free calcium:* 1.15–1.35 mmol/L	• *Hypocalcemia:* Vitamin D deficiency, protein deficiency, hypoparathyroidism, pseudohypoparathyroidism, osteoblastic bone metastases, medullary thyroid carcinoma, hyperphosphatemia (tumor lysis, renal insufficiency), complication of acute pancreatitis, hepatotoxic drugs • *Hypercalcemia:* Primary hyperparathyroidism, hyperthyroidism, pheochromocytoma, osteolytic bone metastases, paraneoplastic (e.g., renal cell carcinoma), overdose with vitamin A or D, medications (thiazides, lithium), sarcoidosis, tuberculosis, immobilization, renal insufficiency
Magnesium	0.7–1.1 mmol/L	• *Hypomagnesemia:* Insufficient intake, gastrointestinal loss, acute pancreatitis, renal loss (Bartter syndrome, polyuria after acute renal failure, diuretics, treatment with aminoglycosides or cisplatin), hyperthyroidism, hyperparathyroidism, hyperaldosteronism or bone metastases • *Hypermagnesemia:* Above 4 mmol/L lead to cardiac and neurological symptoms, iatrogenic (infusions, antacids, laxatives), renal insufficiency, hypothyroidism or adrenocortical insufficiency
Phosphates	0.8–1.5 mmol/L	• *Hypophosphatemia:* Critical levels below 0.35 mmol/L, inadequate intake, alcohol abuse, antacids, malabsorption, vitamin D deficiency, hyperparathyroidism, hyperventilation and respiratory alkalosis, diuretics, insulin therapy for diabetic coma, fast carbohydrate intake in malnutrition or sepsis • *Hyperphosphatemia:* Too low excretion of phosphates (renal insufficiency, hypoparathyroidism, acromegaly, vitamin D overdose) or the release from the intracellular space due to cell death (acidosis, tissue hypoxia, chemotherapy, rhabdomyolysis, hemolysis, immobilization

TABLE 5: Renal function tests.

	Standard value	Differential diagnosis
Creatinine	0.6–1.4 mg/dL (50–130 µmol/L)	• Acute kidney injury and chronic renal insufficiency • Nonrenal causes of creatinine elevation are increased muscle mass, exsiccosis, meat-rich diet, high physical activity
Cystatin C*	0.53–0.95 mg/L	• Acute kidney injury and chronic renal insufficiency • *Nonrenal cause*: Autoimmune diseases
Urea	• 10–50 mg/dL (1.7–8.3 mmol/L) • Blood urea nitrogen (BUN) is easily calculated from the urea concentration: Multiply urea in mg/dL with 0.467#	• *Elevated urea*: Acute kidney injury and chronic renal insufficiency • *Nonrenal causes*: Exsiccosis, high-protein diet and catabolic metabolic situations such as trauma, fever and hunger • *Low urea*: Malnutrition, hepatic insufficiency

*Cystatin C is more sensitive than creatinine to detect mild kidney damage (40–80 mL/min GFR).
#Creatinine can be useful to differentiate prerenal from renal causes when the BUN is increased. In prerenal disease, the ratio is close to 20:1, while in intrinsic renal disease it is closer to 10:1.

EXAMINATION OF BLOOD AND URINE

Plasma Clearance

Plasma clearance is defined as the amount of substance which is cleared from the plasma in a given unit of time. It is also termed as renal clearance and it is based on Fick principle.

Renal functions can be assessed by the following:
- Glomerular filtration rate
- Renal plasma flow
- Renal blood flow

The following values of the following factors are required to determine the plasma clearance of a particular substance:
- Volume of excreted urine
- Concentration of the given substance in urine
- Concentration of the given substance in blood

Measurement of Glomerular Filtration Rate

For calculating the glomerular filtration rate such a substance should be used that is neither secreted nor absorbed in the body. Inulin is one such ideal substance, it is neither absorbed nor secreted and is completely filtered out. Hence Inulin clearance rate can be presumed as GFR. Radioisotopes such as chromium-51 ethylene-diamine-tetra-acetic acid (51 Cr-EDTA) and technetium-99m-labeled diethylenetriamine-pentaacetate (99 Tc-DTPA) can be used as other exogenous markers. Iohexol is the most promising exogenous marker, especially in children.

The normal GFR for an adult male is 90–120 mL/min.

$$GFR/Inulin\ clearance\ rate = UV/P$$

- U = Concentration of the substance in urine
- V = Volume of urine flow
- P = Concentration of the substance in plasma

Creatinine clearance is another method to measure GFR accurately and is easier than inulin clearance, because creatinine is already present in body fluids and its plasma concentration is steady throughout the day. Being a metabolite it is neither reabsorbed nor secreted and is completely filtered out. The normal value of GFR by this method is approximately the same as determined by inulin clearance. This involves the collection of urine over a 24-hour period or preferably over an accurately timed period of 5–8 hours since 24-hour collections are notoriously unreliable.

In the modified diet in renal disease (MDRD) and the CKD-EPI equation, Serum creatinine is also utilized in GFR estimation. These eGFR equations include race, age, and gender variables which make them superior to serum creatinine alone.

Based on the kidney disease, GFR is classified into the following stages. Improving Global Outcomes (KDIGO) stages of chronic kidney disease (CKD):

- *Stage 1*: GFR greater than 90 mL/min/1.73 m^2
- *Stage 2*: GFR between 60 and 89 mL/min/1.73 m^2
- *Stage 3a*: GFR 45–59 mL/min/1.73 m^2
- *Stage 3b*: GFR 30–44 mL/min/1.73 m^2
- *Stage 4*: GFR of 15–29 mL/min/1.73 m^2
- *Stage 5*: GFR less than 15 mL/min/1.73 m^2 (end-stage renal disease)

Measurement of Renal Plasma Flow

To measure renal plasma flow, a substance, which is filtered and secreted but not reabsorbed, needs to be used. One such substance is para-aminohippuric acid (PAH). PAH clearance indicates the amount of plasma which passes through kidneys.

A determined amount of PAH is injected into the body. After sometime, concentration of PAH in plasma and urine and the volume of urine excreted are estimated.

Measurement of Renal Blood Flow

To determine renal blood flow, following values of factors are necessary:

- *Renal plasma flow*: Measured by using PAH
- Percentage of plasma volume in blood indirectly determined by using packed cell volume (PCV).

Calculation of Renal Blood Flow

Renal blood flow is calculated with the values of renal plasma volume and percentage of plasma in blood by using a formula given below.

Renal blood flow = Renal plasma flow/ % of plasma in blood

Urea Clearance Test

This is a clinical test used to assess renal function by using clearance of urea from plasma by kidney every minute. This test requires a blood sample to determine urea level in blood and two urine samples collected at 1 hour interval to determine the urea cleared by kidneys into urine. Normal value of urea clearance is 70 mL/min.

Urea is a waste product formed during protein metabolism and excreted in urine. So, determination of urea clearance forms a specific test to assess renal function.

REFERENCES

1. Okoro RN, Farate VT. The use of nephrotoxic drugs in patients with chronic kidney disease. Int J Clin Pharm. 2019;41(3):767-75.
2. Nwose EU, Obianke J, Richards RS, Bwitit PT, Igumbor EO. Prevalence and correlations of hepatorenal functions in diabetes and cardiovascular disease among stratified adults. Acta Biomed. 2019;90(1):97-103.
3. Damiati S. A Pilot Study to assess kidney functions and toxic dimethylarginines as risk biomarkers in women with low vitamin D levels. J Med Biochem. 2019;38(2):145-52.
4. Rodríguez-Cubillo B, Carnero-Alcázar M, Cobiella-Carnicer J, Rodríguez-Moreno A, Alswies A, Velo-Plaza M, et al. Impact of postoperative acute kidney failure in long-term survival after heart valve surgery. Interact Cardiovasc Thorac Surg. 2019;29(1):35-42.
5. Gounden V, Jialal I. Renal Function Tests. Treasure Island (FL): StatPearls Publishing; 2019.
6. Guder WG, Nolte J. Das Laborbuch für Klinik und Praxis. New York: Urban Fischer; 2009.
7. Siegenthaler W. Differentialdiagnose innerer Krankheiten. New York: Georg Thieme Verlag, Stuttgart; 1988.

History and Clinical Assessment of Lower Urinary Tract Symptoms

CHAPTER 5

Shreyas Nagaraj

INTRODUCTION

The lower urinary tract (LUT) consists of a group of closely related structures which together function and allow an efficient and low-pressure filling of the bladder, storage of urine with good continence and regular complete voluntary expulsion of urine.

LOWER URINARY TRACT SYMPTOMS

Lower urinary tract symptoms (LUTS) are often classified into storage symptoms, voiding symptoms, and postvoid symptoms. The functional classification of LUTS and the classification system proposed by the International Continence Society (ICS) are given in **Tables 1 and 2**, respectively.

TABLE 1: Expanded functional classifications.

Failure of Storage	
Because of the bladder	**Because of the outlet**

1. Overactivity:
   a. *Involuntary contractions (detrusor overactivity):*
     i. Neurologic disease, injury or degeneration
     ii. Increased afferent input or sensitivity
     iii. Inflammation
     iv. Increased neurotransmitter release
     v. Increased sensitivity to transmitter
     vi. Decreased inhibitory pelvic floor activity
     vii. Idiopathic
   b. *Decreased compliance:*
     i. Neurologic disease or injury
     ii. Fibrosis
     iii. Bladder muscle hypertrophy
     iv. Idiopathic
   c. *Combination*
2. Hypersensitivity:
   a. Inflammatory/infectious
   b. Neurologic
   c. Increased neurotransmitter release or sensitivity
   d. Psychological
   e. Idiopathic
3. Under activity (with retention and overflow incontinence)
4. Combination
	1. Genuine stress urinary incontinence:
	   a. Lack of suburethral support
	   b. Pelvic floor laxity, hypermobility
	
	2. Intrinsic sphincter deficiency:
	   a. Neurologic disease or injury
	   b. Fibrosis
	
	3. Combination (genuine stress urinary incontinence and intrinsic sphincter deficiency)
	
	4. Combination (bladder and outlet factors)
	5. Fistula

Failure of Voiding	
Because of the bladder	**Because of the outlet**

1. Neurogenic
2. Myogenic
3. Psychogenic
4. Idiopathic
	1. Anatomic:
	   a. Urethral stricture
	   b. External urethral compression, fibrosis
	2. Functional:
	   a. Striated sphincter dyssynergia (neurogenic)
	   b. Smooth sphincter dyssynergia or dysfunction (bladder neck dysfunction)
	   c. Dysfunctional voiding (non-neurogenic)

The important terms related to incontinence are described in **Table 3**.

Storage failure	Voiding failure
Due to bladder	Due to bladder
Due to outlet	Due to outlet

TABLE 2: International Continence Society Classification.

Storage phase	Voiding phase
Bladder function:	Bladder function:
• Detrusor activity:	• Detrusor activity:
– Normal or stable	– Normal
– Overactive:	– Underactive
- Neurogenic	– Acontractile
- Idiopathic	– Areflexic
• Bladder sensation:	Urethral function:
– Normal	• Normal
– Increased or hypersensitive	• Abnormal:
– Reduced or hyposensitive	– Mechanical obstruction
– Absent	– Overactivity
• Bladder compliance:	– Dysfunctional voiding
– Normal	– Detrusor sphincter dyssynergia
– High	– Nonrelaxing urethral sphincter dysfunction
– Low	
Urethral function:	
• Normal closure mechanism	
• Incompetent closure mechanism	

URINARY INCONTINENCE (FLOWCHART 1)

History

History of Present Illness

The urinary incontinence needs to be categorized based on its association with/without:

- Associated physical activity
- Associated urgency
- Associated sensory awareness

When patient gives a history of mixed urinary incontinence, it is important to ascertain which is more bothersome and dominant.

Wherever possible, the leak will need to be quantified by the number of clothing changed/number of sanitary pads used per day. This helps in assessment of response to treatment.

Next, the frequency of voiding during the day and night needs to be elicited and a note needs to be made of associated hesitancy/urgency/obstructive symptoms, if any. Patient should also be asked whether they need to strain or alter the posture in order to facilitate complete bladder emptying.

Any preceding trauma such as fall, spine/lower back surgery, previous LUT instrumentation with history of pregnancy

TABLE 3: Definitions of various types of incontinence.

Terminology	Description
Urinary incontinence	Complaint of any involuntary leakage of urine
Stress urinary incontinence	Complaint of involuntary leakage on effort or exertion or on sneezing or coughing
Urgency	Complaint of a sudden compelling desire to pass urine, which is difficult to defer
Urgency incontinence	Complaint of involuntary leakage accompanied by or immediately preceded by urgency
Postural incontinence	Complaint of voluntary loss of urine associated with change of body position (e.g., rising from a seated or lying position)
Nocturnal enuresis	Complaint of involuntary loss of urine that occurs during sleep
Mixed incontinence	Complaint of involuntary leakage associated with urgency and also with exertion, effort, sneezing or coughing
Continuous urinary incontinence	Complaint of continuous leakage
Insensible incontinence	Complaint of urinary incontinence in which the woman is unaware of how it occurred
Coital incontinence	Complaint of involuntary loss of urine with coitus

and details of delivery with postoperative stay details need to be noted.

Associated neurological symptoms such as tremors, numbness and tingling sensation in the toes, difficulty in balance and coordination and blurry vision need to be noted.

Coexisting pelvic organ prolapse (POP) history should also be elicited including practice of reducing mass to empty bladder completely.

History of Comorbidities

This is vital as neurological conditions such as Parkinson's, myelodysplasia, medulla spinalis injury, multiple sclerosis, stroke, dementia, and back surgery can affect the functioning of the LUT.

Diabetes mellitus can again affect the continence mechanism.

Past radiation, trauma mostly causes obstructive symptoms.

Note should be made of if the patient is pre-, peri- or postmenopausal, and usage of any oral contraceptive pills (OCPs)/hormone replacement therapy (HRT)—local or systemic.

History of surgery especially to the back, prolapse surgery, hysterectomy and previous anti-incontinence repairs can all lead to a host of LUTS.

History of Medication Intake

Antihypertensive drugs such as labetalol (sympatholytic) can increase stress urinary incontinence (SUI) as it decreases outlet resistance. Drugs used for bronchial asthma such as salbutamol, phenylephrine (sympathomimetics) can precipitate urinary retention. Diuretics do not affect bladder directly but aggravate incontinence due to increased urine production. Pharmacologic agents that can affect the LUT are described in **Table 4**.

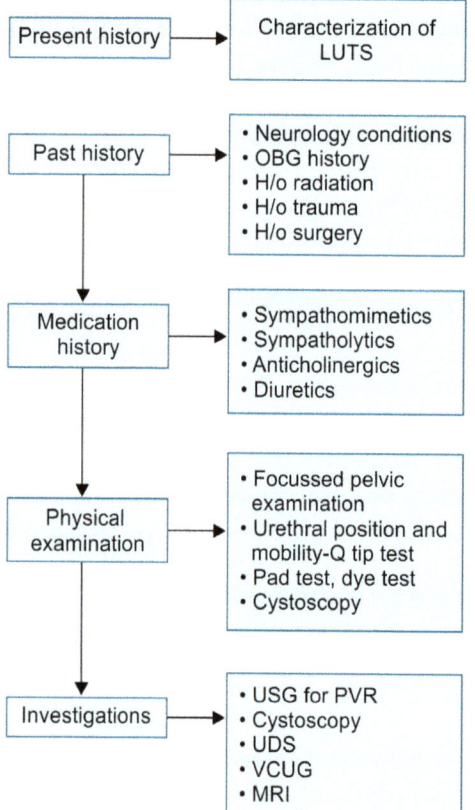

Flowchart 1: Management algorithm for urinary incontinence (LUTS).

TABLE 4: Pharmacologic agents that can affect the lower urinary tract.

Pharmacologic effects	Potential effects on urinary tract
Sympathomimetics (e.g., Amphetamines, Phenylephrine, Salbutamol)	• Can increase outlet resistance and exacerbate obstructive symptoms/overactive bladder symptoms • Can decrease detrusor contractility and precipitate retention
Sympatholytics (e.g., Propranolol, Esmolol, labetalol)	Can decrease outlet resistance and exacerbate stress incontinence
Anticholinergics (e.g., Carbochol, Bethenochol, Hyoscine)	Can contribute to urinary retention, particularly in patients with outlet obstruction
Diuretics (e.g. Furosemide, Torsemide)	Do not affect bladder directly, but because of increased urine production, can aggravate incontinence prolems

Examination

General Examination

Here note needs to be made of the posture and gait of the patient to assess neurological status.

Abdomen Examination

Any previous surgical scars, hernia and organomegaly causing pressure symptoms need to be looked for.

Local Examination

The external genitalia should be examined with particular attention to general appearance, lesions, size of labia, estrogen status and presence of adhesions.

The status of estrogen is often evaluated by whether a urethral caruncle is present or absent, urethral prolapse and labial adhesions. The presence or any or all of the abovementioned, may indicate deficiency of estrogen. Paying attention to the examination of the color and general tissue appearance is important. If the vaginal tissue is deficient in hormones it appears pale, flat and dry with no rugae, as opposed to the pink, healthy tissue with rugae—signs of good estrogenization.

Any associated prolapse should be evaluated and assessed for in detail is described in the *Chapter 22 (Genital Prolapse)*.

Mobility of the urethra and its position should be assessed at rest and with coughing and straining. The Q-tip test objectively demonstrates urethral hypermobility but is now obsolete.

Pad Tests

The recommendation of the ICS is to perform both a pad weight test and a bladder diary (3 days) as proper measure to quantify symptoms in evaluating incontinence **(Box 1)**.

BOX 1: 1-hour pad test.

0 minute:
- Apply preweighed pad
- Drink 500 cc sodium-free liquid
- Sit and rest

30 minutes: Walk and stairs climbing

45 minutes:
- Activities: Sit/stand × 10
- Cough × 10
- Run in place for 1 minute
- Picking up objects from the floor
- Washing hands under running water × 1 minute

60 minutes:
- Collect and weigh pad
- Patient voids, volume measured

Source: Abrams P, Blaivas JG, Stanton SL, Andersen JT. The standardisation of terminology of lower urinary tract function. The International Continence Society Committee on Standardisation of Terminology. Scand J Urol Nephrol. 1988;114(Suppl):5-19.

Dye Testing

Dye testing helps to confirm and verify if the leakage is of urine or whether it is any other fluid like peritoneal fluid or vaginal discharge and also to confirm the diagnosis of urinary tract fistulae.

Cystoscopy

Passing a cystoscope and examining the bladder is important as a means of evaluating whether any pathology in the bladder or the urethra is contributing to the patient's symptoms.

Urine Analysis

Presence of blood cells, pus cells, glucose or proteins in the urine may indicate presence of conditions, which may cause secondary urinary incontinence.

Postvoid Residual Urine

The residual urine stored in the bladder after routine voiding is termed the postvoid residual (PVR). More than 50 mL or more than 10% of the prevoid volume is considered significant.

The 2012 American Urological Association (AUA)/Society of Urodynamics, Female Pelvic Medicine and Urogenital Reconstruction (SUFU) SUI guidelines state that clinicians considering invasive therapy in patients with SUI should assess PVR to gauge bladder emptying, because patients with elevated PVRs preoperatively are at increased risk for developing voiding difficulties postoperatively.

Urodynamic Study

Urodynamic study (UDS) is indicated in patients who are considering invasive, potentially morbid or irreversible surgery; have had prior pelvic floor reconstructive surgery; or have mixed incontinence, urgency of urine or symptoms of urinary obstruction and in patients who have significantly increased PVR urine or neurologic disease.

Imaging

Radiographic Imaging

Voiding cystourethrogram: It is important to do imaging of the upper and lower urinary tracts of patients who have pelvic pathology or have had renal damage **(Figs. 1A to H)**. In patients with recurrent urinary tract infections (UTIs), voiding cystourethrogram (VCUG) is optional.

Ultrasonography

Imaging of the upper urinary tract is recommended in patients with chronic retention of

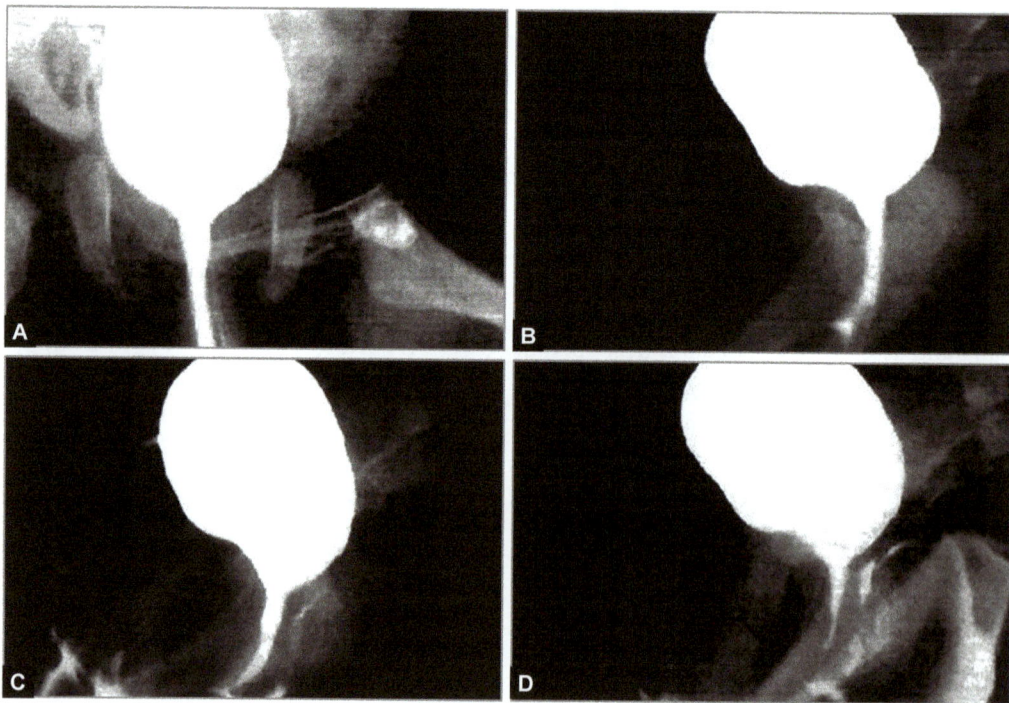

Figs. 1A to D

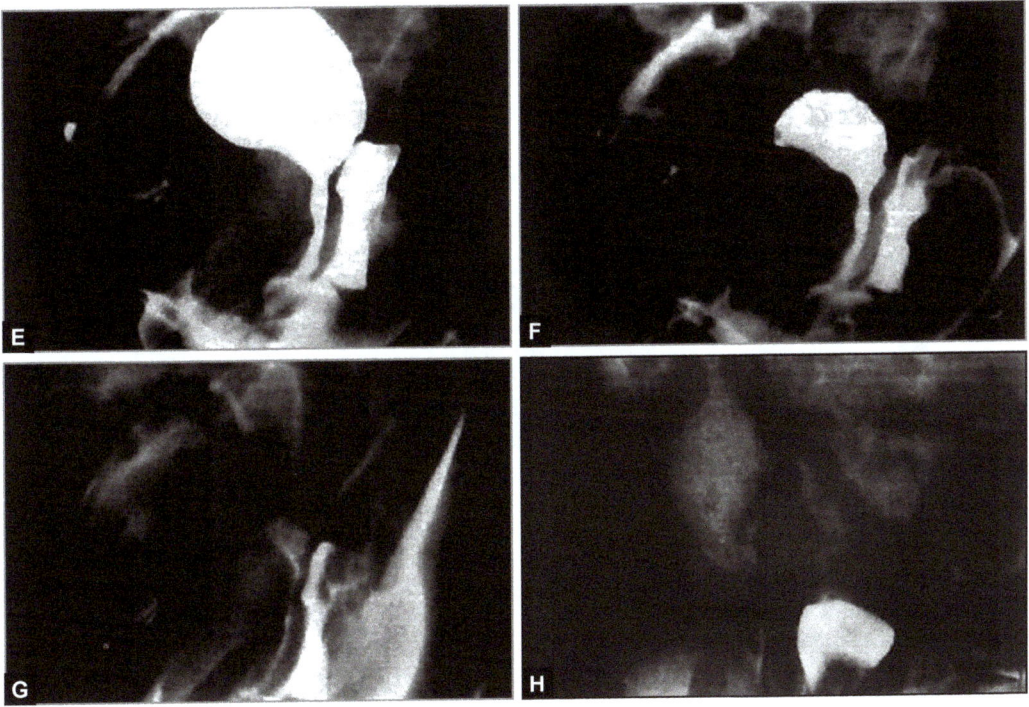

Figs. 1E to H

Figs. 1A to H: Voiding cystourethrogram demonstrating a voiding sequence in an infant girl. (A) Cystogram, frontal projection. The catheter is still in the urethra; (B) Cystogram, lateral projection; (C) Catheter withdrawn; voiding starts. The trigonal canal is formed, and the vagina starts to fill; (D to G) The vagina continues to fill as the bladder empties; (H) Film in the frontal projection. The bladder is empty whereas the vagina remains filled.

urine, suspected extra urethral incontinence, stage III/IV POP (untreated) and neurogenic dysfunction of the detrusor as they are considered to be at high risk for kidney damage **(Fig. 2)**.

Magnetic Resonance Imaging

Magnetic resonance imaging (MRI) is an ideal imaging option to study the urethra and the bladder neck and their anatomy and its correlation with their function **(Figs. 3A and B)**.

MRI has also been advised to evaluate the relaxation of the pelvic floor and POP,

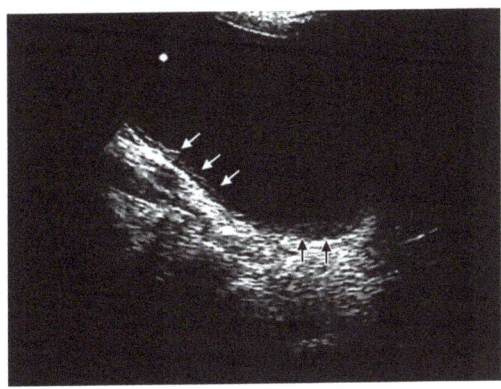

Fig. 2: A sagittal image of the bladder from a patient with recurrent cystitis reveals irregular thickening of the bladder wall (white arrows) and dependent layering debris (black arrows).

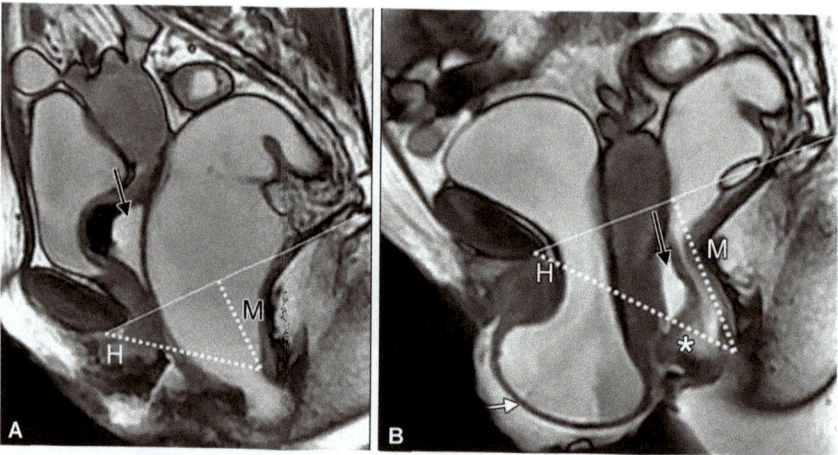

Figs. 3A and B: Cross-sectional images of the pelvic organs during rest and straining, demonstrating prolapse of pelvic organ: (A) Rest; (B) Straining (arrows and asterisk denote prolapse).

particularly in those patients who are undergoing evaluation for complex multi-compartmental pelvic floor reconstruction.

REFERENCES

1. Abrams P, Cardozo L, Khoury S, et al. Incontinence, 5th edition. Paris: International Consultation on Urological Diseases and European Association of Urology; 2013.
2. Townsend MK, Curhan GC, Resnick NM, et al. Postmenopausal hormone therapy and incident urinary incontinence in middle-aged women. Am J Obstet Gynecol. 2009;200:86.e105.
3. Lose G, Rosenkilde P, Gammelgaard J, et al. Pad-weighing test performed with standardized bladder volume. Urology. 1988;23:78-80.
4. Tubaro A, Artibani W, Bertram C, et al. Imaging and other investigations. In: Abrams P, Cardozo L, Khoury S, et al. (Eds). Incontinence. Third International Consultation on Incontinence. Plymouth, UK: Health Publication; 2005.
5. Artibani W, Andersen JT, Gajewski JB. Imaging and other investigations. In: Abrams P, Cardozo L, Khoury S, et al. (Eds). Incontinence. Plymouth, UK: Plymbridge Distributors; 2002. pp. 425-78.
6. Martin DR, Salman K, Wilmot CC, et al. MR imaging evaluation of the pelvic floor for the assessment of vaginal prolapse and urinary incontinence. Magn Reson Imaging Clin N Am. 2006;14:523-35.
7. Macura KJ, Genadry RR, Bluemke DA. MR imaging of the female urethra and supporting ligaments in assessment of urinary incontinence: spectrum of abnormalities. Radiographics. 2006;26:1135-49.
8. Holroyd-Leduc JM, Tannenbaum C, Thorpe KE, et al. What type of urinary incontinence does this woman have? JAMA. 2008;299:1446-56.

CHAPTER 6

Imaging in Urogynecology

Chander P Lulla, Selvapriya Saravanan

INTRODUCTION

A wide array of urogynecological problems requires imaging investigations. Conditions such as genitourinary prolapse and urinary incontinence are particularly important in the ageing female. Ultrasound (USG) has now turned out to be a reliable and possibly superior investigation to magnetic resonance imaging (MRI).[1]

The first step is to justify the investigation to be performed. Unless there is an expectation of significant improvement in patient management following the addition of imaging, it is of no use as an adjunct.[2]

Unlike other modalities, sonography is sometimes endocavitary, which can be kept to a minimum by adopting a transabdominal or perineal approach.[3] The additional concern of sonography being an intrusive procedure is also to be taken into account while counseling a patient for further investigation.[4]

Three-dimensional (3D) reconstruction has revolutionized the way imaging was used in the evaluation of the pelvis.[5]

Both USG and MRI based 3D algorithms are accurate in depicting muscular deficits and pelvic organ prolapse.[6,7]

MRI has an added advantage of giving more information regarding pathology and related anatomy. New dynamic techniques enable the evaluation of stress-induced pathologies.[8]

USG has a clear advantage over MRI because of its ease of operation in the dynamic assessment.[9] Further research and advancements in computer-aided processing have enabled the use of ultrasound and MRI which are comparable or sometimes better than physical examination.[10]

A lot has changed and improved in the field of imaging since the time of the Green classification. With further understanding of the anatomical relationship of the pelvic organs, MRI and ultrasound have taken center stage.

The era of X-rays and contrast conventional radiography has been completely replaced with ultrasound and MRI.

IMAGING OF UPPER GENITOURINARY TRACT

Scanning Techniques and Imaging Modalities

Scanning Technique

- *Patient position*: Supine or lateral decubitus
- *Approach*: Mid-axillary, subcostal or lower intercostal approach
- 3.5–5 MHz probe

Normal Sonographic Appearance (Fig. 1)

- Renal cortex is less echogenic than liver
- Renal sinus (fat and pelvicalyceal system) is more echogenic than the cortex
- Pyramids (if seen) are slightly less echogenic than the cortex
- Renal pelvis may appear as a central slit of anechoic fluid at the hilum

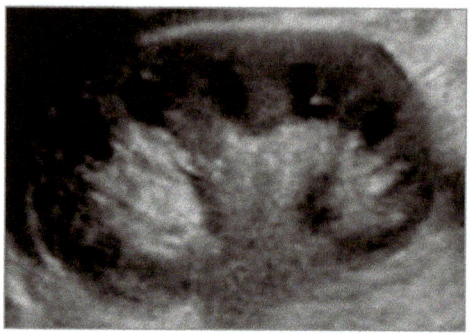

Fig. 1: Normal sonographic appearance of kidney.

Imaging Modalities

Previously conventional radiography using intravenous contrast in the form of intravenous urogram (IVU) was the first-line imaging modality, which is now replaced by computed tomography (CT) and USG.[11] The different intravenous urogram images are shown in **Table 1**.

CT and MRI give better imaging definition, enable to view anomalous drainage pathways

TABLE 1: Intravenous urogram.

Nephrogram (5 min)

- Renal parenchyma = Cortex + Medulla
- Renal pelvicalyceal system:
    - Minor calyx
    - Calyceal cupping by papillae
    - Infundibulum
    - Major calyx
    - Renal pelvis

Compression

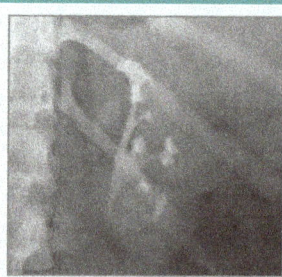

Pyelogram (10 min)

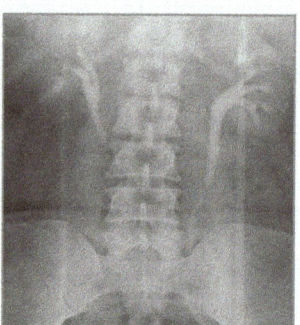

Prevoid

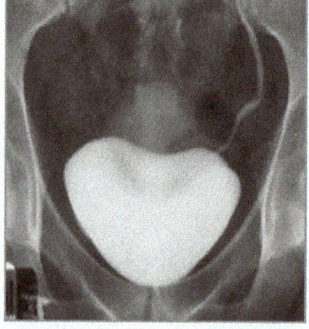

Compression

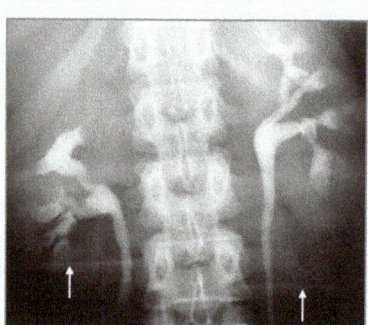

Postvoid

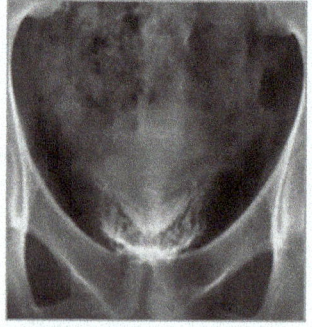

and pinpoint the site of obstruction. Addition of contrast allows assessment of the rest of the organs.[12]

Computed Tomography Scan

- *Plain non-contrast computerized tomography (NCCT)*: The presence of stones
- *Multiphasic*: In the setting of tumors, arterial phase imaging is essential to demonstrate hyperenhancement.
- *Urethra*: Voiding urethrogram can also be performed

Noncontrast phase **(Fig. 2)**:
- Calcification
- To look for calculi along the urinary tract
- Baseline for density measurement

Nephrographic phase (NP)—Abdomen **(Fig. 3)**:
- 60 sec after contrast injection
- Ideal phase for detection of mild parenchymal lesions
- Homogeneous enhancement of renal parenchyma
- Certain hyperenhancing lesions are missed due to delay in acquisition, especially vascular tumors

Excretory phase (EP)—abdomen and pelvis:
- 5 min after contrast injection
- Opacification of urinary system
- Renal pelvis—ureteric
  - Ureteric bud (UB) anomalies or pathologies

Especially in cases where a primary pelvic pathology results in an upstream obstructive dilation due to infiltration or occlusion, which are made out better than other imaging modalities.

Magnetic Resonance Imaging

MRI is the gold standard for visualizing diverticulum of bladder.[13]

Static-fluid MR urography **(Fig. 4)**: Non-contrast images are acquired as the patient holds urine for 4–6 hours allowing the bladder to be full. Heavily T2-weighted images are acquired which gives information only about the excretory system with more contrast. The fundamental idea is similar to that of an MRCP.

Excretory MR urography:[14] Excretory phase of enhancement after IV administration of gadolinium-based contrast material.

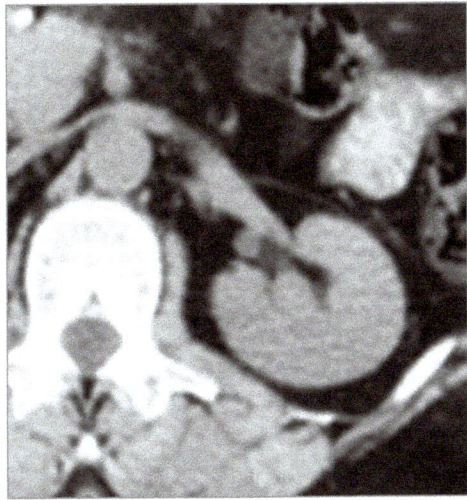

Fig. 2: Noncontrast phase.

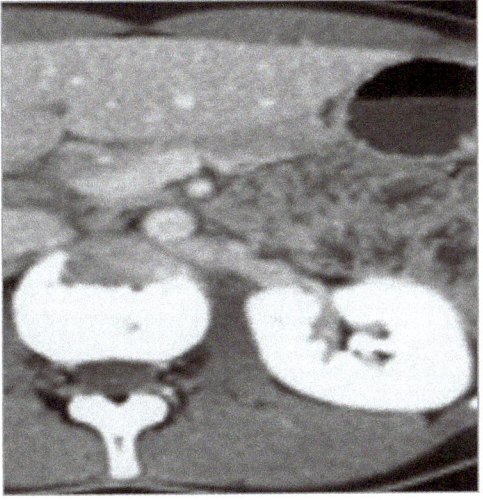

Fig. 3: Nephrographic phase—abdomen.

Video urodynamics is a hybrid of retrograde and voiding cystourethrography with cystometry.

ANATOMICAL ABERRATIONS

Duplex System

This occurs because of fusion not completing between the lower and pole moieties of the kidney resulting in duplications (both complete and incomplete) of the collecting system.

Duplex Kidney

Here there are two pelvicalyceal systems draining a single renal parenchyma **(Figs. 5 and 6)**:

Duplex kidney draining into:
- *Single ureter:* Where the duplicated systems fuse at the pelviureteric junction
- *Bifid ureter (bifid collecting system):* Two ureters fuse before they empty into the bladder
- *Double ureter (double collecting system):* Two ureters that each drain into the bladder on their own

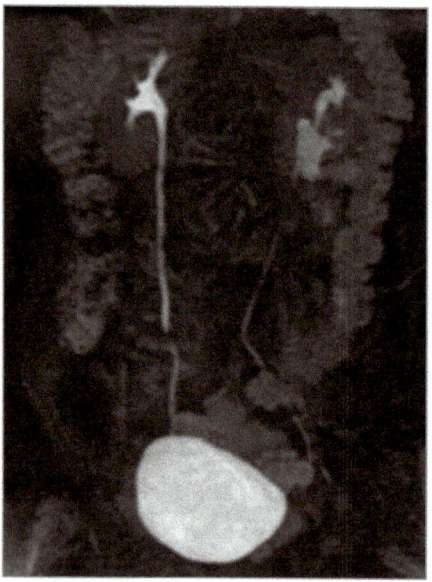

Fig. 4: Static-fluid MR urography.

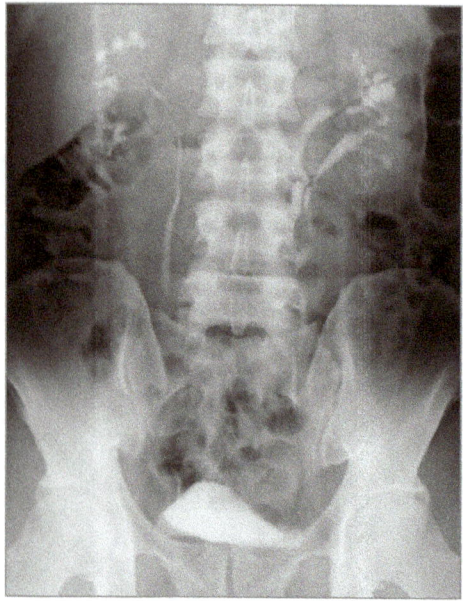

Fig. 5: Intravenous pyelography in a 25-year-old patient with urinary incontinence. The intravenous pyelogram shows a complete duplex system on the left side.

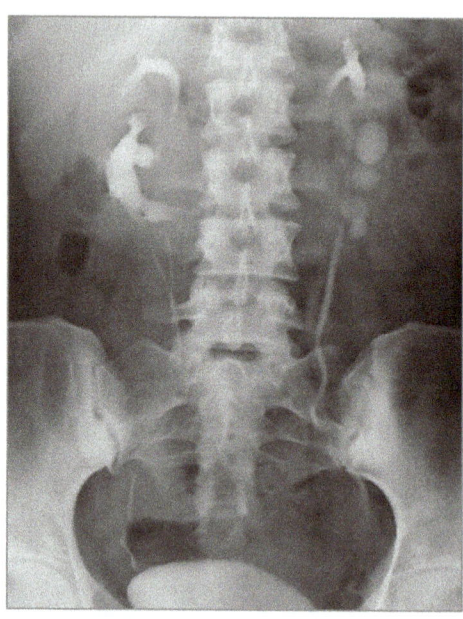

Fig. 6: An 18-year-old girl presenting with the pain in abdomen. Her IVP shows a horseshoe kidney with duplication of the excretory system.

Imaging in Urogynecology

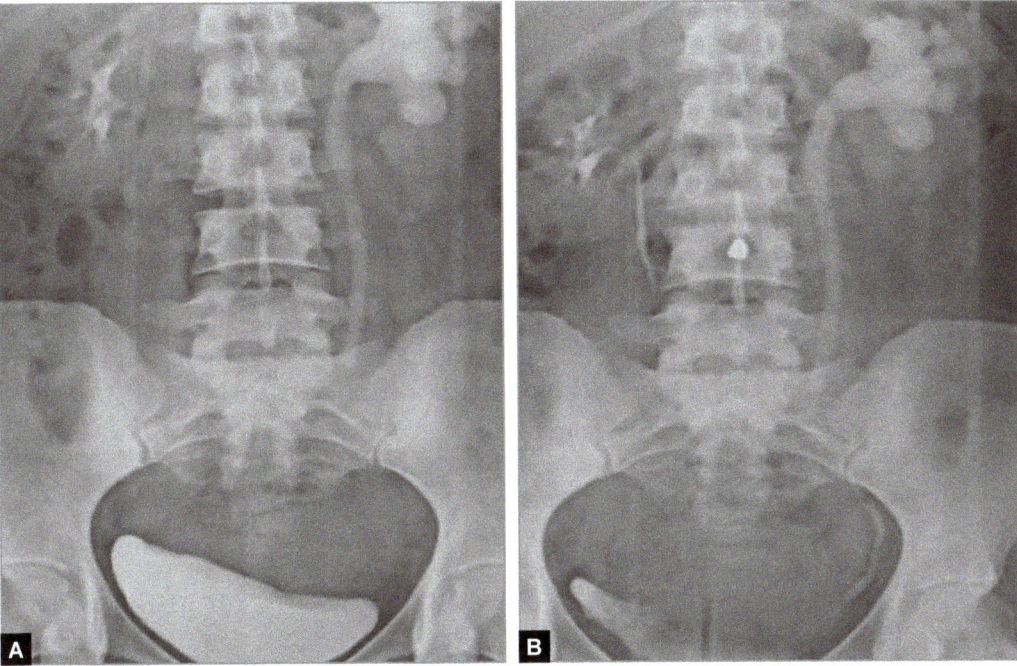

Figs. 7A and B: Prevoid and postvoid images show a persistent left sided hydroureteronephrosis.

Weigert-Meyer Rule (Figs. 7A and B)

Upper Pole Moiety

Ureter inserts heterotopic: Medial and caudal to normal ureter.[15] Ureterocele → Obstruction → Hydroureteronephrosis → Downward and lateral displacement of the functional lower moiety collecting system → Appearing radiographically as "drooping lily" sign.

Lower Pole Moiety

Ureter inserts orthotropic: Normal ureteric orifice (vesicoureteric reflux).

SONOGRAPHY

Ultrasound **(Fig. 8)** is a fast and readily available cheap modality for imaging the kidneys, which shows the presence of obstruction. It not only shows the degree of dilation but also the level of obstruction. CT is better at picking up radiodense calculi which are seen as shadows and artifacts in USG.[16]

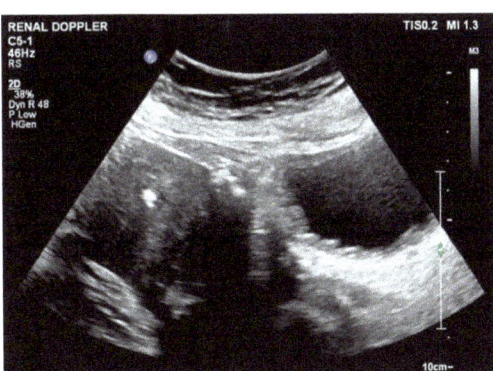

Fig. 8: A partially empty bladder is seen in a 40-year-old diabetic female with the uterus lying posteriorly. A partial image of the IUCD is seen within the endometrium at the fundus.

Care should be taken while doing an introital ultrasound, simple measures such as using warm jelly will prevent tightening of the perineal musculature.[17] The patient can be examined in a semi-reclining position instead of standing position as this would make no difference in a dynamic assessment of the bladder neck **(Fig. 9)**.[18]

Studies are performed during contractions, while coughing, while exerting pressure and Valsalva maneuver **(Fig. 10)**.[19]

The posterior urethrovesical (PUV) angle is the angle between two lines passing along the posterior urethra and trigone;[8] normal is 110–115° on an average.[22] Usually, the posterior urethrovesical angle is 96.8° at rest and 110 while straining. The distance between the bladder neck and lower edge of the pubic symphysis is 20.6 mm at rest and 14.0 mm while straining. The angle between the proximal urethral axis and the vertical plane is the urethral inclination angle which varies with pelvic inclination, although cutoff values of <45° or >45° have been described.[22] The urethropelvic angle is defined as the angle between a line through the middle of the internal urethral orifice and the urethral genu and a line through the posterior surface of the symphysis and the lowermost part of the obturator foramen closest to the film (cutoff of 70° is diagnostic of bladder descent) **(Fig. 11)**.[23]

Bladder wall thickness is best measured after micturition in a lithotomy position with a transvaginal image.[24] These measurements are taken at the thickest part of the trigone, dome and anterior wall of the urinary bladder.

The symphysis orifice (SO) distance is measured at rest as the distance on a horizontal line from the symphysis to the internal urethral orifice (in anterior bladder suspension defects or bladder base insufficiency—values <20 mm are the cutoff points for descent).[25] In incontinent women, the urethral axis at rest (UAR) was found to be related to age (R2 = 0.28); patients with UI had a mean UAR of 25° and a mean urethral angle at straining (UAS) of 43°. Showalter et al.

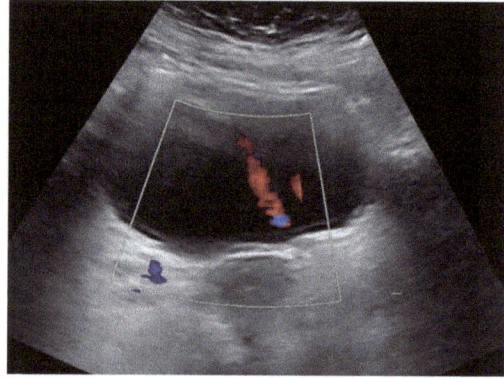

Fig. 10: Right-sided vesicoureteric junction (VUJ) calculus demonstrating pseudo color (twinkling artifact). Left VUJ shows a normal urine jet into the bladder on color Doppler imaging. The measurements are made both at rest and during contraction.[20,21]

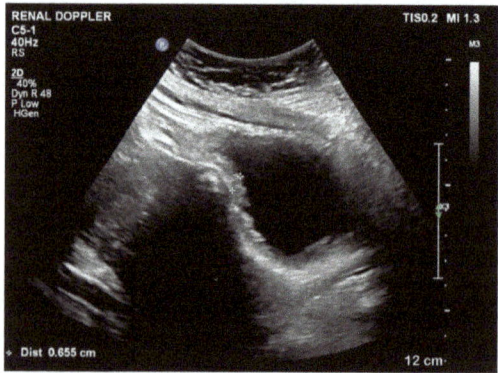

Fig. 9: The patient is suffering from a neurogenic bladder showing the classic trabeculated appearance, with undulating mucosal walls of the bladder marked by the callipers. Mild thickening is demonstrated.

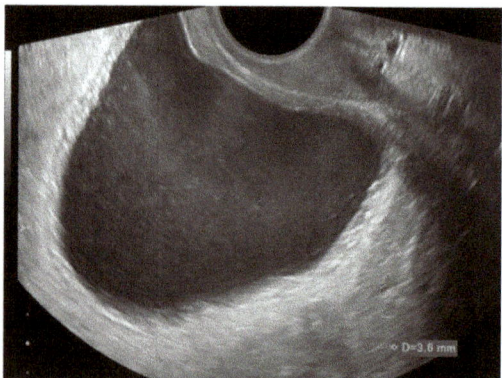

Fig. 11: Demonstration of bladder descent by measurement of urethropelvic angle.

measured UAR and UAS before and after surgery showing that both angles returned to near normal after surgery suggesting a correlation between the correction of the defective bladder support and cure.[26]

The funneling of the proximal urethra, the flatness of the bladder base, and the most dependent portion of the bladder base are important qualitative parameters estimated on straining films. Improper position of the patient or imaging technique does not adequately demonstrate funneling.

URETHRAL DIVERTICULUM

Urethral diverticula (UD) are outpouching of the urethral mucosa into the periurethral fascia. These diverticula maintain communication with the urethral lumen. It is seen in 0.6–6% of women and though it can occur at any age, is mostly seen in the 3rd to 5th decades **(Figs. 12 and 13)**.

Acquired Diverticulum

This is the most common etiology of urethral diverticula. The most widely accepted hypothesis involves rupture of a chronically obstructed and infected periurethral gland into the urethral lumen.

This outpouching epithelializes over time and becomes a true diverticulum lined with urothelium.

Escherichia coli and, less often, chlamydia and gonorrhea are the most common infectious causes.

Congenital Diverticulum

This is rare and usually is seen in the pediatric age group.

Clinical "Triad of Ds": Dysuria, Dyspareunia, and postvoid Dribbling.

Complications of Urethral Diverticulum

- *Infected urethral diverticulum:*
  - *T1*: hyperintense signal
  - *T2*: fluid/fluid level
- Calculus formation occurs in 10% of patients. This can be detected on ultrasound as an echogenic shadow within the urethral diverticulum. On MRI, it appears as a hypointense focus on both T1- and T2-weighted images.
- *Malignancy*: This is extremely rare and so far, there have only been fewer than 100 cases reported.

Even though the most common malignancy encountered in the female urethra is

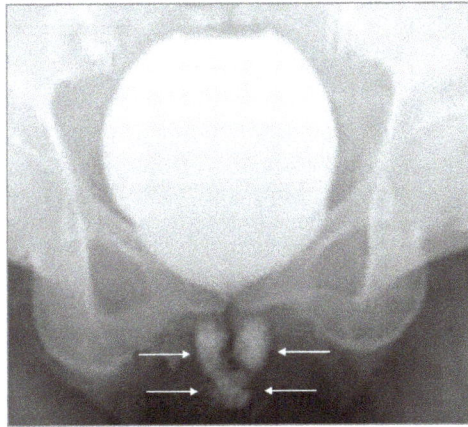

Fig. 12: Voiding cystourethrogram showing a multilocular diverticulum filled with contrast agent (arrows) at the level of the mid-urethra.

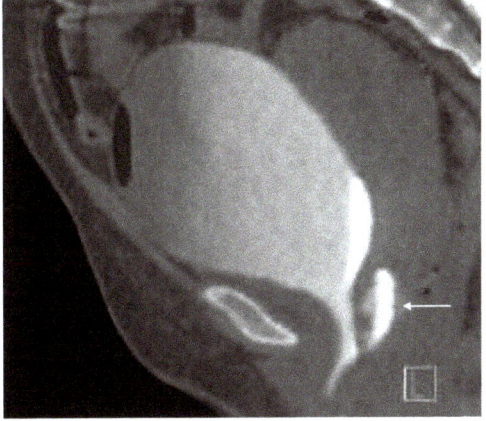

Fig. 13: CT voiding cystourethrogram shows a better-seen communication between the urethral lumen and urethral diverticulum filled with contrast agent (arrow).

squamous cell carcinoma (SCC), however, adenocarcinoma forms the majority (60%) of tumors arising from urethral diverticula.

Other conditions of importance are:
- Rectocele
- Cystocele
- Fistula
- Prolapse
- Incontinence
- Ureterocele
- Ectopic insertion of ureter into the vagina
- Postpartum fistulas and incontinence

REFERENCES

1. Pantazis K, Freeman RM. Investigation and treatment of urinary incontinence. Current Obstet Gynecol. 2006;16(6):344-52.
2. Shah W, Honeck P, Kwon ST, Badawi JK, Alken P, Bross S. The role of perineal ultrasound compared to lateral cystourethrogram in urogynecological evaluations. Aktuelle Urol. 2007;38:144–7.
3. Broekhuis SR, Kluivers KB, Hendriks JC, Fütterer JJ, Barentsz JO, Vierhout ME. POP-Q, dynamic MR imaging, and perineal ultrasonography: Do they agree in the quantification of female pelvic organ prolapse? Int Urogynecol J Pelvic Floor Dysfunct. 2009;20:541-9.
4. Wise BG, Burton G, Cutner A, Cardozo LD. Effect of vaginal ultrasound probe on lower urinary tract function. Br J Urol. 1992;70:12-6.
5. Umek WH, Obermair A, Stutterecker D, Häusler G, Leodolter S, Hanzal E. Three-dimensional ultrasound of the female urethra: comparing transvaginal and transrectal scanning. Ultrasound Obstet Gynecol. 2001;17:425-30.
6. Athanasiou S, Khullar V, Boos K, Salvatore S, Cardozo L. Imaging the urethral sphincter with three-dimensional ultrasound. Obstet Gynecol. 1999;94:295-301.
7. Toozs-Hobson H, Khullar V, Cardozo L. Three-dimensional ultrasound: a novel technique for investigating the urethral sphincter in the third trimester of pregnancy. Ultrasound Obstet Gynecol. 2001;17:421-4.
8. Lockhart ME, Fielding JR, Richter HE, Brubaker L, Salomon CG, Ye W, et al. Reproducibility of dynamic MR imaging pelvic measurements: a multi-institutional study. Radiology. 2008;249:534-40.
9. Majida M, Braekken IH, Umek W, Bø K, Saltyte Benth J, Ellstrøm Engh M. Interobserver repeatability of three and four-dimensional transperineal ultrasound assessment of pelvic floor muscle anatomy and function. Ultrasound Obstet Gynecol. 2009;33:567-73.
10. Weinstein MM, Jung SA, Pretorius DH, Nager CW, den Boer DJ, Mittal RK. The reliability of puborectalis muscle measurements with 3-dimensional ultrasound imaging. Am J Obstet Gynecol. 2007;197:68.e1-68.e6.
11. Platt JF, Rubin JM, Ellis JH. Distinction between obstructive and nonobstructive pyelocaliectasis with duplex Doppler sonography. Am J Roentgenol. 1989;153:997-1000.
12. Gufler H, DeGregorio G, Allmann KH, Kundt G, Dohnicht S. Comparison of cystourethrography and dynamic MRI in bladder neck descent. J Comput Assist Tomogr. 2000;24:382-8.
13. Leyendecker JR, Barnes CE, Zagoria RJ. MR urography: techniques and clinical applications. Radiographics. 2008;28:23-47.
14. Grobner T. Gadolinium—a specific trigger for the development of nephrogenic fibrosing dermopathy and nephrogenic systemic fibrosis? Nephrol Dial Transplant. 2006;21:1104-8.
15. Kolbl H, Bernaschek G, Wolf G. A comparative study of perineal ultrasound scanning and urethrocystography in patients with genuine stress incontinence. Arch Gynecol Obstet. 1988;244:39-45.
16. Martan A, Masata J, Halaska M, Voigt R. Ultrasound imaging of the lower urinary system in women after burch colposuspension. Ultrasound Obstet Gynecol. 2001;17:58–64.
17. White RD, McQuown D, McCarthy TA, Ostergard DR. Real-time ultrasonography in the evaluation of urinary stress incontinence. Am J Obstet Gynecol. 1980;138(2):235-7.
18. Schaer G, Koelbl H, Voigt R, Merz E, Anthuber C, Niemeyer R, et al. Recommendations of the German Association of Urogynecology on functional sonography of the lower female urinary tract. Int Urogynecol J Pelvic Floor Dysfunct. 1996;7(2):105-8.
19. Tunn R, Petri E. Introital and transvaginal ultrasound as the main tool in the assessment of urogenital and pelvic floor dysfunction: an imaging panel and practical approach. Ultrasound Obstet Gynecol. 2003;22(2):205-13.
20. Bader W, Degenhardt F, Kauffels W, Nehls K, Schneider J. Ultrasound morphologic parameters of female stress incontinence. Ultraschall Med. 1995;16(4):180-5.

21. Schaer G, Koelbl H, Voigt R, Merz E, Anthuber C, Niemeyer R, et al. Recommendations of the German Association of Urogynecology on functional sonography of the lower female urinary tract. Int Urogynecol J Pelvic Floor Dysfunct. 1996;7(2):105-8.
22. Green TH, Jr. Development of a plan for the diagnosis and treatment of urinary stress incontinence. Am J Obstet Gynecol. 1962;83:632-48.
23. Mikulicz-Radecki F. Röntgenologische studien zur ätiologie der urethralen inkontinenz. Zbl Gynäk. 1931;55:795-810.
24. Khullar V, Salvatore S, Cardozo L, Bourne TH, Abbott D, Kelleher C. A novel technique for measuring bladder wall thickness in women using transvaginal ultrasound. Ultrasound Obstet Gynecol. 1994;4(3):220-3.
25. Gjorup T. Reliability of diagnostic tests. Acta Obstet Gynecol Scand. 1997;166(Suppl):9-14.
26. Showalter PR, Zimmern PE, Roehrborn CG, Lemack GE. Standing cystourethrogram: an outcome measure after anti-incontinence procedures and cystocele repair in women. Urology. 2001;58:33-7.

7. Basics of Urodynamics

Premkumar Krishnappa

INTRODUCTION

Urinary bladder has twofold function, storage and voiding. Bladder acts as a reservoir of urine during the filling phase and as a pump during the voiding phase.

Storage of urine requires:
- Accommodation of increasing volumes of urine at low intravesical pressure and with appropriate sensation.
- A bladder outlet that is closed at rest and remains closed with increased intra-abdominal pressures.
- Absence of involuntary abnormal contractions of detrusor during the filling.

Bladder emptying requires:
- Coordinated contraction of the bladder smooth muscles for an adequate magnitude and duration
- Simultaneous lowering of the resistance at the level of smooth and striated sphincters
- Absence of anatomical obstruction during the flow

The whole process of bladder filling and emptying is controlled and coordinated by the autonomic nervous system through sympathetic and parasympathetic nerves (**Fig. 1**).

As always, sympathetic system helps in retaining of urine and parasympathetic system regulates the coordinated emptying.[1]

Urodynamics, as the name suggests, is a study of the "Dynamics of Micturition."

It is a series of investigations, which reproduces the patient's lower urinary tract functions more objectively and helps to identify the pathophysiology of the symptoms involved and guide treatment plan for the same. These

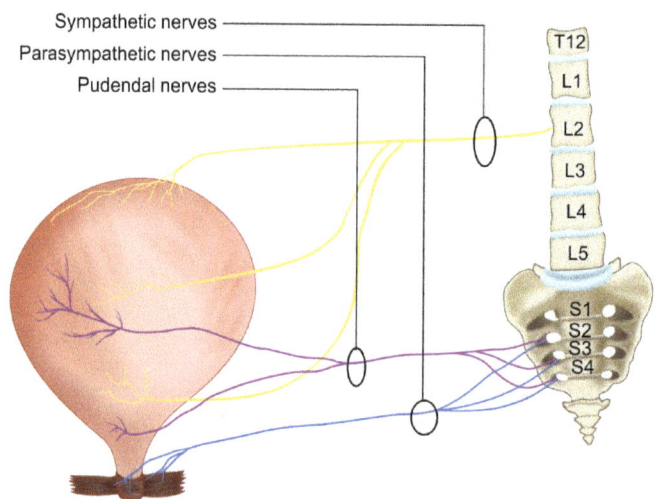

Fig. 1: Bladder innervation.

involve few very basic tests, which does not involve catheterization or high-end equipment and also some invasive assessment, involving catheterization and assistance from radiology with high-end equipment.

THE NEED FOR THE URODYNAMIC EVALUATION

Urodynamic assessment is used to understand the pathophysiology of the symptoms of the patient, which is either not clearly understood, prolonged, or nonresponsive to basic treatments. It is also useful to evaluate patients with neurological problems. The concept of urodynamics is, objectively identifying the natural process of bladder filling and emptying, with or without a note of activities in the bladder, abdomen, and the sphincters.

PREREQUISITES FOR URODYNAMICS

Clinical Information

This is more than vital for the urodynamic evaluation. The symptoms have to be elaborately known, so that we actually know what we are expecting, or ruling out, in the urodynamics.

Symptoms and clinical data should include:
- *Irritative symptoms*: Frequency, urgency, and incontinence (stress/urge and its severity).
- *Obstructive symptoms*: Poor stream of urine, hesitancy, and straining to void.
- *Neurological symptoms or disorders if any*: Surgical intervention on lower urinary tracts, prolapse of pelvic organs, multiple or complicated/prolonged deliveries. Make a note of any medications the patient is on, that may influence the lower urinary tract functioning. Bladder diary is useful if the symptoms are predominantly irritative, for objective assessment. A sample of the same is shown in **Table 1**.[2]

Physical Findings

Abdominal examination is done for surgical scars, location of the external urethral meatus, and its caliber (meatal stenosis). Pelvic examination is done for identifying vaginal prolapse and tone of the perineal body along with neurological examination of superficial and deep sacral reflexes.

Investigations
- Urinalysis, urine culture
- Ultrasonography of the urinary system and pelvis

CONTRAINDICATIONS FOR URODYNAMICS
- Patient with cognitive impairment who cannot understand the instructions
- Mechanical urethral obstructions (stricture, stenosis)
- Presence of urinary tract infection
- Urodynamics unlikely to change the management plan[3]

THE URODYNAMIC STUDIES

Noninvasive Assessments
- Uroflowmetry
- Postvoid residual urine (PVRU)

Invasive Assessments
- Cystometry
- Pressure-flow study
- Leak point pressures (abdominal and detrusor)
- Electromyography (EMG)
- Urethral pressure profile
- Video urodynamics (with fluoroscopy and/or ultrasound assistance)
- Ambulatory urodynamics

Equipment Required

Noninvasive Tests
- *Uroflowmetry machine*: Types—gravimetric method, rotating disk, and electronic dipstick **(Fig. 2)**.
- Ultrasonography for evaluation of the residual urine.

Basics of Urodynamics

TABLE 1: Daily bladder diary for objective assessment.

Time	Liquid intake		Bathroom visits		Urine leakage	Urgency to urinate	What were you doing at the time of leak?
Sample	Juice	100 mL	Two times	250 mL	Once small volume	Yes/No	Running
6–7							
7–8							
8–9							
9–10							
10–11							
11–12							
12–1							
1–2							
2–3							
3–4							
4–5							
5–6							
6–7							
7–8							
8–9							
9–10							
10–11							
11–12							
12–1							
1–2							
2–3							
3–4							
4–5							
5–6							

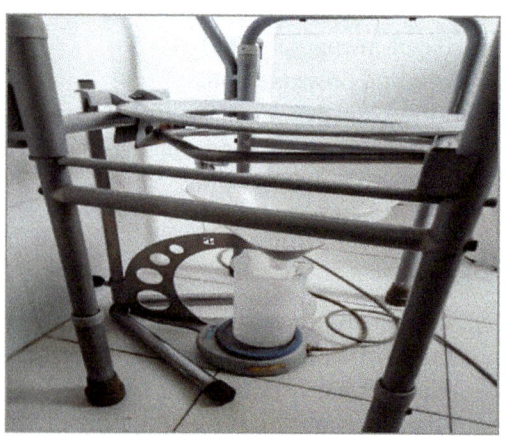

Fig. 2: Uroflowmetry machine.

Invasive Urodynamics

Basic equipment required are catheters, normal saline for filling the bladder, pressure transducers, computer with the specific software for assessment, seating/standing facility during the test, uroflowmetry instrument connected to the computer.

- *Catheters*: Two single lumen or one double lumen catheter (for insertion into the bladder, one to record the pressures inside the bladder and one for filling the bladder). The catheter sizes vary depending on the institution. The general

Basics of Urodynamics 45

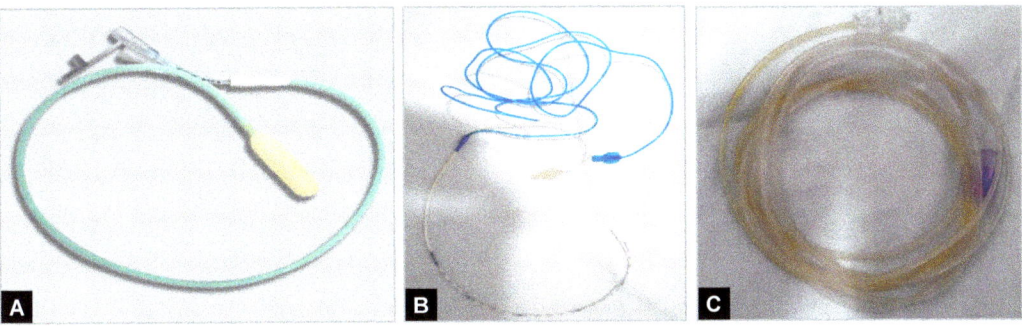

Figs. 3A to C: Different types of catheter.

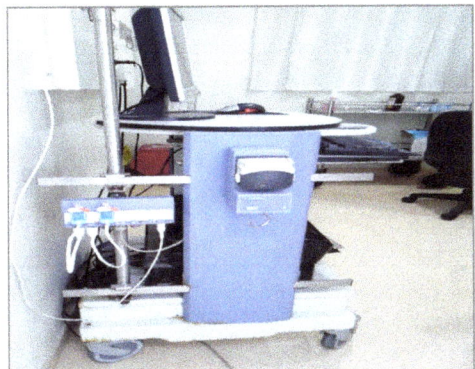

Fig. 4: Transducer setup.

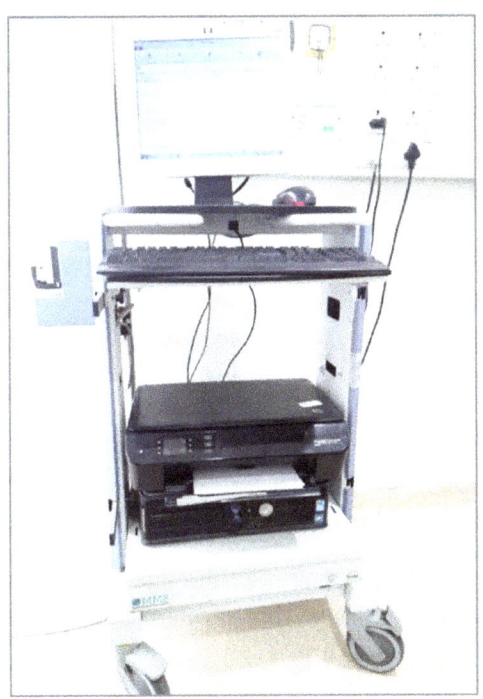

Fig. 5: Computer with software for urodynamics.

agreement is a catheter size between 6 and 10 fr **(Figs. 3A to C)**.

- *Rectal catheter*: It is placed for measurement of indirect pressures in the abdominal cavity.
- *Transducers*: These barometric instruments measure the pressures generated in the catheter lumen either at the end of the catheter or on tips of the tip-loaded transducers. The information is transmitted to the software which projects these pressures in the form of a graph and gives the real-time values with changes in all the pressures **(Fig. 4)**.
- *Software and computer*: The computer is loaded with the specific software for projecting and visualizing all the pressures with graphical representation and numbers and also a real-time assessment of the changes in the same **(Fig. 5)**.

Noninvasive Urodynamics

Uroflowmetry: It was traditionally done by visual inspection of the act of micturition. The other simpler method is to check the voided volume over a given time using a timer. The problem with these methods is, they do not give a proper estimation of speed and other useful parameters, and are predominantly subjective. It is modified for privacy and convenience with a machine—uroflowmeter.

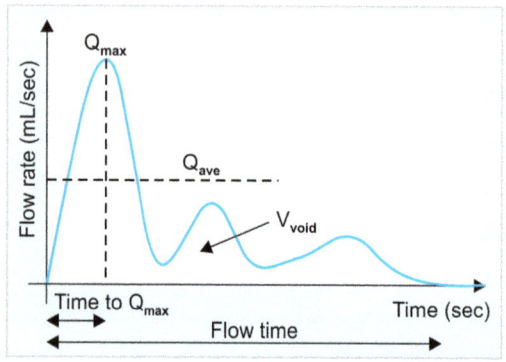

Fig. 6: Uroflowmetry parameters.

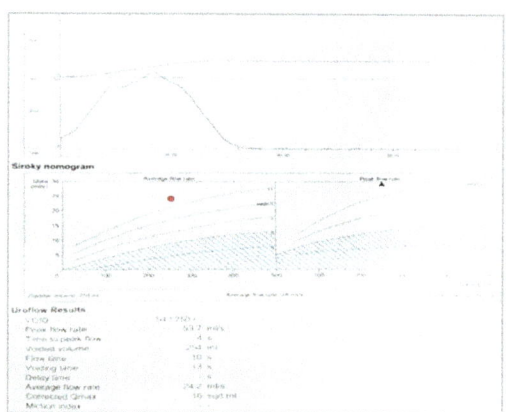

Fig. 7: Normal uroflowmetry curve.

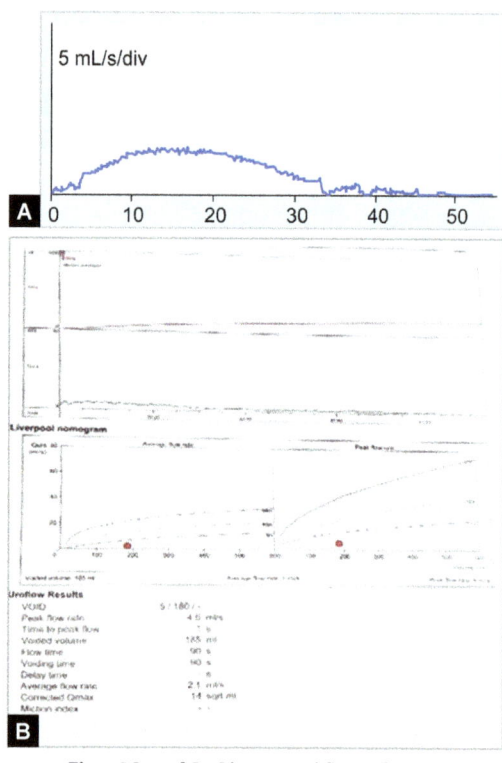

Figs. 8A and B: Obstructed flow of urine.

The usual equipment used is based on a gravimetric method which takes into account the volume of the liquid falling on the sensor and calculates the speed of the fall. Though there are many more methods, it is away from the scope of this article to discuss in detail about them. The parameters assessed by uroflowmetry are:
- The maximum speed of the flow—Q_{max}
- The average speed of the flow—Q_{ave}
- Time duration of voiding, volume voided—V_{void} **(Fig. 6)**

The curve of the flow, duration of the flow, and pattern of the flow are other relevant findings.

The authenticity of the test is only considered when the voided volume is more than 150 mL, since any lower volumes will not mimic the natural volumes for voiding.

Though the normal findings are extensively debated, usual accepted values are: A Bell-shaped curve, Q_{max}—15 mL/s or above, Q_{ave}—7 mL/s or above, voiding time—30 seconds, and time to Q_{max}—5 seconds.

A normal uroflowmetry: It varies physiologically with volume voided, age, time of the day, and patient's psychological status and the interpretation is based on the clinical feedback **(Fig. 7)**.

Abnormal patterns of uroflowmetry and their interpretation: **Figures 8 to 10** show abnormal patterns of uroflowmetry and their interpretation.

Postvoid residual urine: It is the remaining intravesical fluid volume determined directly after completion of the voiding. The technique (e.g., ultrasound or catheter) used to measure the volume is usually specified on reporting.

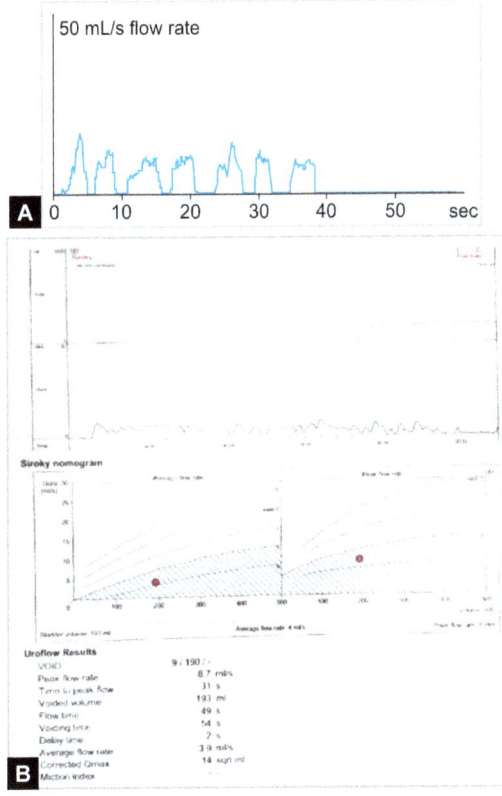

Figs. 9A and B: Interrupted flow—bladder hypocontractility/obstruction/abdominal strain.

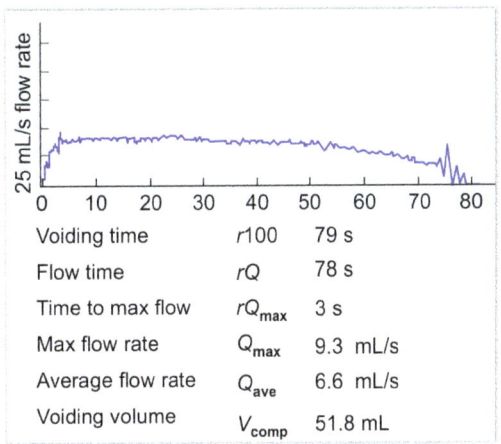

Fig. 10: Urethral stricture/meatal stenosis.

Voided percentage (Void%): It is the numerical description of the voiding efficacy, i.e., the proportion of bladder content emptied at a given time. Calculation: [(volume voided/ volume voided + PVR) × 100]. It is suggested solely for the purpose of standardization— that the term voided percentage with the abbreviation Void% is preferred.[4]

Indications of Invasive Urodynamic Evaluation

- Lower urinary tract symptoms (LUTS) not fitting into any clear urological diagnosis.
- Any surgical intervention planned for LUTS and urodynamic results influencing the intervention.
- When there are overlapping symptoms of LUTS (i.e., obstruction with overactivity).
- Associated neurological problems which may be influencing the LUTS.
- Postsurgical persistence of LUTS or appearance of new symptoms.

Preparations for the Test

To begin, the patient is informed in detail about the procedure before the study. Patient is fully awake and aware during the procedure except if there is a requirement to have a sedation as in case of small children. Patient is usually evaluated in the natural voiding posture— standing in males and sitting in females. Supine position is sometimes used in neurologically affected patients which is an important information to be provided while reporting.

The person conducting the test should be aware of the clinical scenario to understand the basic problem and probable findings which may be expected during the study. As an example, if the patient has severe urgency and incontinence as a symptom with no or minimal residue in the bladder, filling the bladder has to be at a very slow rate and expect a leak at the early part of the test. Each variation during the test has to be meticulously noted, as it affects the decision making for the clinical problem. The patient has to be communicated to give proper feedback throughout the test and cooperate for proper conclusions. As mentioned earlier, measurement of pressure is the most important aspect of the test.

The patient will have the catheters inserted in the bladder (double lumen or two separate catheters) and in the rectum/colostomies as the case may be. The bladder catheters are opened up to empty the residual urine, before the transducers are connected. The catheters are then connected to the specified transducers. The transducers may be water pressure based, in which case the catheters are open ended or air pressure based, in which case the catheters are closed systems with air filled balloons at the bladder end. Usually the water pressure-based strain gauge is employed. One catheter in the bladder is connected to the transducer and the other to the controlled irrigation system which fills the bladder. The irrigation channel is connected to the flow monitor which controls the speed of fluid going into the bladder.

The transducers are always placed at the level of the pubic symphysis to start with and all the pressures are zeroed on the computer software. To validate the proper placement of the catheters and to check the patency, the patient is asked to cough at the start of the procedure and every 1 minute or after 50 mL of filling and at the end of the procedure. The graph is checked for consistent changes on cough all through.

Pressures

Measurement of pressures in the bladder and the abdomen is a crucial step in the interpretation of the investigation. The difference between the bladder and the abdominal pressures gives an inferred pressure which is the detrusor pressure. The vesical, abdominal, and the detrusor pressures are symbolized as P_{ves}, P_{abd}, and P_{det}, respectively.

- *Intravesical pressure*: P_{ves} is the pressure on the liquid present within the bladder. This pressure is a resultant of the pressure exerted by the bladder muscle (P_{det}) and the adjoining abdominal organs (P_{abd}). So practically $P_{ves} = P_{det} + P_{abd}$. All the pressures are calculated at the level of symphysis pubis and zeroing all at the start of the procedure at this level.
- *Abdominal pressure*: P_{abd} is in true sense the pressure of the abdominal organs on the fluid inside the bladder. It is approximated by measuring the rectal (ideal) or vaginal or colostomy pressure. As said earlier the pressure is measured at the level of pubic symphysis.
- *Detrusor pressure*: P_{det}, as shown in the equation above, is deduced as $P_{det} = P_{ves} - P_{abd}$. At the start of the test, since both P_{ves} and P_{abd} are zeroed, P_{det} is also zero. Any changes in the abdominal pressures will cancel with the vesicular pressure and P_{det} will ideally be zero, unless the P_{ves} shows higher pressure that is contributed by the detrusor and in such cases, P_{det} will rise.
- *Urethral pressure*: Pura is practically the pressure required by fluid to open up the urethra for voiding. It is done for specific indications and is performed by infusing fluid through the side hole of the catheter in the urethra which is held in place by balloons at bladder neck and external meatus.

CONDUCTING THE TEST AND INTERPRETATION

Cystometry

It is a continuous real-time monitoring of pressure/volume relation of the bladder. Mainly assessing the filling aspect of the bladder, it is useful to reproduce the symptom of incontinence and diagnose the anatomical reason for the same. It involves the filling of the bladder with a small-sized catheter and simultaneously monitoring the pressures of the detrusor, bladder, and the abdomen, as described earlier. The rate of filling varies depending on what the initial clinical diagnosis is and can be a slow fill if severe overactivity is suspected or a fast fill when provocation associated bladder activity is required to be assessed.

The bladder filling volume is usually about 300–600 mL in adults. For children the volume is calculated as 60 mL + 60 mL × age = volume (<2 years old), 180 mL + 15 × age = volume (>2 years old).

Leak Point Pressures

It is, in simple terms, the pressure in the bladder (P_{det}) or the abdomen (P_{abd}) at which there is leakage of urine from the bladder during filling. The assessment of both the pressures is done after at least half the bladder capacity (200–300 mL) is filled.

Types

Detrusor leak point pressure (DLPP): It is the value of the P_{det} at which there is a leak of urine with an absence of P_{abd}. The significance is, a higher value carries a high chance of upper tract reflux and subsequent pathology. A value of above 40 cmH$_2$O carries a higher risk of vesicoureteral reflux.

Abdominal leak point pressure (ALPP): It is the value of the P_{abd} at which there is a leakage of urine in the absence of P_{det}. It can be obtained by Valsalva (VLPP) or cough (CLPP). It is the direct measure of the urethral contribution for the continence. Values <60 cmH$_2$O is severe stress incontinence and is because of intrinsic sphincter deficiency. Pressures >90 cmH$_2$O implies a pelvic floor weakness and descent of the bladder base.

Pressure-flow Study of Voiding

It is a study of the relation of the pressures to the flow of urine and is mainly the assessment of the voiding phase of micturition. The parameters of concern are the maximum flow rate (Q_{max}), P_{det} at this maximum flow (P_{det} at Q_{max}), contribution of abdominal straining, volume voided, PVRU, and the flow pattern. Pressure-flow studies are predominantly ordered to confirm or rule out obstructed urine flow and detrusor contractions. Obstruction may be due to structural causes or dynamic causes.

- *Structural:* Urethral stricture, meatal stenosis, or bladder neck contracture
- *Dynamic:* Overactive urethral closure due to voluntary or involuntary behavioral (dysfunctional voiding), neurological lesion (detrusor sphincter dyssynergia)

Detrusor pressures can be very weak, weak, normal, or strong depending on which nomogram is followed.

There are a lot of nomograms which help in concluding the test result in terms of presence or absence of obstruction.

International Continence Society (ICS) nomogram is one of them. These nomograms are prepared for men. Since the anatomical considerations in male and female are different there are attempts to define obstruction specific to females. As a general rule, flow rate <12–15 mL/s with a P_{det} of >20 cmH$_2$O is considered mild obstruction in females.[5] Obstruction is considered severe if the detrusor pressures are >50 cmH$_2$O.

Electromyography

Urethral sphincter muscle plays an important role in the maintenance of the continence. Normally, sphincter shows increasing activity in the filling phase and is completely silent (sphincter relaxation) during the voiding phase. During the course of the pressure-flow studies, the activity of the urethral sphincter is assessed to know the activity of the urethral sphincter muscle. It is identified by the surface electrodes placed on the urethral sphincter region or anterior vaginal wall. The needle or wire electrodes are avoided because of the uncomfortable procedure and artifacts because of direct muscle stimulation.

The usefulness of EMG is in identifying a dyssynergic sphincter and sphincter muscle weakness. It is also used for biofeedback treatment.

Urethral Pressure Profile

Maintenance of continence is the function of urethra. Urethral closure pressure or resistance is the difference between the urethral pressure and the corresponding vesicle pressure. Urethral pressure is the pressure required to just open up the opposed urethral lumen. Urethral pressure profile is the relation of the pressure to the length of the urethra. There are many techniques such as perfusion technique, catheter-mounted transducer, or balloons connected to transducers to determine the same but none are without artifacts. The microtransducer method has shown great reproducibility. Typically the urethral pressure is high during bladder filling phase and decreases during voiding. The significance is that, during Valsalva or cough, there is a sharp increase in the urethral pressure and contributes for the continence.

Types of Urethral Pressure Recording

Resting urethral pressure: Maximum urethral closure pressure (MUCP) is typically 40–60 cmH$_2$O **(Fig. 11)**.

Functional urethral length is about 3 cm.

Stress urethral pressure profile is when the pressures are measured with simultaneous Valsalva or cough. Stress MUCP is more accurate and reproducible but still shows variability up to 20–25% in the same subject.[6]

Stress MUCP has more predictability and power in diagnosing urethral incompetence compared to resting pressure profile. But a

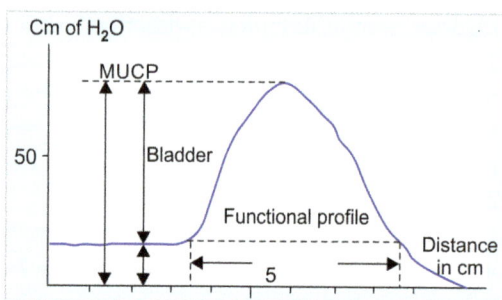

Fig. 11: Maximum urethral closure pressure (MUCP).

variation of the resting urethral pressure (fall of resting MUCP) in excess of 20–25 cmH$_2$O in the absence of detrusor activity, is considered as urethral instability and predicts incontinence.

Video Urodynamics

Video urodynamics is indicated when diagnosis remains unclear after simpler study or when complex pathology is expected. Utilizing radiology studies like image intensifier/X-ray/ultrasonography during the routine urodynamic evaluation is sometimes done for a more accurate diagnosis. It is useful especially in patients with LUTS due to neurological conditions. With the X-ray in place, the filling of the bladder is done with contrast instead of the usual normal saline. The advantages are simultaneous visualization of the anatomical changes and the measurement of pressures. The helpful findings are dyssynergy of sphincter, competence of the bladder neck, location of the urethral obstruction, descent of bladder base, intrinsic sphincter deficiency, and leakage of contrast on fluoroscopy during the study.

The disadvantages with the video urodynamics are the radiation involved and the discomfort on the lower urinary tract.

Ambulatory Urodynamics Monitoring

There are many situations where the patient's symptoms are not reflected in the cystometry, pressure flow, and video urodynamics. In case a patient persists to have a leak, but not during the tests or when medically attended, ambulatory urodynamics gives adequate information. Ambulatory urodynamics monitoring (AUM) is the monitoring of leakage, flow recordings, with pressure recordings of bladder and abdomen with or without pressure in the urethra in an ambulatory setting.

The catheter placements are as usual but they are taped, strapped, or stitched to prevent slippage. Patient is given push buttons to record events such as urgency, leak, and urination. Drinking and regular voiding are also recorded. AUM is usually indicated in failure of treatment, persistent symptoms in absence of abnormality on regular urodynamic evaluation.

CLINICAL APPLICATIONS OF URODYNAMIC STUDY

Urodynamic study is sought when the diagnosis is in dilemma based on the regular investigations. It helps in predicting the outcome of treatment, reason for failure of treatment, and to plan treatment for the same.

The approach as to what aspects are to be looked into in urodynamics is decided before ordering a study. This is based on the clinical symptom, extent of the problem, response of basic treatment given, and the impact it makes on surgical or nonsurgical treatment options.

Stress Incontinence

The indication of urodynamics in stress incontinence is when it is associated with symptoms of urgency, to rule out overactivity and underactivity before a surgical plan is made. A combined evaluation with MUCP, ALPP, and additional video urodynamics will give a clear definition of the type of stress incontinence.

- *Type 1*: Stress incontinence with <2 cm descent of the bladder base
- *Type 2*: Stress leak with >2 cm descent of bladder base:
  - *Type 2a*: Descent only when provoked
  - *Type 2b*: Permanent descent
- *Type 3*: Stress leak with bladder neck and proximal urethra fully open at rest

Type 2 is because of hypermobility and types 1 and 3 are because of intrinsic sphincter deficiency.

Urge Incontinence

The diagnosis of urge incontinence approaches 70–100% with urodynamic evaluation. If a nonsurgical approach is planned, then treatment can be started based on clinical symptoms of urge incontinence, especially if the stress component is absent.

Mixed Incontinence

When symptoms are of both stress and urge incontinence, urodynamics gives the component of each and helps plan management.

Voiding Difficulty with Incontinence

With additional voiding difficulty or history of anti-incontinence surgery, urodynamics plays an important role in diagnosis. Video urodynamics has a proven advantage over the cystometry and pressure-flow studies.

Neurogenic Lower Urinary Tract Symptoms

Any lesions along the nervous system can have its impact on micturition. The symptoms cannot be accurately predicted based on the lesion in many cases. The spectrum of impact may be from:

- *Bladder*: Acontractile detrusor to hyperactive detrusor
- *Sphincter*: Incompetent to hyperactive sphincters
- Coordinated bladder and sphincter activity to dyssynergic bladder and sphincter activity

The above needs to be properly defined to make a treatment plan which is physiologically and socially acceptable. One important precaution during the tests is to be aware of the autonomic dysreflexia which is commonly seen in high spinal cord injury patients.

SPECIAL CASES

Children

Though the test protocol is the same, the indications are different in children. It may be neurogenic bladder dysfunction, anatomical abnormality, and its impact on the urination, habitual, or late maturation of the nervous system with impact on bowel and bladder function.

Elderly Patients

Most elderly patients will have physiological detrusor overactivity. In frail patients, urodynamic evaluation is significant only if the residual urine is high which would require intermittent catheterization. Low volume residue with incontinence can be managed with anticholinergics. A bedside simple cystometry may be sufficient to take decisions in very frail patients, when regular urodynamics is unavailable or impractical.

REFERENCES

1. Vignoli G (Ed). Physiology of Micturition in Female. In: Urodynamics for Urogynecologists. Springer: Cham; 2018.
2. Daily bladder diary, urology topics, urologic diseases. National Institute of Diabetes and Digestive and Kidney diseases. [online] Available from: www.niddk.nih.gov/-/media/CFF38717ADB04D14B079828A52422A35.ashx [Last accessed on April, 2021].
3. Mc Kertich K. Urodynamics. Aust Fam Physician. 2011;40(6):389-91.
4. Rosier PFWM, Schaefer W, Lose G, Goldman HB, Guralnick M, Eustice S, et al. International Continence Society Good Urodynamic Practices and Terms 2016: Urodynamics, uroflowmetry, cystometry, and pressure-flow study. Neurourol Urodynam. 2017;36(5):1243-60.
5. Groutz A, Blaivas JG, Chaikin DC. Bladder outlet obstruction in women: definition and characteristics. Neurourol Urodyn. 2000;19(3):213-20.
6. Homma Y, Batista J, Bauer S, Griffiths D, Hilton P, Kramer G, et al. Chapter 7, Urodynamics. 2nd International Consultation on Incontinence, 2nd edition, 2001, July. Paris; 2002.

Stress Urinary Incontinence: Assessment and Management

Nita Thakre, Anuj Thakre

INTRODUCTION

International Continence Society defines urinary incontinence as the involuntary loss of urine that represents a hygienic or social problem to the individual.

Urinary incontinence is many times an underdiagnosed health issue that has a direct relationship with age. It affects around 50–80% of the elderly and is more common in females.

On most occasions, patients seek diagnosis and treatment with a delay of 6–9 years as a result of social stigma and a belief that it is a part of the ageing process. An estimated 50–70% of women are affected with urinary incontinence and out of them only 5% receive appropriate diagnosis and treatment.[1] It is imperative to create more awareness among the general population and medical professionals regarding this treatable condition which affects the quality of the affected.

TYPES OF URINARY INCONTINENCE[2]

Stress: A type of leakage which occurs following physical stressors which increase the intra-abdominal pressure, such as coughing, sneezing, laughing, climbing stairs and exercising.[3,4]

In patients with genital prolapse the stress urinary incontinence (SUI) may remain undiscovered. It has been proposed that the prolapse leads to kinking of the urethra. This mechanism contributes to the continence. Such SUI can be observed after reduction of the prolapse. This is known as *occult or latent SUI*.

Urge: It is a type of urinary leakage where the incontinence is immediately preceded by a strong urge to urinate.

Mixed: It is a combination of stress and urge incontinence.

Overflow: It is a type of incontinence secondary to incomplete evacuation due to a bladder outlet obstruction or poor detrusor contractility. The incontinence occurs once the bladder exceeds its capacity to store.[5]

Functional: The inability to maintain continence due to causes other than lower urinary tract or neurological pathology, such as psychiatric disorders, infection of lower urinary tract, impaired mobility, etc.[6,7] Functional incontinence is considered a fifth type of incontinence.[4,5,8]

PATHOPHYSIOLOGY

Any activity which causes an increase in the intra-abdominal pressure such as, laughing, sneezing, coughing, climbing stairs, also increases the pressure inside the bladder, exceeding the urethral resistance, causing urine to leak.

In women with SUI, the pathophysiology can be urethral hypermobility and/or intrinsic sphincter deficiency (ISD). These may present in varying proportions.

Urethral hypermobility occurs as a result of a combination of damage to the pelvic floor connective tissue, levator ani muscle complex tear and denervation injury to pelvic/pudendal nerves. These injuries ultimately lead to loss of urethral support and intrinsic sphincter tone after many years. It may occur during delivery, delivery requiring instrumentation, prolonged labor, chronic constipation, chronic bronchitis, and uncontrolled factors such as age and menopause. The injury during childbirth is the most important factor. During increased intra-abdominal pressure, the proximal urethra and the bladder neck descend and rotate away and come out of the pelvis and become extra-abdominal. Thus intraurethral pressure becomes less than the bladder pressure, resulting in urine leakage (**Fig. 1**).

Intrinsic sphincter deficiency, is a less common cause. Here the urethral sphincter is unable to coapt and the resting urethral resistance is inadequate to maintain continence. This occurs due to devascularization and/or denervation of bladder neck and proximal urethra. The urethral rigidity (lead pipe urethra) can occur due to postoperative fibrosis following pelvic surgery, pelvic radiation, neurologic injury and lack of estrogen. In such cases, the incontinence is usually severe as leakage occurs at marginal increases in intra-abdominal pressures. In patients with ISD, leakage also occurs with changing positions (**Fig. 2**). Many patients may experience continuous urinary leakage requiring use of diapers.

According to hammock theory by Delancey, optimal urethral compression does not take place if the endopelvic connective tissue is detached from its normal lateral points of origin at the arcus tendineus from the lateral pelvic wall (**Fig. 3**).

According to another theory, the posterior urethral wall moves further down as compared to the anterior wall during stress maneuvers in patients with SUI which results in funneling of the proximal urethra.

Stress incontinence worsens during sports and activities such as golf, tennis, or aerobic exercises. Leakage is more common while standing than supine position. In most cases the amount of urine leakage is very less,

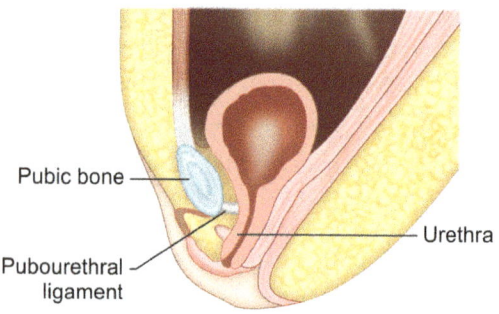

Fig. 1: Pubourethral ligament supporting proximal urethra.

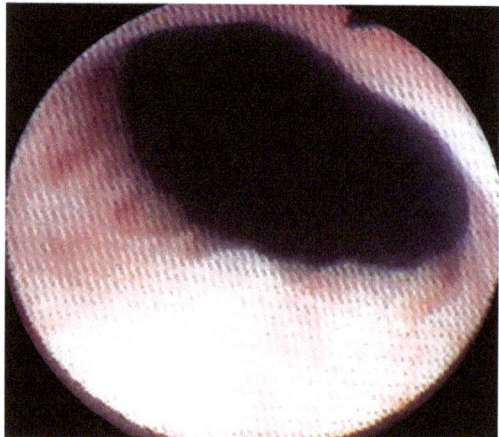

Fig. 2: Intrinsic sphincter deficiency on cystoscopy shows an open bladder neck.

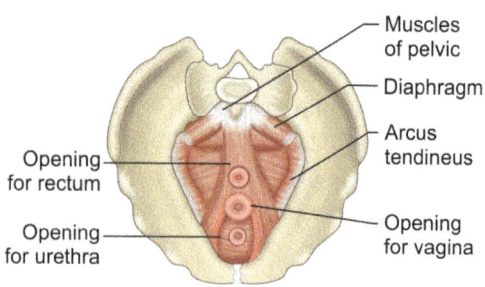

Fig. 3: Levator ani muscle complex.

unless the condition is severe. In SUI due to ISD, the volume of leakage is high.

Female SUI broadly subcategorized into the following three types:
1. *Type I:* SUI without urethral hypermobility. It is mild in severity
2. *Type II (Genuine SUI):* SUI with urethral hypermobility
3. *Type III:* SUI due to intrinsic sphincter deficiency. It is a severe and complex form of SUI.

DIAGNOSIS

Questionnaires are used to assess the quality of life of women with incontinence.[9] They are easy to use, valid, and reliable. These are filled up by patients before they enter the office. It also helps in evaluating the post-treatment outcome.
- Kelleher Questionnaire
- Urinary Distress Inventory (UDI)-6
- Incontinence Quality of Life (IQoL) Questionnaire

EVALUATION

History

The questions are asked in local language.
- Severity and quantity of urine leakage
- Frequency
- Onset, duration and progress
- Exacerbating factors such as coughing, sneezing, lifting, sexual activity, bending, sound of running water, and sound of key in the door
- Constant dribbling or not
- With or without frequency, urgency, dysuria, pain on full bladder
- History of (H/o) urinary tract infections (UTI)
- Associated with fecal incontinence or pelvic organ prolapse (POP)
- Obstetrical history details such as prolonged labor, difficult deliveries, forceps delivery, multiparity, obstetrical tears, and large baby
- Patients with POP may c/o heaviness, pain, and a bulging sensation in pelvic area.
- H/o reduction of bulge before urination and defecation
- H/o incontinence procedures, hysterectomy, or pelvic floor reconstructive procedures or any urologic procedures
- H/o spinal and brain surgery
- H/o smoking, alcohol or caffeine intake, and occupational history
- H/o pre-existing medical conditions, e.g., chronic UTI, urolithiasis, chronic cough, chronic obstructive pulmonary disease (COPD), congestive cardiac failure (CCF), diabetes mellitus (DM), Obesity, central nervous system (CNS) or spinal cord issues
- *H/o medications*: Diuretics, muscle relaxants, cholinergic or anticholinergic drugs, alpha-blockers, beta-mimetics, sedatives, angiotensin converting enzyme (ACE) inhibitors.

Morbidity

- Skin irritation
- Candidal infections
- Cellulitis
- Falls and fractures
- Decreased sleep

Psychological Morbidity
- Depression
- Poor self-esteem
- Social withdrawal
- Curtailed social and recreational activities
- Sexual dysfunction from embarrassment

Focused Physical Examination

- BP and weight
- Urinalysis and culture

- Tell patient to collect the urine voided and measure it
- Measure PVR (postvoid residue) either by catheterization or ultrasound

Abdominal Examination

- Surgical scars, hernias are suggestive of connective tissue weakness
- Distended bladder after voiding
- The back should be inspected.

Neurologic Examination

Gait, power, sensation, and deep tendon reflexes (DTR) of the lower limbs

Sensation of the Perineum and Perianal Area

- Examine for soft touch and light prick sensations
- Elicit the anal wink reflex using a cotton swab
- Elicit the bulbocavernosus reflex by gently tapping the clitoris with a cotton swab to rule out pudendal neuropathy

Pelvic Floor Examination

- Examine the external genitalia and urethral meatus
- Look for vaginal atrophy, urethral caruncle (hypoestrogenism)
- Palpate and look for urethral diverticulum
- Look for any watery or purulent discharge
- Elicit urethral and trigonal tenderness, suggestive of urethritis, urethral syndrome, or interstitial cystitis
- Look for fistula opening
- Look for signs of pelvic organ prolapse and quantify it by POP-Q
- Examine the perineal muscle tone by asking the patient squeeze the examining finger by performing Valsalva maneuver

An examination is performed, inspecting the anterior vaginal wall during straining with the posterior wall retracted with speculum. If a cystocele is observed, then a sponge holding forceps or similar instrument is inserted over the speculum blade and opened to support the lateral vagina. The tips of the sponge holding forceps should be against the bilateral ischial spines. If the cystocele is present with the patient straining and the lateral vagina supported, then a midline defect exists either in isolation or with a paravaginal defect.

Another clue to a midline defect is the loss of rugae with straining. If the cystocele is no longer present with lateral support, then a pure paravaginal defect is present.

Another clue to paravaginal defects is collapsing side walls during bivalve speculum examination. If anterior wall prolapse is present with lateral support, then the next maneuver is to use the closed ring forceps to provide midline anterior vaginal support while the patient is straining again. If some cystocele is still noted, then a combined central and paravaginal cystocele is present. If no bulge is noted, then the defect is purely central.

Next, attention is turned to the posterior vaginal wall. The half speculum is used to retract the anterior wall of the vagina, while the posterior wall is examined during Valsalva maneuver. The presence or absence of a rectocele should be noted. If a double bump is observed when the patient strains, an enterocele may be present in addition to the rectocele.

Next, the perineal body is inspected. The height and thickness of the tissue is noted. A badly compromised perineal body may be short and consist of mostly skin with little or no underlying muscle. The levator muscles are palpated, and the resting tone is noted. Then, the patient is instructed to squeeze the examining fingers, and the levator strength can be appreciated. A rectovaginal examination is performed to determine the thickness of the rectovaginal septum.

The patient is asked to strain. Tissue felt sliding through the examining fingers may indicate an enterocele. Resting and squeezing rectal sphincter tone is noted. As the rectal finger is withdrawn, the external anal sphincter should be palpated between this finger and the thumb. The absence or attenuation of this body of muscle indicates a sphincter laceration.

If any doubt remains about pelvic organ prolapse, examine the patient in the standing position. Instruct the patient to stand with legs apart and one foot resting on a step stool. When the patient performs the Valsalva maneuver, the force of gravity helps the pelvic organs (e.g., uterus, bladder) descend down the vagina and helps in diagnostic capability but practically difficult to perform.

Advanced Evaluation

Voiding Diary

A patient is asked to maintain a record of volume, type and time of fluid intake. She is asked to record the time and volume of each voiding episode. She is also asked to record any episode of incontinence, its triggering factors or any episode of nocturia is a separate column. This should be done for at least 3 days.

Cotton Swab Test

It is a screening test performed to look for urethral hypermobility. A change of angle greater than 30° indicates the latter.

Cough Stress Test

It is used to evaluate stress-induced leakage when a bladder is reasonably full. Patient is examined in lithotomy and asked to cough. If the patient fails to leak in the lithotomy position, the cough stress test is elicited in standing position. Immediate leakage of a few drops or a spurt of urine is indicative of SUI. A delayed and prolonged leak is indicative of *stress-induced detrusor instability*.

In patients with prolapse, speculum examination should be performed after reducing the prolapse and asking the patient to cough while supporting the prolapse with fingers and not compressing the urethra to elicit occult SUI.

It has been suggested that patients with pure stress incontinence, a simple cough stress test may be more useful than the complex urodynamic profiles.[10]

As a final step the patient is asked to empty the bladder, and an empty-supine cough stress test is performed. A positive result is suggestive of ISD. These patients further require Urodynamic testing to evaluate the chances of procedural outcome and prognosis.

Marshall and Boney's Test

An index finger and the second finger are placed on either side of the bladder neck. This supports the proximal urethra. With the bladder relatively full, instruct the patient to perform Valsalva or cough. The absence of leakage with bladder neck elevation and the presence of leakage after withdrawing the bladder neck support confirms stress urinary incontinence due to urethral hypermobility. This also suggests a favorable outcome of the surgical treatments, such as sling procedures or Burch procedure.

Urine analysis and culture to rule out UTI. Postmenopausal women are more susceptible due to hypoestrogenism.

BUN and creatinine is routinely done and may disclose a case of *obstruction*.

Blood sugar to rule out diabetes.

Measure PVR urine volume using a catheter or ultrasound, depending on availability.

A high PVR volume is suggestive of acontractile bladder or bladder outlet obstruction.

Cystoscopy

Indications for performing cystoscopy: hematuria, persistent irritative voiding symptoms such as frequency, urgency, dysuria due to cystitis or stone, voiding dysfunction, fistula, bladder diverticulum, suspected malignancy, and treatment failure.

Urodynamic Studies

Urodynamic studies evaluate the pressure-flow relationship between the bladder and urethra. It gives information regarding the functional status of the lower urinary tract. It is an adjunct to clinical diagnosis. It may help to confirm diagnosis, predict treatment outcome, or facilitate discussion during counseling. It has a high positive predictive value at the lowest cost with minimal inconvenience to the patient.[11] It is not recommended in all patients of SUI.

Indications include the recurrence of incontinence, associated voiding difficulties, increased PVR, suspected neurological dysfunction and in patients with upper urinary tract changes.

MANAGEMENT

Management of urinary incontinence must be *tailored* according to its type and cause.

Diapers and pads may be used temporarily or long-term to keep the perineum dry.

Medical management have been beneficial, especially in cases of urge and mixed incontinence.

Anticholinergic agents such as Oxybutynin, Tolterodine, Trospium, Solifenacin, Darifenacin, and Fesoterodine have shown beneficial outcomes. Beta-3 agonists such as Mirabegron approved in 2012 and Solabegron currently in Phase 2 clinical trials. *Antispasmodic* drugs such as Flavoxate can be used safely in elderly due to lack of anticholinergic side-effects. Tricyclic antidepressants such as Imipramine and Amitriptyline have shown beneficial results in some cases.

Serotonin/norepinephrine reuptake inhibitor, i.e., Duloxetine is the first drug developed and marketed for SUI. Duloxetine is approved in Europe, but is not approved by the US FDA. The dose is 40 mg twice a day.

The side effects are nausea, vomiting, worsening of hypertension, headache, constipation and dry mouth. It is mainly offered for a short time, to patients who are waiting to get their surgical treatment.

Estrogen

It is indicated in perimenopausal and postmenopausal women with stress and urge incontinence, and patients with vaginal atrophy due to genitourinary syndrome of menopause. Topical estrogen cream is preferred and takes about 3 months to show treatment benefit.[12,13] Oral estrogen therapy is not recommended.

Investigational Agents

Kuismanen et al in a pilot study states that adipose stem cells (ASCs) and collagen, when injected in urethra has demonstrated subjective improvement. It is a nonsurgical alternative to sling procedures.[14,15]

Behavioral Therapies

Behavioral therapy has been found to be more effective than pharmacologic interventions.[9] A drawback to this is the requirement of high patient motivation.

Pelvic Floor Muscle Training or Kegel's Exercises

It is an effective noninvasive treatment[16] with a success rate of 75–80% which can be achieved by properly performing Kegel's exercises in women with mild stress urinary incontinence with urethral hypermobility without vaginal prolapse. Patients are advised to perform pelvic floor muscle training (PFMT) by controlling urination or defecation with minimal contraction of abdominal, buttock, or inner-thigh muscles. This helps strengthen the levator ani muscles complex. Contraction of the pelvic floor reduces detrusor pressure and increases the urethral pressure and thus enhances continence. The doctor should help the patient identify the correct muscle complex by asking the patient to squeeze the intravaginal or intrarectal finger while examining the patient **(Fig. 4)**. PFMT may be used alone, with vaginal cones, biofeedback therapy, or with electrical stimulation.[17]

Vaginal Cones

Vaginal cones are useful in progressively increasing the strength of the pelvic floor muscles. A single cone is inserted into the vagina and is held in place by tightening the levator ani muscles for as long as 15 minutes. They are available in sets of five, with increasing weights. Patient is advised to perform it twice a day.

Biofeedback

Biofeedback therapy is a rehabilitation therapy where an electronic device provides a feedback when the patient contracts the correct levator ani muscle. It is useful for people having difficulty identifying the pelvic floor muscles. It has been found to be beneficial for all types of urinary incontinence.

Electrical Stimulation

It is the stimulation of levator ani muscles using *painless* electric currents.

Acupuncture

Electroacupuncture involving the lumbosacral region (18 sessions over 6 weeks) has found to reduce urine leakage.[18]

Extracorporeal Magnetic Resonance Therapy

The patient is asked to sit on a *chair* containing the magnetic device.

Dietary Modifications and Weight Loss

Patients are advised to avoid of bladder stimulants such as tea, coffee, alcohol, soft drinks, sugary and spices (bladder diet). The patients are advised to restrict fluid intake to 6–8 glasses of per day. Weight loss has also improved urine incontinence.[19]

Bladder Training and Timed Bladder Emptying

This is mainly useful for patients with urgency, urge and mixed incontinence. Patients are advised to start with voiding intervals of 1 hour and increased by 15–30 min per week. A voiding diary kept by the patient is helpful for assessing the progress. Distraction and relaxation techniques help in delaying the voiding.

Anticipatory Pelvic Floor Contractions

The patient is taught to perform a strong rapid intentional pelvic floor contraction just before anticipated episodes of increased intra-abdominal pressure such as cough or sneeze. This is called *Knack maneuver*.

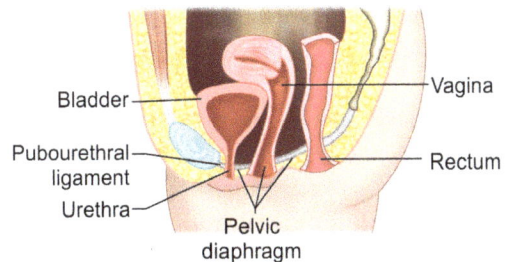

Fig. 4: Pelvic floor supporting pelvic organs.

Modification of Activity

Aerobics can be substituted with another fitness activity. Patients are advised to stop smoking. Any underlying medical conditions, such as asthma, COPD and chronic constipation should be adequately treated.

Urethral Occlusive Devices and Pessary

These can be tried as a palliative measure. Urethral occlusive devices are currently unavailable in India. Drawbacks include high cost and difficulty in usage. A pessary is a ring- or dish-shaped devices, which are inserted in the area under the bladder neck/proximal urethra.

Surgical Care

Patients not responding to conservative and medical treatment may be offered surgical treatment. In severe cases which are correctable surgically, medical therapy is not mandatory. It includes the treatment of bladder or uterine prolapse. Surgical treatment principle is based on increasing urethral outlet resistance.

Surgical treatment options are:[20,21]
- Midurethral slings (synthetic)
- Pubovaginal sling using autologous fascia
- Bladder neck suspension (Burch Colposuspension)
- Periurethral bulking agent therapy
- Artificial urinary sphincter

Midurethral Slings

It can be *transobturator or retropubic*.[22] The patient should be offered the procedure that surgeon is well versed with, so that he or she can give the best result. Surgeon's experience in performing specific types of surgery plays an important role.

Tension-free vaginal tape (TVT) is a polypropylene (prolene) mesh in the size of 1.1 cm by 40 cm which is covered by a plastic sheath which is attached to two stainless steel needles on both ends **(Fig. 5)**. TVT is placed retropubically and TVT-O is placed transobturator, at the level of midurethra.[22,23] TVT can be placed from below or above. TVT-O can be placed inside-out or outside-in.

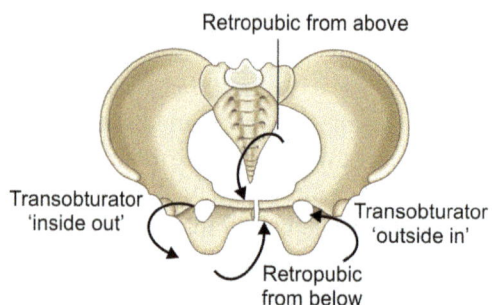

Fig. 5: Graphical presentation of types of midurethral sling placement.

Tension-free Vaginal Tape

Anesthesia: Spinal (preferable) or general anesthesia

Position: Lithotomy

Incisions: One vaginal and two suprapubic incisions two finger breadth away from midline on either side.

Procedure: Bladder is catheterized. Make a 2–2.5 cm vertical incision at the midurethra level on the anterior vaginal wall. Dissect paraurethrally to reach the endopelvic fascia. The direction of the point of the scissor should be facing the axilla of the same side. With the help of rigid catheter guide, deviate the bladder neck to the opposite side. The handle of the catheter guide should be placed on the same side of the needle insertion.

Now, the TVT needle is placed paraurethrally, and it should puncture the endopelvic fascia and reach the space of Retzius. The needle should come out of abdominal wall at the incision site. Make sure the needle hugs the posterior wall of pubic symphysis during its passage to avoid injury to any major vessels or tissues.

Cystoscopy is performed after filling up the bladder with at least 250 mL of normal saline. It is done by keeping the TVT needle in-situ to rule out any injury to bladder and urethra. Advance the needle and the tape. Leave the needle in the abdomen. Repeat the same procedure on the contralateral side after emptying the bladder.

Avoid twists of the tape during insertion. Take out both the needles from the abdominal wound after confirming bladder and urethral integrity by cystoscopy. Cut the tape at both abdominal ends, and leave the plastic sheath in place.

Adjusting the tension on the tape is the most crucial step in the whole procedure. Titrate the tension by tightening and loosening the tape. It should be tension-free. Place an artery forceps between the urethra and the tape while tightening the tape.

Fill up the bladder with about 250 mL of normal saline and ask the patient to cough. Make sure that the patient leaks a few drops of urine **(Fig. 6)**.

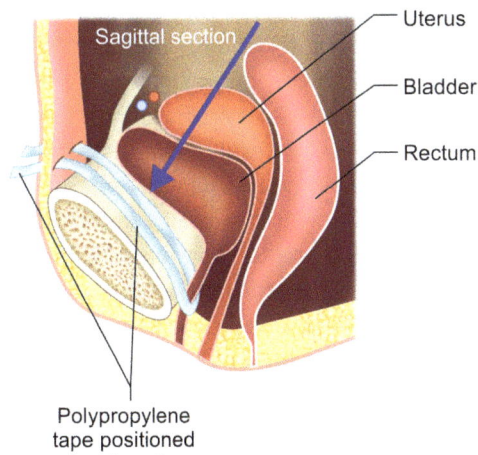

Fig. 6: Graphical presentation of retropubic sling placement at midurethra.

After adjusting the sling, carefully remove the plastic sheath. Now close the vaginal and abdominal incisions. Make sure, while pulling out the plastic sheath the tape is not pulled up along with it.

Transobturator Tape Sling (TVT-O)

In the transobturator tape (TOT) sling procedure, the needles are passed from the medial portion of the obturator canal at the level of the clitoris, inside the groin folds. These are of two types: (1) *inside-out;* (2) *outside-in.* Outside-in is preferred as the point of entry in the groin is fixed. Tightening of sling is performed in much the same way as with TVT, and is placed in a tension-free manner. Make sure while placing the needle that there is no "buttonholing" of the lateral vaginal wall. Retropubic MUS has more suppression efficiency compared to transobturator approach.

Immediate postoperative care: Patient is given IV antibiotics for 24 hours. Next day, remove the vaginal pack. Give a trial of voiding. Discharge the patient from the hospital with pain medications and oral antibiotics. If a patient is unable to void, make sure she is pain-free. We may need to reinsert the catheter if she is unable to void. Keep the catheter for 2–3 weeks and follow-up for removal of catheter and voiding trial.

Complications: Sling erosion into the vagina or bladder/urethra.[24] Retention of urine may occur if sling is too snug to the urethra. If urethral obstruction secondary to TVT occurs, urethrolysis, i.e., incision of sling and freeing of the urethra should be performed within the 3–6 weeks. Partial obstruction manifests with voiding symptoms such as hesitancy, straining, urgency, urge incontinence. Infection, bleeding, hematoma formation are perioperative and immediate postoperative complications.[25]

Expected outcomes: For the tension-free vaginal tape procedure, the long-term cure rate is 84% at a mean follow-up of over 10 years. Reich et al. found an objective cure rate of 89.8% at a mean follow-up of more than 7 years.[26,27] The subjective cure rate was 82.4%. According to Barber MD, Kleeman S, Karram MM, et al., it was observed that, transobturator tape (TOT) procedures have good durability on 5-year follow-up. Short-term studies have confirmed that TOT is not inferior to TVT procedures.[28] However, Schierlitz et al. found that retropubic TVT was more effective than TOT sling in women with urodynamic SUI and ISD.[29]

Pubovaginal Sling

Indications include genuine and severe SUI and occult SUI in a prolapse repair patient. In this procedure, sling is placed at the level of bladder neck proximal urethra or midurethra. By doing this procedure, the descent of bladder neck and urethra is prevented. It is designed to restore the bladder neck and urethra to their anatomically correct positions. It also improves the resting urethral closure pressure with increase in intra-abdominal pressure during physical activity.

Contraindications: Urge incontinence and poor detrusor function.

Sling material: Autologous (fascia lata, rectus sheath, and anterior vaginal wall) or allogeneic (uncommon) or synthetic (polypropylene) material. Sling should be tension-free and biocompatible.

Preoperative counseling: Patient should be counseled about the risks and complications.

Anesthesia: General/spinal

Position: Lithotomy

Sling sizes:
- Classic pubovaginal slings (2 × 14 cm)
- Hemislings (2 × 7 cm)
- Patch slings (2 × 4 cm)
- Rectus fascia pubovaginal sling
- Fascia lata pubovaginal sling
- Rectus fascia suburethral sling
- Fascia lata suburethral sling
- Vaginal wall suburethral sling

Complications: Bleeding, urethral and/or bladder injury, infection, urinary retention, de novo urge incontinence, worsening of already existing urge incontinence and sling erosion through bladder or vagina.

Those patients who are selected for a pubovaginal sling should be counseled for a possible requirement of self-catheterization and voiding dysfunction postoperatively.

Burch Colposuspension

In Burch retropubic urethropexy, the basic mechanism is intra-abdominal placement of the urethrovesical junction (UVJ) and proximal urethra. Due to this anatomic placement the intra-abdominal pressure and proximal urethral pressure becomes equal. This helps in restoration of continence.

The surgery can be performed by an open or laparoscopic approach. The open procedure is preferred over the laparoscopic technique but should be performed when a concomitant open surgery is planned for other indications. Laparoscopic Burch if performed by an experienced surgeon has provided satisfactory outcomes as well.

Patients with type III stress urinary incontinence having a fixed, rigid and nonfunctioning proximal urethra (ISD) are not offered a Burch procedure. As they do not have hypermobile urethra, which needs correction.[30] These patients are better served by a midurethral sling procedure.[31]

Pregnancy can disrupt pelvic support so the procedure should be offered only to those who have completed childbearing.

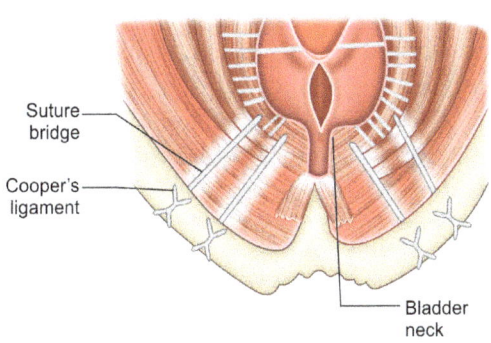

Fig. 7: Graphical presentation of placement of Burch sutures.

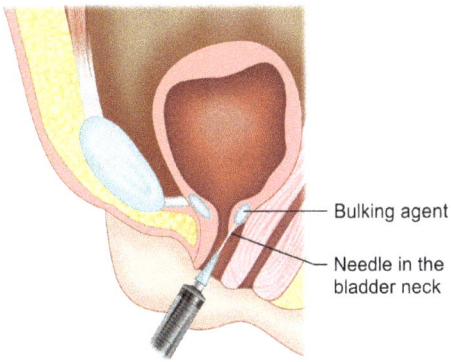

Fig. 8: Injecting paraurethral bulking agent.

Procedure: The first suture is placed at the level of the bladder neck about 2 cm lateral to it. Two to three sutures are placed in the fascia and anterior vaginal wall proximal to the bladder neck about 1 cm apart **(Fig. 7)**. The sutures are placed into corresponding sites on Cooper's ligament. Make sure that there is no excessive tension on the sutures. Create a "suture bridge" on either sides as shown in the **Figure 7**. An assistant should elevate the vagina before tying the sutures. Cystoscopy is performed after sutures are tied, rule out injury to the urinary tract.

Expected outcomes: A Cochrane review compared Burch colposuspension with synthetic tapes and found no difference in efficacy.[32] SISTEr trial compared Burch with autologous sling. It was observed that slings were more effective.

Another Cochrane review compared tapes with autologous slings and it was found that both had equivalent operative time and rate of complications but de novo detrusor overactivity was less with tapes.

Paraurethral Bulking Agents

It is mainly opted in patients who are medically compromised and elderly who cannot tolerate surgery. The mechanism of action usually is an improved seal effect or an obstructive effect. Bovine GAX collagen, Teflon, autologous tissues such as fat and cartilages are tried. An ideal agent is yet to be identified. Bulkamid hydrogel is an injectable hydrogel is consisted of 97.5% water and 2.5% of cross-linked polyacrylamide.[33] It is non-degradable, homogeneous and migration resistant **(Fig. 8)**.[34,35] It is easily administered under local anesthesia. It is 1 year results suggest that 92% patients are cured or improved and it does not have any serious adverse effects.[36]

Mixed Urinary Incontinence

Always treat urgency first if it is predominant. If SUI is predominant, correct it first with the discussion of need of postoperative anticholinergic therapy. In some patients, SUI itself can present as urgency, which is likely to resolve after surgery.

LATEST GUIDELINES FOR MESH FOR INCONTINENCE FROM NICE, OCTOBER 2018

1. In July, the Government issued a national "pause" in England on the use of vaginal mesh implants following preliminary recommendations from an independent review which heard that thousands

of women had experienced disabling conditions as a result of the treatment.
2. Women should be offered a full range of nonsurgical treatment before the use of surgical procedures including mesh or tape.
3. Surgical mesh and surgical tape should only be used as a treatment of last resort.
4. National database to record all procedures was advised to set up.

An investigative report in The BMJ said mesh manufacturers had "hustled" their products into widespread use, while an editorial in the same journal described the era of mesh implants as "shameful".

In India, the government has not banned the use of sling. It is up to us as a treating surgeon to use it judiciously for the right patients, for the right indications and by a well-trained experienced surgeon for providing the best outcome to our patients.

FUTURE DIRECTIONS AND CONTROVERSIES

Pubovaginal sling surgery can be a treatment of choice for all types of SUI. The chances of one having some serious complications from sling surgery are uncommon. It is upon the surgeon's preference looking into the patient's previous surgical history, vitality of host tissue/fascia, choice of a particular material and procedure that usually drives the decision for the type of the surgery offered to the patient. The ideal choice of the sling material and procedure are controversial. The patient's choice for a particular procedure is to be considered as well.

In the cases of recurrent SUI, use of classic pubovaginal or hemislings constructed with rectus fascia is a better option; otherwise, one can offer to use the synthetic retropubic TVT placed retrograde or antegrade with sufficiently good outcome.[21]

As better insight into the relationship between the sling materials and the host response is elucidated, the success rates of sling surgery will continue to improve. At present, synthetic polypropylene mesh midurethral slings seem to have some of the best durability with the least problems; they will be hard to improve on in the future. Perhaps tissue engineering using autologous stem cells is the next step in the evolution of pubovaginal slings for definitive correction of female SUI.[21]

REFERENCES

1. Erdem N, Chu FM. Management of overactive bladder and urge urinary incontinence in the elderly patient. Am J Med. 2006;119(3 Suppl 1): 29-36.
2. Abrams P, Cardozo L, Fall M, Griffiths D, Rosier P, Ulmsten U, et al. The standardisation of terminology of lower urinary tract function: report from the Standardisation Sub-committee of the International Continence Society. Neurourol Urodyn. 2002;21(2):167-78.
3. American College of Obstetricians and Gynecologists. Practice Bulletin No. 155: Urinary Incontinence in Women. Obstet Gynecol. 2016;127 (5):e66-81.
4. Rogers RG. Clinical practice. Urinary stress incontinence in women. N Engl J Med. 2008;358(10):1029-36.
5. Delancey JO, Ashton-Miller JA. Pathophysiology of adult urinary incontinence. Gastroenterology. 2004;126(1 Suppl 1):S23-32.
6. Chutka DS, Fleming KC, Evans MP, Evans JM, Andrews KL. Urinary incontinence in the elderly population. Mayo Clin Proc. 1996;71(1):93-101.
7. Gibbs CF, Johnson TM 2nd, Ouslander JG. Office management of geriatric urinary incontinence. Am J Med. 2007;120(3):211-20.
8. Kelleher CJ, Cardozo LD, Khullar V, Salvatore S. A new questionnaire to assess the quality of life of urinary incontinent women. Br J Obstet Gynaecol. 1997;104(12):1374-9.
9. Balk EM, Rofeberg VN, Adam GP, Kimmel HJ, Trikalinos TA, Jeppson PC. Pharmacologic and nonpharmacologic treatments for urinary

incontinence in women: a systematic review and network meta-analysis of clinical outcomes. Ann Intern Med. 2019;170(7):465-79.
10. Swift SE, Yoon EA. Test-retest reliability of the cough stress test in the evaluation of urinary incontinence. Obstet Gynecol. 1999; 94(1):99-102.
11. Summitt RL Jr, Stovall TG, Bent AE, Ostergard DR. Urinary incontinence: correlation of history and brief office evaluation with multichannel urodynamic testing. Am J Obstet Gynecol. 1992;166(6 Pt 1):1835-44.
12. Grady D, Brown JS, Vittinghoff E, Applegate W, Varner E, Snyder T. Postmenopausal hormones and incontinence: the Heart and Estrogen/Progestin Replacement Study. Obstet Gynecol. 2001;97(1):116-20.
13. Hendrix SL, Cochrane BB, Nygaard IE, Handa VL, Barnabei VM, Iglesia C, et al. Effects of estrogen with and without progestin on urinary incontinence. JAMA. 2005;293(8):935-48.
14. Waknine Y. Adipose Stem Cells: Potential Option for Female SUI. Medscape Med News. 2014:2-9.
15. Kuismanen K, Sartoneva R, Haimi S, Mannerström B, Tomás E, Miettinen S, et al. Autologous adipose stem cells in treatment of female stress urinary incontinence: results of a pilot study. Stem Cells Transl Med. 2014;3(8):936-41.
16. Qaseem A, Dallas P, Forciea MA, Starkey M, Denberg TD, Shekelle P, et al. Nonsurgical management of urinary incontinence in women: a clinical practice guideline from the American College of Physicians. Ann Intern Med. 2014;161(6):429-40.
17. Dumoulin C, Cacciari LP, Hay-Smith EJC. Pelvic floor muscle training versus no treatment, or inactive control treatments, for urinary incontinence in women. Cochrane Database Syst Rev. 2018;10:CD005654.
18. Liu Z, Liu Y, Xu H, He L, Chen Y, Fu L, et al. Effect of Electroacupuncture on Urinary Leakage Among Women With Stress Urinary Incontinence: a Randomized Clinical Trial. JAMA. 2017;317 (24):2493-501.
19. Subak LL, Wing R, West DS, Franklin F, Vittinghoff E, Creasman JM, et al. Weight loss to treat urinary incontinence in overweight and obese women. N Engl J Med. 2009;360(5):481-90.
20. American Urological Association. Surgical Treatment of Female Stress Urinary Incontinence (SUI): AUA/SUFU Guideline. [online] Available from: https://www.auanet.org/education/guidelines/incontinence.cfm. [Last accessed on April, 2021].
21. MedScape. Urinary Incontinence. [online] Available from: https://emedicine.medscape.com/article/452289-overview. [Last accessed on April, 2021].
22. Rackley RR, Abdelmalak JB, Tchetgen MB, Madjar S, Jones S, Noble M. Tension-free vaginal tape and percutaneous vaginal tape sling procedures. Tech Urol. 2001;7(2):90-100.
23. Mostafa A, Agur W, Abdel-All M, Guerrero K, Lim C, Allam M, et al. Multicenter prospective randomized study of single-incision mini-sling vs tension-free vaginal tape-obturator in management of female stress urinary incontinence: a minimum of 1-year follow-up. Urology. 2013;82 (3):552-9.
24. Madjar S, Tchetgen MB, Van Antwerp A. urethral erosion of tension-free vaginal tape. Urology. 2002;59(4):601.
25. Olsson I, Kroon U. A three-year postoperative evaluation of tension-free vaginal tape. Gynecol Obstet Invest. 1999;48(4):267-9.
26. Zhang P, Fan B, Zhang P, Han H, Xu Y, Wang B, et al. Meta-analysis of female stress urinary incontinence treatments with adjustable single-incision mini-slings and transobturator tension-free vaginal tape surgeries. BMC Urol. 2015;15:64.
27. Reich A, Kohorst F, Kreienberg R, Flock F. Long-term results of the tension-free vaginal tape procedure in an unselected group: a 7-year follow-up study. urology. 2011;78(4): 774-7.
28. Barber MD, Kleeman S, Karram MM, Paraiso MF, Walters MD, Vasavada S, et al. Transobturator tape compared with tension-free vaginal tape for the treatment of stress urinary incontinence: a randomized controlled trial. Obstet Gynecol. 2008;111(3):611-21.
29. Schierlitz L, Dwyer PL, Rosamilia A, Murray C, Thomas E, De Souza A, et al. Effectiveness of tension-free vaginal tape compared with transobturator tape in women with stress urinary incontinence and intrinsic sphincter deficiency: a randomized controlled trial. Obstet Gynecol. 2008;112(6):1253-61.

30. Amaye-Obu FA, Drutz HP. Surgical management of recurrent stress urinary incontinence: a 12-year experience. Am J Obstet Gynecol. 1999;181(6):1296-307.
31. Bergman A, Koonings PP, Ballard CA. Negative Q-tip test as a risk factor for failed incontinence surgery in women. J Reprod Med. 1989;34(3):193-7.
32. Tanagho EA. Colpocystourethropexy: the way we do it. J Urol. 1978;116:751-3.
33. Pai A, Al-Singary W. Durability, safety and efficacy of polyacrylamide hydrogel (Bulkamid®) in the management of stress and mixed urinary incontinence: three year follow-up outcomes. Cent European J Urol. 2015;68(4):428-33.
34. Kirchin V, Page T, Keegan PE, Atiemo K, Cody JD, McClinton S. Urethral injection therapy for urinary incontinence in women. Cochrane Database Syst Rev. 2012;2:CD003881.
35. Cornu JN, Peyrat L, Haab F. Update in management of male urinary incontinence: injectables, balloons, minimally invasive approaches. Curr Opin Urol. 2013;23(6):536-9.
36. Davis NF, Kheradmand F, Creagh T. Injectable biomaterials for the treatment of stress urinary incontinence: their potential and pitfalls as urethral bulking agents. Int Urogynecol J. 2013;24(6):913-9.

Tension-free Vaginal Tape

Shakir Tabrez Z

INTRODUCTION

Tension-free vaginal tape (TVT) was introduced in 1996 by Ulmsten et al. for the management of stress urinary incontinence (SUI).

It has, since then, achieved comparable rates of success to the earlier gold standard, Burch colposuspension. It also has a shorter learning curve with comparably lesser complications as proven by several peer reviewed articles.

STRESS URINARY INCONTINENCE

As per the definitions formulated by the International Continence Society (ICS), stress urinary incontinence (SUI) is defined as "the complaint of any involuntary loss of urine on effort or physical exertion or on sneezing or coughing".[1] An accidental leakage of urine, which occurs with a sudden elevation of abdominal pressure without detrusor contraction, is stress urinary incontinence.

DIAGNOSTIC WORKUP

This has been dealt with elaborately in the previous chapter on Stress Urinary Incontinence. The important aspects being a detailed history include bladder diary and a systematic examination include assessing neurological factors.

Investigations, which should not be missed, include an ultrasound for measurement of residual urine. A urodynamic evaluation is not always necessary except in mixed urinary incontinence where associated Detrusor pathology is suspected. Transperineal ultrasound is gaining popularity for its precise delineation of anatomical defects.[2] Cystoscopy, though it has arisen in certain conditions, is not a routine necessity prior to the procedure.

CONSERVATIVE MANAGEMENT

This includes lifestyle modification, intravaginal estrogen creams, trial of pessaries and most importantly, pelvic floor rehabilitation in a supervised manner with bladder training for a minimum period of 12 weeks.

When all the above options fail, surgery is the choice of treatment.

Tension free transvaginal tape is a form of urethropexy based on the "Integral theory" and hence is designed to simulate the pubourethral ligament. While counseling the patient preoperatively for surgery, the factors which need to be considered include future child bearing and need for combining other surgeries to repair associated pelvic floor defects, if any.

TVT Sling Material Properties

The sling material used needs to comply with the NICE guideline, which recommends a Type 1, monofilament, macroporous, polypropylene mesh. The quality of the mesh decides the outcome of the surgery, both short-term and long-term. Loosely woven material appears to better integrate into the host tissue.

The standard TVT system consists of an approximately 45 cm long and 1 cm wide mesh attached to stainless steel needles on either side, covered in a plastic sheath. There is also a reusable TVT introducer and a rigid catheter guide.

Surgical Steps

- Local/regional anesthesia should suffice unless patient's comorbidities necessitate General anesthesia.
- In a dorsal lithotomy position, an 18 F Foley catheter is inserted into the bladder.
- After hydrodissection, grasp the anterior vaginal wall with two Allis forceps, 1.5 cm incision is made on the anterior vaginal wall, 1 cm away from the proximal urethral meatus.
- After initial sharp dissection paraurethrally, blunt dissection is done in the endopelvic fascia, taking care to direct the dissection in the direction of the patient's axilla.
- The rigid catheter guide is introduced into the Foley catheter and this helps to make sure urethra is not injured when the insertion needles are passed paraurethrally.
- The handle of the guide is pulled to the surgeon's left side to expose the patient's right fascia and vice versa.
- The needle is then inserted where it punctures the endopelvic fascia, traverses the space of Retzius (in the direction of the patient's ipsilateral midaxillary plane) and exits through a stab puncture on the anterior abdominal wall just above the pubic bone. Care should be taken to avoid the inferior epigastric vessels on the anterior abdominal wall.
- Utmost care must be maintained to ensure the needle clings to the pubic bone during this maneuver.
- With the needle *in situ*, cystoscopy is performed to rule out bladder and urethral injuries. Special attention should be given to the 7-11 o'clock and similarly, 1-5 o'clock areas on either side.
- After ruling out injuries, the needle is advanced and the tape is pulled out through the abdominal wall and left there.
- After emptying the bladder, the same steps are repeated on the contralateral side.
- After ensuring the tape has not twisted and tension is not too tight by placing a Metzenbaum scissors between the tape and the urethra at the mid urethral level, the tape tension is adjusted and the needles are cut.
- The plastic sheath is cut after adjusting the tension (as doing so prematurely makes it difficult to move the tape) and removed from the vaginal end after which the abdominal and vaginal ends are closed.

COMPLICATIONS

The intraoperative complications include hemorrhage and injury to the bladder or urethra.

The hemorrhage is usually controlled with pressure. In case of injury to the bladder noticed during cystoscopy, the needle can be removed and reinserted with postoperative bladder drainage for 7 days to ensure bladder injury healing. In case of urethral injury, the injury is sutured, sling procedure abandoned and suprapubic bladder drainage ensued for 14 days minimum. Rare complications include injury to large vessels or bowel.

Postoperative complications include:

- Acute urinary retention, which is due to excess tension. Here tape mobilization and continuous bladder drainage can be given a short trial, failing which tape division will be required which needs to be decided within 2 weeks of surgery, failing which patient can end up with bladder outlet obstruction.

- De novo urgency is a known side effect after anti-incontinence procedures for which the patient needs to be counseled preoperatively.
- Wound infection, dyspareunia
- Sling erosion (into either the vagina or bladder/urethra)[3,4] and urethral sloughing are rare.

Reich et al. found an objective cure rate of 89.8% at a mean follow-up of 7 years and subjective cure rate was 82.4%.

REFERENCES

1. Haylen BT, de Ridder D, Freeman RM, Swift SE, Berghmans B, Lee J, et al. An International Urogynecological Association (IUGA)/International Continence Society (ICS) joint report on the terminology for female pelvic floor dysfunction. Int Urogynecol J. 2010; 21(1):5-26.
2. Viereck V, Bader W, Lobodasch K, Pauli F, Bentler R, Kölbl H. Guideline-based strategies in the surgical treatment of female urinary incontinence: the New Gold Standard is almost the same as the Old One. Geburtshilfe und Frauenheilkunde. 2016;76(8):865-8.
3. Zhang P, Fan B, Zhang P, Han H, Xu Y, Wang B, et al. Meta-analysis of female stress urinary incontinence treatments with adjustable single-incision mini-slings and transobturator tension-free vaginal tape surgeries. BMC Urol. 2015;15:64.
4. Kurien A, Narang S, Han HC. Tension-free vaginal tape-Abbrevo procedure for female stress urinary incontinence: a prospective analysis over 22 months. Singapore Med J. 2017;58(6):338-42.

Tension-free Transobturator Tape Insertion

CHAPTER 10

Ashish Kale

EVIDENCE-BASED PERSPECTIVES

Transobturator tape (TOT) procedure is well-documented in literature surgical treatment of primary stress urinary incontinence (SUI). However, the optimal management of persistent SUI poses a dilemma to the gynecologist. Moreover, there is paucity of the data with limited studies. The study group led by Hassonah et al. from Toronto[1] studied and compared the outcome of the laparoscopic two-team sling procedure, tension-free vaginal tape (TVT) insertion and TOT insertion in the treatment of recurrent SUI in women. Specifically, the complications were evaluated in both the short-term and the long-term. This was a study done on a small sample size of 46 patients, which found out that there were no statistically significant differences between the three groups as regards the outcome. The reason attributed for the non-statistically significant difference was due to the small group of patients evaluated.

Urinary retention is a known complication of sling procedures. The likely cause for this is the tape being placed under too much tension.[2]

As per the studies from California led by Ho MH et al.,[3] reviewing the recently available data in the treatment of female SUI with TOT, it has been proven that the complication rate decreases significantly with TOT as compared to the other sling surgeries as the intrapelvic and retropubic passage is avoided.

SURGICAL STEPS

Here, there are two approaches which are as follows:
1. *The outside-inside approach*: Here the tape is inserted from the obturator foramen and directed into the vaginal incision.
2. *The inside-out approach*: Here the tape is directed from the vaginal incision to the obturator foramen.

The effectiveness of this approach is almost like that of tension-free vaginal tape, at least on short-term follow-up. It is important to develop a standardized technique for the surgical procedure. The knowledge and practice of tips and tricks from experts is vital as it would help make this technique easier to learn and practice for beginners and help reduce incidence of the most frequent complications.

The French group has assessed 10 rational steps in the procedure to standardize the surgical procedure. The standardization of this technique is described in 10 steps that include the following:[4]

1. Ergonomy of the patient
2. Infiltration of the anesthetic
3. Single incision in the vagina
4. Creating a pathway to place the device
5. Placing of the device
6. Checking the position of the tape (flat position)
7. Ensuring the right tension of the mesh
8. The excess lateral arms of the mesh emerging out of the skin need to be cut

9. Drainage of urine to ensure no stenosis
10. Suturing the mucosa of the vagina and the skin

LANDMARK COMPARATIVE STUDIES

The recent study published in 2018 by the Austrian Urogynecology Working Group[5] compared outcomes of the retropubic versus the transobturator tension-free vaginal tape (TVT vs. TVT-O) at 5 years. This was done in a total of 569 women undergoing surgery for primary stress incontinence, who were randomized to receive a TVT or TVT-O. Importantly, both the primary and the secondary outcomes were evaluated in detail. The primary outcome measure was continence defined as a negative cough stress test at a volume of 300 mL. Additionally, they have been comparable in that the results demonstrate comparable outcomes between TVT and TVT-O especially for postoperative continence and quality of life (QoL). There was hardly any difference for the perioperative problems.[6]

CONCLUSION

It has been proved beyond doubt that the safety and effectiveness of TOT is comparable to TVT, at least in the short-term follow-up. The study-to-study variability in the rate of perforation derives from three factors: (1) technique, (2) training, and (3) experience.

REFERENCES

1. Hassonah S, Medel S, Lovatsis D, Drutz HP, Alarab M. Outcome of the laparoscopic two-team sling procedure, tension-free vaginal tape insertion, and transobturator tape insertion in women with recurrent stress urinary incontinence. J Obstet Gynaecol Can. 2013;35(11):1004-9.
2. Imoh-Ita F, Ross C. Management of high urinary residual following insertion of a tension free transobturator tape: an innovative approach. J Obstet Gynaecol. 2012;32(8):812.
3. Ho MH, Lin LL, Haessler AL, Bhatia NN. Tension-free transobturator tape procedure for stress urinary incontinence. Curr Opin Obstet Gynecol. 2006;18(5):567-74.
4. Mangano E, Campagne-Loiseau S, Curinier S, Botchrosvili R, Canis M, Chauvet P, et al. Transobturator vaginal tape in 10 steps. J Minim Invasive Gynecol. 2020;27(1):27-8.
5. Tammaa A, Aigmüller T, Hanzal E, Umek W, Kropshofer S, Lang PFJ, et al. Retropubic versus transobturator tension-free vaginal tape (TVT vs TVT-O): five-year results of the Austrian randomized trial. Neurourol Urodyn. 2018;37(1):331-8.
6. Aigmüller T, Tammaa A, Tamussino K, Hanzal E, Umek W, Kölle D, et al. Retropubic vs. transobturator tension-free vaginal tape for female stress urinary incontinence: 3-month results of a randomized controlled trial. Int Urogynecol J. 2014;25(8):1023-30.

11 Autologous Rectus Fascia Sling

T Srikala Prasad

INTRODUCTION

Stress urinary incontinence (SUI) is defined as "the complaint of any involuntary leakage of urine on effort or exertion or on sneezing or coughing".[1,2]

Pubovaginal sling (PVS) using autologous rectus fascia is an excellent procedure in the surgical management of women suffering from all forms of SUI. This is an abdomino-vaginal surgery in which the fascia harvested from the rectus sheath is used as a support for the proximal urethra with a fixation overlying the rectus sheath. This was first popularized by McGuire and Lytton in 1978.[3] Blaivas and Olsson (1998) were modified McGuire's technique by reducing the length of the rectus fascia graft.[4] This procedure effectively corrected both urethral hypermobility and intrinsic sphincter deficiency (ISD). Hence this was the procedure commonly used by all urologists to surgically correct SUI. Ulmsten et al. in the year 1996 introduced a very effective midurethral procedure which was minimally invasive and easy to perform (Tension-free Vaginal Tape).[5] This procedure and its modifications revolutionized the surgical management of SUI making the synthetic midurethral slings the surgery of choice for majority of cases and restricting PVS for selected indications. The beneficial effects of using autologous fascial slings and the complications associated with the use of synthetic mesh have resulted in more surgeons preferring this procedure to other techniques.

HOW PUBOVAGINAL SLING PREVENT URINARY LEAK?

The sling placed at proximal urethra and bladder neck increases the bladder outlet resistance and restores the urethrovesical junction. When there is an increase in intra-abdominal pressure, the bladder outlet resistance gets increased as the sling gets pulled up anteriorly and it compresses the posterior urethra by rotating the bladder base posteroinferiorly which decreases the urinary leak.[6]

CLINICAL ASSESSMENT

The clinical assessment including history taking, clinical examination and investigations including urodynamic evaluation have been discussed in detail in the earlier chapters.

INDICATIONS FOR PUBOVAGINAL SLING

- Intrinsic sphincter deficiency
- Urethral hypermobility
- Mixed urinary incontinence
- Midurethral complex deficiency
- Neurogenic incontinence (Myelodysplasia, sacral agenesis, T12-S1 spinal cord injury). PVS may not completely correct incontinence in these patients, even though it will augment outlet resistance. These patients also suffer from incomplete bladder emptying either because of a hypotonic bladder or an atonic bladder which leads to overflow incontinence. However, since these patients who are

suffering from neurogenic bladder require lifetime clean intermittent catheterization (CIC), PVS using autologous fascia is very useful to them as they are prone for mesh erosion, in case synthetic slings are used.
- *Recurrent SUI after a failed midurethral sling*: Many of these patients on repeat evaluation have been found to be suffering from ISD and PVS is an ideal choice.
- *Synthetic mesh erosion*: These patients are best managed by removal of the offending mesh and a PVS placement as there is a possible urethral tissue loss.
- *Concomitant urethral procedure*: In patients who are undergoing a surgical repair for urethral diverticulum, urethrovaginal fistula or urethroplasty for severe urethral stricture, PVS as a concomitant procedure gives an extra support to the repair.
- *Concomitant abdominal procedure*: Patients undergoing abdominal procedures for any other problem such as fibroid, ovarian cyst or incisional hernia repair (rectus fascia harvested in these patients also is good enough) who also require surgical management of SUI.

Contraindications to Midurethral Slings

Previous pelvic irradiation, chronic pelvic pain, dyspareunia, immunosuppressed states and chronic corticosteroid therapy.[6]

OPERATIVE PROCEDURE[7]

The patient is fully evaluated and explained about the procedure, the risks, and benefits including the possibility of temporary voiding dysfunction and wound complications such as seroma. Sterile urine is ensured by treating asymptomatic bacteriuria prior to the procedure. Antibiotics such as cephalosporin are administered as a prophylactic measure an hour before the procedure. The surgery is performed using regional or general anesthesia.

The patient is put in a low modified dorsal lithotomy position using Allen stirrups. An 18 Fr Foley catheter is placed with 15–20 mL of distilled water in the balloon. This will help us to identify the bladder neck. A Pfannenstiel incision of 8 cm length is made 3 cm above the pubic symphysis and the wound is deepened till the rectus sheath. Abdominal flaps are raised above and below. Defattening of the rectus sheath is done to reduce the thickness of the graft and facilitate smooth transfer for its placement **(Figs. 1A and B)**.

The proposed rectus fascial graft is marked with a marker pen to the required size of 8 × 2 cm and the edges can be tapered. Using sharp dissection, the rectus fascial sling is harvested and safeguarded in saline **(Fig. 2)**. The upper and lower flaps of the rectus sheath are mobilized from the underlying muscle to facilitate tension-free

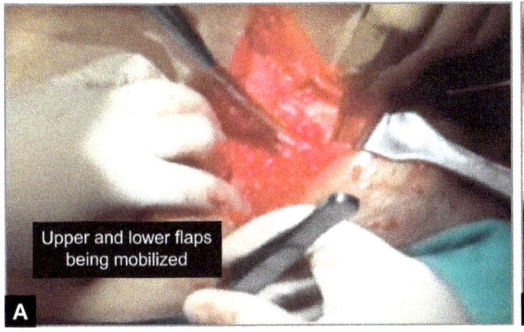
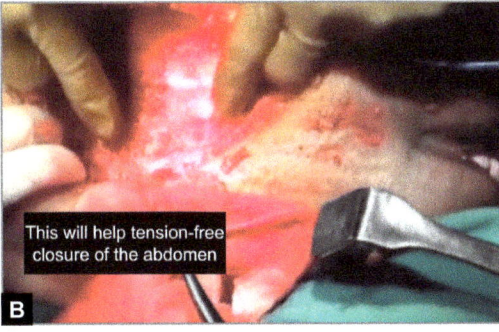

Figs. 1A and B: Defattening of the rectus sheath.

closure of the rectus sheath. The ends of the sling are anchored separately with a running stitch using 2-0 polypropylene and the polypropylene thread is left long (around 15 cm) to facilitate easy transfer and passage of the sling **(Figs. 3A and B)**.

The retropubic space is dissected lateral to the lateral border of the rectus muscle where yellow fat will identify the cleft. A finger introduced through the dissected space perforates the fascia, hugs the bone and traverses the retropubic space.[7] This is normally a simple procedure but difficulty can be encountered in previously operated patients. The procedure is repeated on the opposite side also **(Figs. 4A to D)**.

The proximal urethra is now exposed after hydrodissection with normal saline. The first Allis clamp is held 2 cm from the external urinary meatus. The second Allis clamp is held almost at the level of the bladder neck. The anterior vaginal wall is reflected from the underlying periurethral fascia using scissors angled towards the ipsilateral shoulder and thick flaps are created on both sides. The retropubic space is approached from below also with the help of the Metzenbaum scissors perforating the endopelvic fascia using a careful "push and spread technique". This is done on the opposite side also.

The Foley catheter ensures that the bladder is empty. A finger introduced through the dissected space from above should meet the finger introduced through the dissected space from below. If the fingers touch without the feel of an intervening structure such as the bladder, the ligature carrier can be safely introduced from above downward through the dissected space in the vagina **(Figs. 5A to D)**.

A check cystoscopy is done with a full bladder both with the 30° and 70° lenses with the ligature carrier inside, to ensure that there is no inadvertent entry of the instrument into the bladder **(Fig. 6)**. Movement of the ligature carrier will demonstrate the movements being transmitted, without the needle entry into the bladder.[8]

If a bladder perforation occurs, it is often located in between the 1 and 11 o'clock position.[8] In that situation, the ligature carrier is safely retrieved and carefully reintroduced

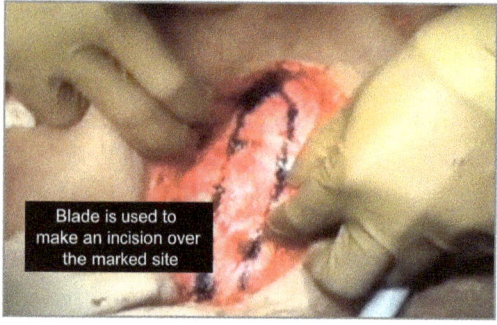

Fig. 2: Marking for the sling harvest.

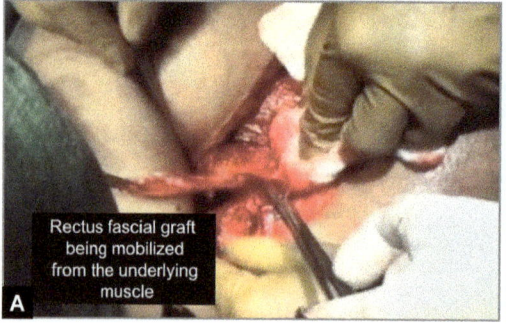
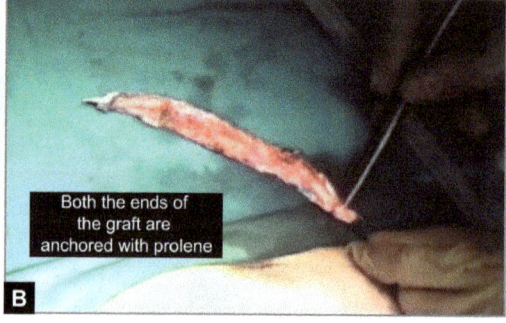

Figs. 3A and B: Mobilization and anchoring of the sling.

Autologous Rectus Fascia Sling

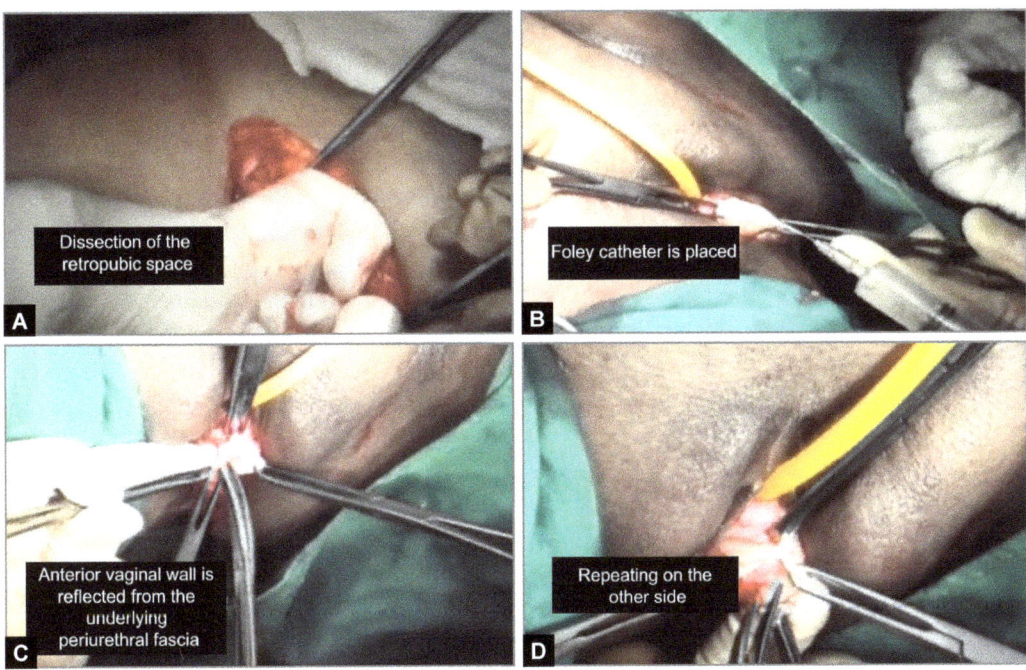

Figs. 4A to D: Initial steps of retropubic space dissection.

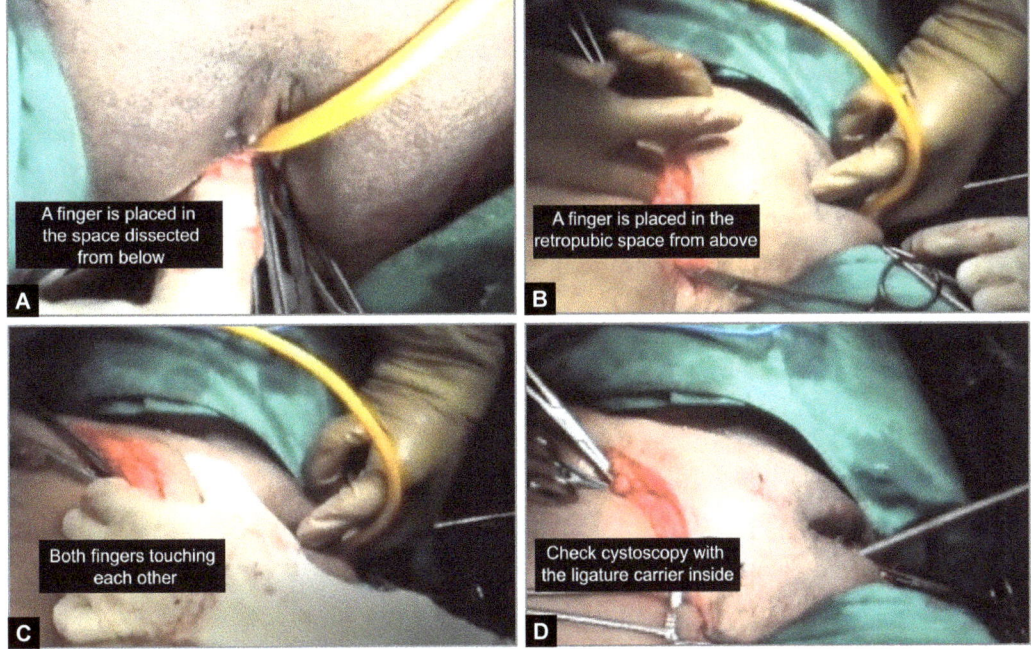

Figs. 5A to D: Final steps of retropubic dissection.

following the guidelines described. Check cystoscopy is repeated again to confirm that there is no bladder entry now. The bladder is catheterized with a 22 Fr Foley catheter. The Polypropylene thread attached sling is now fed into the ligature carrier and the sling is brought through the retropubic space into the abdomen. The procedure is repeated on the opposite side and the sling is placed under the proximal urethra. The important step is the incorporation of the sling into the endopelvic fascia and subsequent fibrosis.

The 2 cm wide sling also ensures that it provides the needed urethral support. The sling is fixed to the underlying periurethral tissues with a fine delayed absorbable suture in the midline supporting proximal urethra **(Fig. 7)**. This ensures that the sling stays correctly. The anterior vaginal wall is now closed **(Fig. 8)**.

The polypropylene threads attached to the edges of the sling are brought out of the rectus sheath by making a small perforation on both sides **(Figs. 9A and B)**.

The rectus sheath can now be comfortably closed with 1-Polypropylene suture.

Fig. 6: Check cystoscopy.

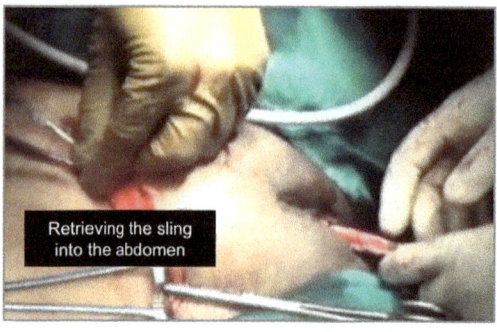

Fig. 7: Sling passage and retrieval.

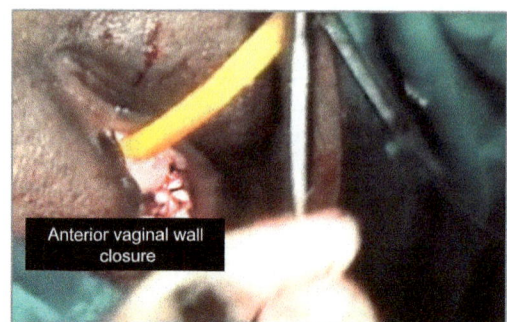

Fig. 8: Closure of anterior vaginal wall.

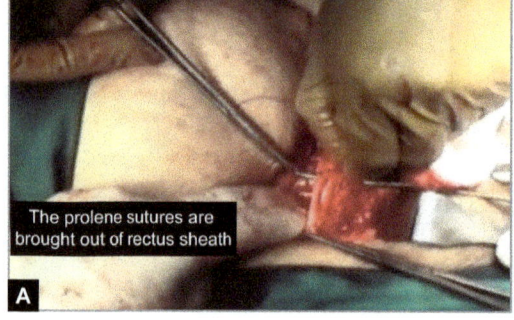

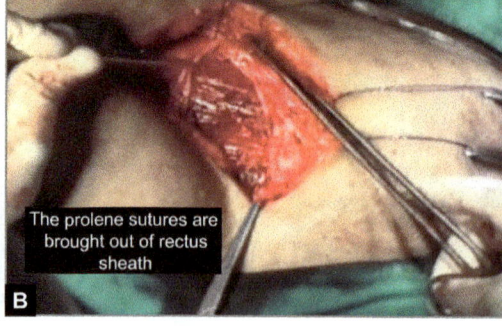

Figs. 9A and B: Retrieval of prolene sutures through the rectus sheath.

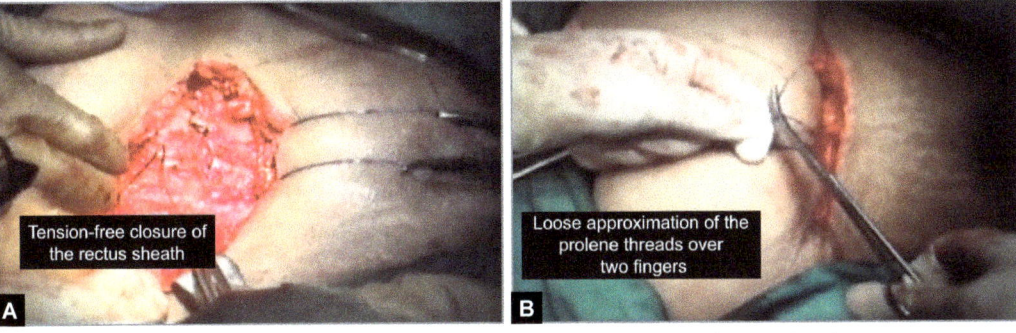

Figs. 10A and B: Tension-free fixation of sling and closure of rectus sheath.

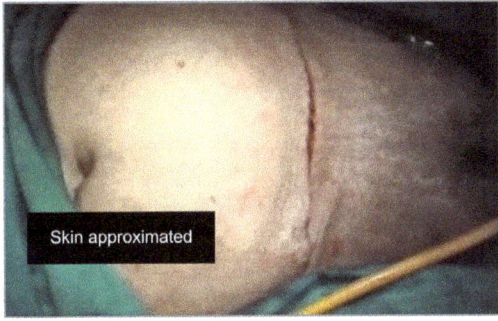

Fig. 11: Final result.

The polypropylene threads attached to both ends of the sling are now loosely tied in the midline **(Figs. 10A and B)**. Two fingers can be placed under the knot so as to avoid over tightening and obstructive voiding.

An Australian study[9] concluded that "a lax sling height of less than 40 mm was associated with a higher risk of postoperative urinary retention and the need for intermittent self-catheterization and urethrolysis". A subcutaneous drain is kept especially in obese women and the skin is closed **(Fig. 11)**.

AUTOLOGOUS FASCIAL SLING WITH STAMEY NEEDLE/LIGATURE CARRIER[4,10]

A 6-7 cm Pfannenstiel incision is used to harvest a strip of rectus fascia of 8 × 2 cm and is safeguarded in saline after placing Polypropylene sutures on either end. The incision in the rectus sheath is closed.

An 18 Fr Foley catheter is inserted into the bladder and the proximal urethra is now exposed after hydrodissection by a midline vertical incision over the proximal urethra and the retropubic space is dissected from below. Stamey needle is inserted from above downward into the retropubic space and guided through the vaginal incision. Check cystoscopy is now done to rule out inadvertent bladder entry. The polypropylene suture is guided through the eye of the needle and brought into the abdomen. The procedure is now repeated on the opposite side. The fascial sling is now anchored in the midline over the periurethral fascia. The polypropylene sutures are tied in the midline over two fingers kept under the sutures thereby avoiding obstructive voiding. Incision is closed in the same way using absorbable sutures **(Fig. 12)**.

Fascia Lata as an Autologous Sling[4,8,11,12]

Autologous fascia lata sling (AFLS) would be a good choice in patients in whom harvest of rectus fascia would be particularly challenging as in patients suffering from morbid obesity (where we are concerned about the increased possibility of wound infection, wound seroma), prior abdominal procedures including abdominoplasty and mesh hernia repairs (where we do not wish to compromise a good repair).

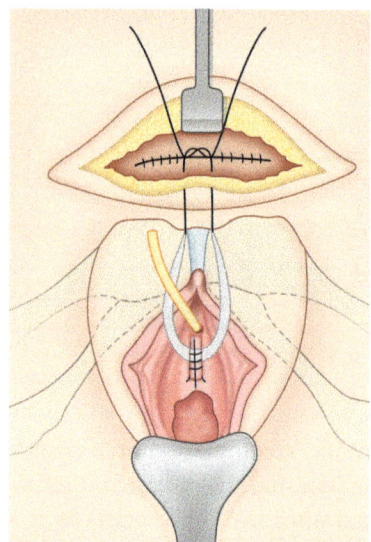

Fig. 12: Autologous fascial sling with Stamey needle.

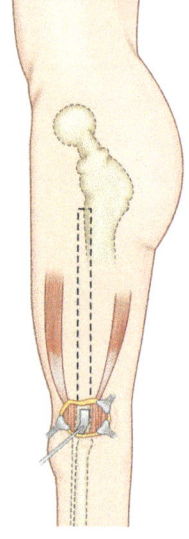

Fig. 13: Fascia Lata harvesting.

The postoperative recovery is faster and there is a marked decrease in the possibility of hernia occurring. However, this procedure is not advocated by many, because of unfamiliar territory, the need to reposition the patient and the increased time required to operate.

Technique of Fascia Lata Harvest[4,8,12,13]

This is also done under regional or general anesthesia. Patient is placed in the lateral position. The anterolateral aspect of the thigh from the greater trochanter to the patella distally is exposed. The greater trochanter is the proximal attachment and the lateral condyle of the femur is the distal attachment of the fascia lata **(Fig. 13)**. The knee is elevated and the leg is internally rotated at the hip and secured and fixed using adhesive plaster.

A 3 cm transverse incision is made just above the patella over the iliotibial band. Incision is deepened down till the level of the fascia lata. Two parallel, longitudinal incisions which are 2 cm apart are made on the fascia lata perpendicular to the skin incision in the direction of fascial fiber. The incision is deepened and the proximal portion of the graft is mobilized from the underlying muscle and lifted for transection. This free end is now secured with polypropylene suture. The fascia lata is now separated from the adipose tissue above and the muscle below.[5] A graft of 2 × 8 cm is harvested using a Crawford fascial stripper.

As the length of fascial sling is now reduced to 8 cm, a simpler technique is now followed. Two transverse incisions of around 3 cm are made. The first incision is made 4–6 cm superior to the lateral femoral condyle and the next incision is made 8 cm cranial to the first. Incision is deepened down till the level of the fascia lata on both ends. The fascia lata graft is harvested by making two longitudinal incisions 2 cm apart. Finger dissection aided with retractors is now used to mobilize graft of size 8 × 2 cm. Both ends are secured with a Polypropylene suture and safeguarded in saline. Compression to the thigh is applied immediately to constrict the perforating vessels and hemostasis is ensured. Thigh closure is done in layers without closing the fascia lata. Wound is released after 8 hours and a sterile dressing applied. This fascia lata graft can be used to perform a PVS in either of the ways described earlier.

Autologous Retropubic Midurethral Sling[14]

The usual surgical technique of autologous fascial PVS has been associated with voiding dysfunction, de novo overactive bladder symptoms, wound infection, and increased recovery time.

To overcome this problem, autologous midurethral placement was tried as an alternative.

The technique involves the use of a small suprapubic incision, harvesting of 8 cm rectus fascial sling loaded as a "sling-on-a string", a modified reusable retropubic needle and midurethral positioning in a tension-free fashion. A good subjective medium-term cure rate with acceptable patient reported satisfaction scores was achieved. Moreover de novo overactive bladder symptoms such as urgency were low, with no cases of erosion and chronic pelvic, groin or vaginal pain.

Autologous transobturator midurethral sling is an alternative therapy for SUI.[15]

A midline incision is made in the anterior vaginal wall in the region of the mid urethra after hydrodissection with normal saline. The anterior vaginal wall is reflected from the underlying periurethral fascia. Dissection was carried to the obturator foramen bilaterally. A transverse abdominal incision was made and an 8 × 1 cm strip of rectus fascia was harvested and prepared with two stay sutures on each end of the fascial sling. This sling was used to perform a transobturator midurethral sling through an "outside in approach" just like with a synthetic sling. The sling was secured proximally and distally with interrupted sutures. Careful attention was paid to tensioning the sling, which was left flush with the urethra. The stay sutures were then tied down and cut flush with the skin level. The anterior vaginal wall and skin incisions were then closed.

COMPLICATIONS

- *Voiding dysfunction*: Some patients have a temporary voiding dysfunction postoperatively. They may be taught CIC or if unwilling, put on an indwelling catheter for another 10 days during which time the edema around the bladder neck is likely to settle and the patient will be able pass urine normally.

  Obstructive urinary symptoms persisting beyond 3–6 months occur in less than 5% of the patients and they may require surgical help.[16] Even then, it is not necessary to cut the sling. The abdominal wound can be opened in the midline and the knot in the polypropylene thread can be cut. This will facilitate relief of obstructive voiding. Since the sling has gone through the retropubic space and fibrosis has occurred on both sides by now, there is usually no recurrence of SUI. This procedure can be done under local infiltration anesthesia alone or supplemented with intravenous anesthesia. In case the patient is still unable to void, she will require cystoscopy and further procedures such as urethrolysis.

  De novo urgency, urgency incontinence, detrusor overactivity or impaired detrusor contractility can also occur.
- Bladder perforation is prevented by following the steps earlier described and tackled accordingly. The patient is kept on

a continuous bladder drainage for 10 days. The American Urological Association (AUA) Guidelines meta-analysis reported a perforation rate of 4%.[17,18]
- Urethral erosion or vaginal extrusion is generally not encountered.[13]
- Wound infection and seroma can occur especially in obese patients and diabetics.
- Urinary tract infections, incisional hernia, pelvic and retropubic hematoma are other complications.

CONCLUSION

Autologous fascial sling is now being increasingly performed because of better cure rates and absence of the complications associated with synthetic mesh. It still remains a gold standard for the surgical treatment of SUI.[11]

PRACTICE POINTS

Pubovaginal sling is an excellent surgery for all patients requiring surgical management of SUI, especially those suffering from ISD.

Urodynamic Study is useful in the diagnosis of ISD. However, certain symptoms such as significant urine leak with even minimal stress, like clearing the throat may be a marker of ISD.[19] Patients with ISD also leak urine during vehicular jerks. Some patients give a history of stress leak even after they have just returned from the restroom after emptying the bladder.

While placing the sling, it is preferable to place the underside of the graft on the body side of the patient.[8]

When a concomitant urethral reconstruction along with PVS is planned, it is preferable to harvest the fascia and place the sling over the proximal urethra without tensioning. Urethral reconstruction is performed now and then the sling is fixed in the proximal urethra and tensioned.[8]

Pubovaginal sling is a simple and effective surgery. However, there is an increased incidence of seroma/wound infection in obese/diabetic women and patients may be counseled regarding that.

Postoperative voiding dysfunction, which can occur, can be tackled as explained. However, patients need to be counseled about this complication.

REFERENCES

1. Abrams P, Cardozo L, Fall M, Griffiths D, Rosier P, Ulmsten U, et al. The standardization of terminology of lower urinary tract function: report from the Standardisation Sub-Committee of the International Continence Society. Neurourol Urodyn. 2002;21:167-78.
2. Haylen BT, de Ridder D, Freeman RM, Swift SE, Berghmans B, Lee J, et al. An International Urogynecological Association (IUGA)/ International Continence Society (ICS) joint report on the terminology for female pelvic floor dysfunction. Neurourol Urodyn. 2010;29:4-20.
3. McGuire EJ, Lytton B. Pubovaginal sling procedure for stress incontinence. J Urol. 1978;119:82-4.
4. Dmochowski RR, Osborn DJ, Reynolds WS. In: Campbell-Walsh Urology 11th edition. Gurugram: Elsevier India; 2015.
5. Ulmsten U, Henriksson L, Johnson P, Varhos G. An ambulatory surgical procedure under local anesthesia for treatment of female urinary incontinence. Int Urogynecol J Pelvic Floor Dysfunct. 1996;7:81-5.
6. Plagakis S, T se V. The autologous fascial sling: an update in 2019. Lo Urin Tract Symptoms. 2020;12(1):2-7.
7. Kobashi KC. Evaluation and management of women with urinary incontinence and pelvic prolapse. In: McDougal WS, Wein AJ, Kavoussi LR, Partin AW, Peters CA. Campbell-Walsh Urology, 11th edition. Gurugram: Elsevier India; 2015.
8. Nager CW, Kraus SR, Kenton K, Sirls L, Chai TC, Wai C, et al. Urodynamics, the supine empty bladder stress test, and incontinence severity. Neurourol Urodyn. 2010;29(7):10.
9. Cameron AP, Lewicky-Gauppe C, Edward J. Pubovaginal fascial sling. In: Graham SD, Keane TE. McGuire Glenn's Urologic Surgery, 7th edition. Philadelphia: Lippincott Williams & Wilkins; 2010.

10. Dmochowski RR, Blaivas JM, Gormley EA, Juma S, Karram MM, Lightner DJ, et al. Update of AUA guideline on the surgical management of female stress urinary incontinence. J Urol. 2010;183(5):1906-14.
11. Preece P, Chan G, O`Connell H, Gani J. Optimising the tension of an autologous fascia pubovaginal sling to minimize retentive complications. Neururol Urodyn. 2019;38:1409-16.
12. Karram MM, Bhatia N. Patch procedure: Modified transvaginal fascia lata sling for stress urinary incontinence. Obstet Gynecol. 1990;75(3 Pt 1):461-3.
13. Welk BK, Herschorn S. The autologous fascia pubovaginal sling for complicated female stress incontinence. Can Urol Assoc J. 2012;6(1):36-40.
14. Blaivas JG, Simma-Chiang V, Gul Z, Dayan L, Kalkan S, Daniel M. Surgery for stress urinary incontinence: autologous fascial sling. Urol Clin North Am. 2019;46(1):41-52.
15. de Vries AM, Heesakkers JP. Contemporary autologous fascial sling for female stress urinary incontinence: its role in the era of synthetic midurethral tapes. Asian J Urol. 2017;5(3):141-8.
16. Taha DE, Wadie BS. Pubovaginal sling, the godfather of midurethral slings that remained so. Journal of Acute Disease. 2015;4(2):91-6.
17. Linder B, Elliot DS. Autologous transobturator midurethral sling for female stress urinary incontinence. J Urol. 2015;191(4S):995-6.
18. Leach G, Dmochowski R, Appell R, Blaivas JG, Hadley HR, Luber KM, et al. Female Stress Urinary Incontinence Clinical Guidelines Panel summary report on surgical management of female stress urinary incontinence. The American Urological Association. J Urol. 1997;158:875-80.
19. Dağdeviren H, Cengiz H, Helvacıoğlu Ç, Heydarova U, Kaya C, Ekin M. A comparison of normal and high post-void residual urine and urodynamic parameters in women with overactive bladder. Turk J Obstet Gynecol. 2017;14:210-13.

Urge Urinary Incontinence: Management Options

Urvashi Neelagar, Basavaraj Neelagar

INTRODUCTION

Patients diagnosed to have overactive bladder or urge urinary Incontinence—either clinically or based on urodynamic study—need a multi-modality treatment to achieve the desired results.

BEHAVIORAL THERAPY

These include a set of modifications in the patient's behavior or their environment aimed at improving their symptoms:[1]

- *Explain the condition to the patient*: Many patients are not aware of the physical basis for their symptoms and consider themselves neurotic. Discussing with patients about the problem and reassuring them would help.
- *Bladder diary*: Maintain bladder diary and make necessary changes in intake as per the chart. Encourage timed voiding.[2]
- *Bladder training*: It is an essential part of urge incontinence management:
  - Patients are encouraged to postpone urination once they get the urge to go, which can be gradually increased over days to weeks from 2 to 5 minutes to begin with to almost an hour or till the interval between the visits reaches 3–4 hours.
  - Pelvic floor exercises, counting the numbers from 1 to 100, diverting the mind, would all help in increasing the "hold time" and delay the urination.
  - Drugs would help patients avoid bladder spasms and leak episodes, thus help build their confidence and stick to bladder training exercises.[3]
- *Weight loss*: Obesity is associated with both urge and stress incontinence. Reduction in body weight helps in reducing the symptoms.[4]
- *Dietary changes*: Avoid bladder irritants like caffeine, chocolate, spicy foods, acidic juices, artificial sweeteners, etc.[5]
- *Biofeedback*: It helps in strengthening the pelvic floor muscles. Sensors placed on the skin help in recognizing pelvic muscle contractions by computer graphs or audible tones thus encouraging the patient to continue with pelvic floor muscle training.[6]

MEDICAL THERAPY

Uropharmacology

A brief review of the innervation of the bladder and the lower urinary tract helps in understanding the pharmacological management of overactive bladder **(Fig. 1)**.[7]

Bladder function is controlled by the sympathetic and parasympathetic nervous systems.

Bladder contractions are mediated by acetylcholine-induced stimulation of postganglionic parasympathetic muscarinic cholinergic receptors on bladder smooth muscle. There are five different subtypes of muscarinic receptors named M1 to M5. M3 receptor

Urge Urinary Incontinence: Management Options

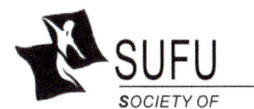

SUFU
SOCIETY OF URODYNAMICS, FEMALE PELVIC MEDICINE & UROGENITAL RECONSTRUCTION

Society of Urodynamics, Female Pelvic Medicine and Urogenital Reconstruction Foundation
Overactive Bladder Clinical Care Pathway

Overactive Bladder Syndrome (OAB):
A clinical syndrome characterized by the presence of urinary urgency, usually accompanied by frequency and nocturia, with or without urgency urinary incontinence in the absence of obvious pathology.

Diagnostic Approach	**Goal:** To document symptoms and signs that characterize OAB and to exclude other disorders that could be cause of patient's symptoms	**Required evaluation:** • History/Assessment of lower urinary tract symptoms (LUTS) – onset, duration, and degree of bother • Contributing comorbidities • Fluid intake • PE • Urinalysis	**Optional evaluation:** Performed at provider's discretion: • Postvoid residual urine (if retention is suspected) • Bladder diary • Urodynamics, cystoscopy and diagnostic renal/bladder ultrasound should not be used in the initial work-up of the uncomplicated patient, but may be used in complicated or refractory patients at provider's discretion	
Patient Education	**Patient discussion:** • Discuss healthy bladder habits • Review normal bladder function • Discuss normal fluid intake and voided volumes • What is normal vs. abnormal frequency?		**Establish treatment plan/Expectations:** • OAB is variable and chronic symptom complex, with no single ideal treatment • Available treatments vary in required patient effort, invasiveness, risks, and reversibility • Most OAB treatments can improve but do not eliminate symptoms	
1st Line or Initial Treatment	**Behavior/Lifestyle:** Should be discussed and offered as first line therapy to all patients	• Urge suppression, PFMT, bladder training • Dietary modification • Therapies may be instituted at any time and combined with pharmacotherapy • Optimal treatment duration/trial 4–8 weeks	**Reassess after 4–8 weeks**	If at any point during treatment the patient is satisfied, continue present treatment. If inadequate symptom relief, consider adding medication, dose escalation, change in medication, combination antimuscarinic and beta-3 agonist medication, consider 3rd line treatments or refer to specialist

2nd Line Treatment (Medication)	**Pharmacotherapy:** Initiate if inadequate improvement with conservative management or at provider's discretion if the symptoms warranted to be bothersome enough	• Current classes of medications include: Antimuscarinics, beta-3 agonist
		• Choice of class or medication depends on age, comorbidities, concomitant medications, formulary restriction:
		– Trial of pharmacotherapy should be at least 4–8 weeks
		– Manage side effects (if present):
		  - Avoid constipation
		  - Adjust fluids, dry mouth aids
		  - Patient medication aid tool*
		  - Medication change or dose adjustment
				*Coming soon

Contd...

Contd...

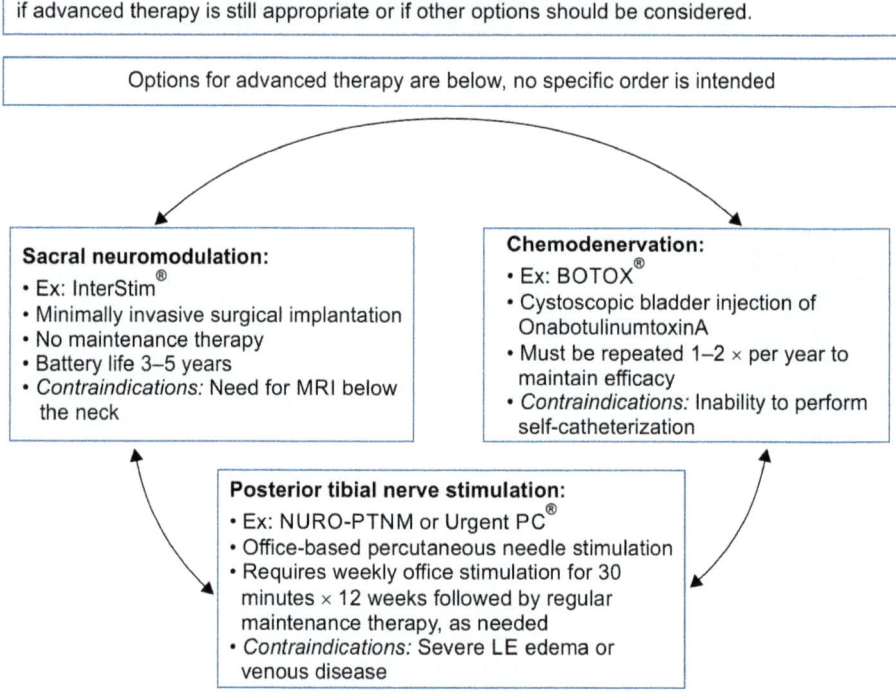

Fig.1: Pharmacological management of overactive bladder.[13]
(PE: physical examination; PFMT: pelvic floor muscle training; CIC: clean intermittent self-catheterization)
Source: Figure reproduced from www.sufuorg.com.

mediates the smooth muscle contractions including bladder smooth muscles. Since most of the antimuscarinics are not highly selective, they act on receptors elsewhere on the body and manifest as side effects that include blurred vision, cognitive dysfunction, dry mouth, pruritus, and constipation.

Stimulation of the sympathetic system through beta adrenoceptors results in bladder wall relaxation. Of the three beta adrenoceptors, beta-3 is the predominant in bladder detrusor muscle. Beta-3 adrenoceptor agonists (mirabegron) were developed based on this concept. They act by relaxing the bladder wall, thus improving the bladder volume.

Adverse effects of beta-3 agonists include increase in heart rate and blood pressure, nausea, and headache. Hence, it is contraindicated in patients with poorly controlled hypertension.

Anticholinergics are the mainstay of treatment of an overactive bladder.[8] These drugs inhibit detrusor muscle contractions by acting on muscarinic receptors (antagonists). Commonly used drugs are discussed here:

- *Tolterodine*: It is a nonselective anticholinergic. Its side effects like dry mouth and constipation are relatively less:
  - *Dosage*: 2–4 mg OD/BD
- *Trospium*: It is a nonselective quaternary amine. Main advantage is it does not cross the blood-brain barrier, hence does not have central nervous system (CNS) side effects like confusion/cognitive dysfunction. It is suitable in elderly:
  - *Dosage*: 20 mg OD/BD
- *Solifenacin*: It is a tertiary amine selective M3 receptor antagonist. It does not bind to receptors in salivary glands. Hence, it has low incidence of dry mouth:
  - *Dosage*: 5–10 mg OD
- *Darifenacin*: It is an another selective M3 receptor antagonist. It is safe in elderly:
  - *Dosage*: 7.5–15 mg OD
  - *Adverse events*: It is contraindicated in active urinary tract infection (UTI), urinary retention, and narrow angle glaucoma.
- *Mirabegron*:[9] Newer drug, a selective beta-3 adrenoceptor agonist, helps in bladder wall relaxation, and improves storage:
  - *Dosage*: 25–100 mg OD/BD
  - *Combination therapy*: In severe/refractory cases, drugs from these two different classes may be combined. Many trials that have used combinations of solifenacin with mirabegron showed a significant improvement in mean volume voided per micturition, and reduction in urinary frequency.
- *Intravesical botulinum toxin*: Patients who are symptomatic despite oral pharmacotherapy or those who do not tolerate the side effects may benefit from intravesical botulinum toxin injection:
  - Botulinum toxin is a neurotoxin produced by Clostridium botulinum—a gram positive, anaerobic bacteria.
  - It acts by blocking the release of acetylcholine at the neuromuscular junction, afferent desensitization effects at the bladder as well as centrally.
  - Only OnabotulinumtoxinA is FDA approved.
  - *Dosage*: 100–300 units
  - *Contraindications*: Active UTI, retention of urine or persistent high post void residue (>200 mL), pregnancy/women planning for pregnancy, known hypersensitivity to the drug, and inability or unwillingness to perform clean intermittent self-catheterization (CIC).
  - *Procedure*: It can be done as a day care procedure. The dry powder in the botulinum toxin vial is reconstituted with 10 mL of 0.9% normal saline and gently mixed by rotating the vial. Vigorous shaking can lead to toxin denaturation. The reconstituted vial may be refrigerated (2–8°C) up to 24 hours.

    The injection procedure is done under suitable anesthesia with rigid/flexible cystoscope under antibiotic cover (avoid aminoglycosides). The special needle used is usually 22–27 gauge with 4 mm long tip. The bladder is optimally distended, and thorough visualization of the bladder is done to rule out any tumor/stone. Ideally, the vial should be opened for reconstitution only after confirming a normal cystoscopy.

The reconstituted drug is injected uniformly throughout the bladder. There are no universally accepted guidelines regarding the location and number of injections. It may be given over 20 sites of 0.5 mL each or 10 sites of 1 mL each and both intradetrusor and submucosal injections are acceptable. Postprocedure, observe the patient for hematuria and urinary retention. The effect of injection is not immediate and may take up to 2 weeks. Patients are continued on oral therapy for 2 weeks and reviewed at 2 weeks with post void residual urine. CIC may be initiated if residue is high (>200 mL).[10]

Electrical Stimulation

- *Sacral neuromodulation*: A temporary electrode is inserted percutaneously under fluoroscopy guidance in the sacral foramen adjacent to a sacral nerve (S3). Stimulation of the nerve results in inhibition of detrusor contractions. The permanent electrode is placed only in those patients who show >50% reduction in their urge incontinence symptoms.
- *Posterior tibial nerve stimulation*: Electrical stimulation of the posterior tibial nerve stimulates the sacral micturition center through S2-S4 sacral nerves. Stimulation is done for 30 minutes for 12 weeks and continued with maintenance therapy through a small needle placed just above the medial malleolus. This treatment is recommended in patients who have not responded to medical therapy.[11]

SURGICAL THERAPY

- *Augmentation cystoplasty (clam cystoplasty)*: It is preferred in neurogenic bladders with small capacity or poor compliance. A detubularized segment of terminal ileum is interposed in the bivalved bladder.
- *Partial detrusor myomectomy (autoaugmentation of bladder)*: A portion of detrusor muscle is incised or excised to create a "pseudo diverticulum" bulge of the bladder mucosa, thus increasing the capacity and also reducing the bladder pressures.
- *Urinary diversion*: It is offered as a last resort. Cystectomy followed by orthotopic neobladder reconstruction or ileal conduit is done.[12]

REFERENCES

1. Subak LL, Quesenberry CP, Posner SF, Cattolica E, Soghikian K. The effect of behavioral therapy on urinary incontinence: a randomized controlled trial. Obstet Gynecol. 2002;100(1):72-8. doi: 10.1016/s0029-7844(02)01993-2. PMID: 12100806.
2. Stav K, Dwyer PL, Rosamilia A. Women over estimate daytime urinary frequency: the importance of the bladder diary. J Urol. 2009;181(5):2176-80. doi: 10.1016/j.juro.2009.01.042. Epub 2009 Mar 17. PMID: 19296975.
3. Roe B, Williams K, Palmer M. Bladder training for urinary incontinence in adults. Cochrane Database Syst Rev. 2000;(2):CD001308. doi: 10.1002/14651858.CD001308. Update in: Cochrane Database Syst Rev. 2004; (1):CD001308. PMID:10796768.
4. Hunskaar S. A systematic review of overweight and obesity as risk factors and targets for clinical intervention for urinary incontinence in women. Neurourol Urodyn. 2008;27(8):749-57. doi: 10.1002/nau.20635. PMID: 18951445.
5. Ernst M, Gonka J, Povcher O, et al. Diet modification for overactive bladder: an evidence-based review. Curr Bladder Dysfunct Rep. 2015;10:25-30. https:// doi.org/10.1007/s11884-014-0285-0.
6. Burgio KL, Goode PS, Locher JL, et al. Behavioral training with and without biofeedback in the treatment of urge incontinence in older women: a randomized controlled trial. JAMA. 2002;288(18):2293-9. doi:10.1001/jama.288.18.2293.
7. Fowler C, Griffiths D, de Groat W. The neural control of micturition. Nat Rev Neurosci.

2008;9:453-66. https://doi.org/10.1038/nrn2401

8. Geoffrion R; UROGYNAECOLOGY COMMITTEE. Treatments for overactive bladder: focus on pharmacotherapy. J Obstet Gynaecol Can. 2012;34(11):1092-101. doi: 10.1016/S1701-2163(16)35440-8. PMID: 23231848.

9. Chapple CR, Cardozo L, Nitti VW, Siddiqui E, Michel MC. Mirabegron in overactive bladder: a review of efficacy, safety, and tolerability. Neurourol Urodyn. 2014;33(1):17-30. doi: 10.1002/nau.22505. Epub 2013 Oct 11. PMID: 24127366.

10. Ferreira RS, D'Ancona CAL, Oelke M, Carneiro MR. Intradetrusor onabotulinumtoxinA injections are significantly more efficacious than oral oxybutynin for treatment of neurogenic detrusor overactivity: results of a randomized, controlled, 24-week trial. einstein (São Paulo). 2018;16(3):eAO4207. https://doi.org/10.1590/S1679-45082018AO4207

11. Schreiner L, Santos TG, Souza AB, Nygaard CC, Silva Filho IG. Electrical stimulation for urinary incontinence in women: a systematic review. Int Braz J Urol. 2013;39(4):454-64. doi: 10.1590/S1677-5538.IBJU.2013.04.02. PMID: 24054395.

12. Vasdev N, Biles BD, Sandher R, Hasan TS. The surgical management of the refractory overactive bladder. Indian J Urol. 2010;26(2):263-9. doi: 10.4103/0970-1591.65402.

13. Society of Urodynamics, Female pelvic medicine and Urogenital reconstruction Foundation: Overactive Bladder Clinical Care Pathway.

CHAPTER 13

Assessment and Management of Patient with Obstructive Lower Urinary Tract Symptoms

Vishal

INTRODUCTION

Nearly about half of all women who are older than 40 years have some form of lower urinary tract symptoms (LUTS). According to the International Continence Society the female lower urinary tract symptoms (FLUTS) include storage symptoms, voiding (obstructive) symptoms and postmicturition symptoms. The probable causes of obstructive lower urinary tract symptoms are enlisted in **Table 1**.[1,2]

Presenting Symptoms

- Poor urinary stream
- Intermittent urinary stream
- Straining to void
- Sensation of incomplete voiding
- Infrequent voiding
- Hesitancy
- Acute retention presenting with pain
- Overflow incontinence or frequency
- Urinary tract infection (UTI) due to urinary stasis

ASSESSMENT

History

History taking should be aimed toward determining the primary cause for the obstructive LUTS. A proper drug intake and medical history including genital and UTI are necessary. History of previous surgery as continence surgery is a well-known causative factor for LUTS.

TABLE 1: Causes of obstructive lower urinary tract symptoms.

Anatomical		*Functional*	
Extrinsic	Pelvic organ prolapse	*Impaired coordination*	Fowler's syndrome
	Post anti-incontinence procedure		Detrusor-external sphincter dyssynergia
	Uterine fibroid or tumor		Primary bladder neck obstruction
Urethral	Meatal stenosis		Neurological disease
	Stricture	*Perioperative*	Pain
	Caruncle		Epidural
	Diverticulum	*Infective/ Inflammatory*	Urinary tract infection
	Skene's gland cyst or abscess		Acute vulvovaginitis
Luminal	Stone		Vaginal lichen planus/sclerosis
	Bladder/urethral tumor		Genital herpes
	Ureterocele	*Pharmacological*	Opiates
Impaired detrusor contractility	Age-related bladder changes		Antipsychotics
			Antidepressants
			Antimuscarinics
			α-adrenergic agonist

Examination

A careful general abdominal and pelvic examination should be performed. Abdominal and pelvic examination should be performed after emptying the bladder and masses palpated for (such as ovarian cyst or fibroids).

Urethra or vulvovaginal area is noted for any inflammation and the urethra is palpated for tenderness and scarring. Infected urethral diverticulum or vaginal cysts are noted, and any genital prolapse demonstrated.

Neurological examination and psychiatric evaluation should be performed. The lumbar region should be examined for the stigmata of an underlying spinal disorder.

INVESTIGATIONS

Investigations required in evaluating a woman with obstructive LUTS are uroflowmetry and ultrasonography. Other investigations such as urodynamic study and evaluating a possible UTI may help in making a more accurate diagnosis.

International Prostate Symptom Score

This score is also valid for the assessment of FLUTS. This helps in assessing the severity of the symptoms as well as its effect on the quality of life of the individual concerned.[3] International Prostate Symptom Score (IPSS) is assessed by taking a history of symptoms in the past month and the severity is graded accordingly **(Tables 2 and 3)**.

Frequency Volume Chart

Record of fluid intake and output which is essential in evaluating LUTS. The intake of fluids in any form is noted with respect to time and noted as well as the amount of urine

TABLE 2: International Prostate Symptom Score (IPSS).

Patient name: _____ Date of birth: _____ Date completed: _____

In the past month	Not at all	Less than 1 in 5 times	Less than half the time	About half the time	More than half the time	Almost always	Your score
1. *Incomplete emptying*: How often have you had the sensation of not emptying your bladder?	0	1	2	3	4	5	
2. *Frequency*: How often have you had to urinate less than every 2 hours?	0	1	2	3	4	5	
3. *Intermittency*: How often have you found you stopped and started again several times when you urinated?	0	1	2	3	4	5	
4. *Urgency*: How often have you found it difficult to postpone urination?	0	1	2	3	4	5	
5. *Weak stream*: How often have you had a weak urinary stream?	0	1	2	3	4	5	
6. *Straining*: How often have you had to strain to start urination?	0	1	2	3	4	5	
		None	1 time	2 times	3 times	4 times	5 times
7. *Nocturia*: How many times did you typically get up at night to urinate?	0		1	2	3	4	5

Total I-PSS

Score: *1–7:* Mild; *8–19:* Moderate; *20–35:* Severe

TABLE 3: Quality of Life Score due to the symptoms.

Quality of life due to urinary symptoms	Delighted	Pleased	Mostly satisfied	Mixed	Mostly dissatisfied	Unhappy	Terrible
If you were to spend the rest of your life with your urinary condition just the way it is now, how would you feel about that?	0	1	2	3	4	5	6

TABLE 4: A typical 3-day frequency volume chart.

	Day 1			Day 2			Day 3		
	Intake	Output	Wet	Intake	Output	Wet	Intake	Output	Wet
7 am									
8 am									
9 am									
10 am									
11 am									
12 pm									
1 pm									
2 pm									
3 pm									
4 pm									
5 pm									
6 pm									
7 pm									
8 pm									
9 pm									
10 pm									
11 pm									
12 am									
1 am									
2 am									
3 am									
4 am									
5 am									
6 am									

and the time at which it was voided are noted down **(Table 4)**.

Uroflowmetry

Uroflowmetry test is the initial screening procedure of choice **(Fig. 1)**. A voided urine volume of at least 150 mL is required for a proper assessment. Uroflowmetry with a consistent peak flow of less than 15 mL/sec with a voided volume of more than 150 mL should suggest bladder outlet obstruction in a female, especially in the absence of gross pelvic organ prolapse.

Flow rates consistently below 15 mL/sec suggest impaired voiding. Obstructed voiding may occur in the presence of normal

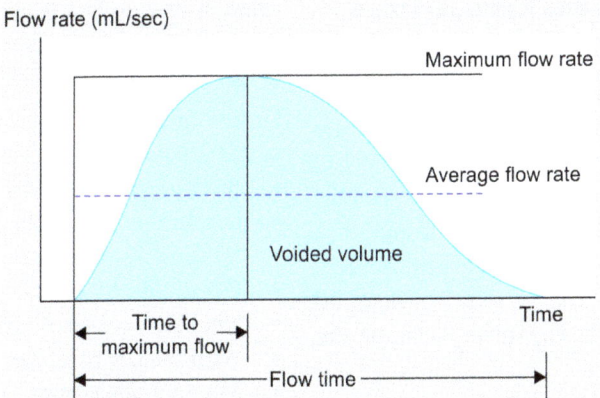

Fig. 1: Normal uroflowmetry graph. International Continence Society recommended nomenclature. Basic elements of maximum flow, mean flow, total flow time, and total voided volume.

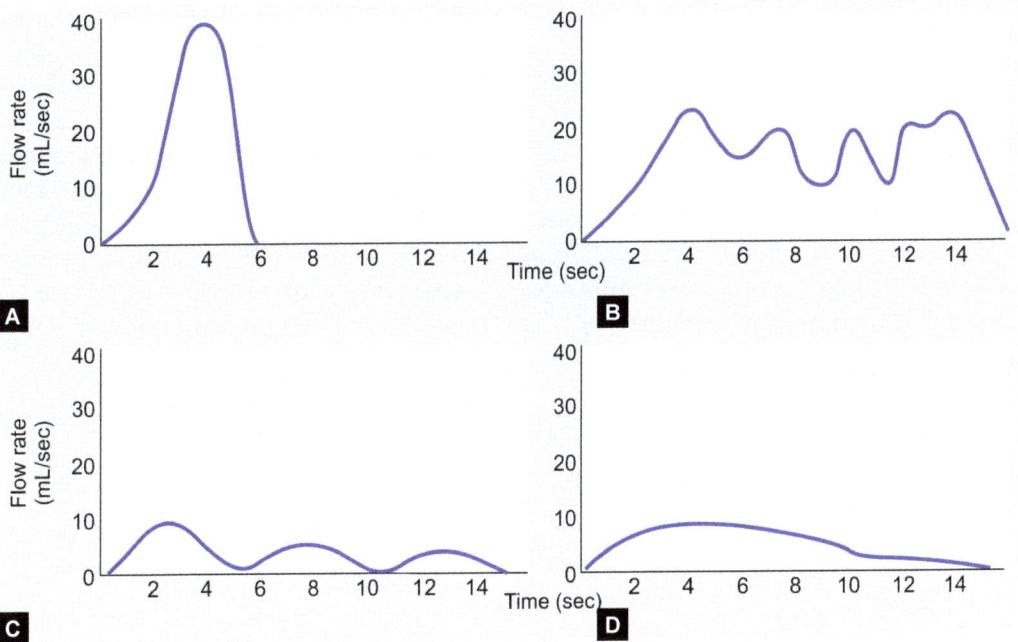

Figs. 2A to D: Various uroflowmetry patterns.

uroflowmetry because the detrusor may compensate by increasing the voiding pressure. Graphical representation of various uroflowmetry patterns are shown in **Figures 2A to D**.

Radiologic Investigation

Lumbosacral X-ray films can demonstrate congenital conditions such as spina bifida occulta or acquired conditions such as intervertebral disc prolapse.

Video cystourethrography can provide additional information at the time of urodynamic study. Using contrast radiographic studies, conditions such as trabeculation, diverticula and ureteric reflux can be identified. Even distal urethral stenosis can be identified.

Ultrasonography and Residual Urine

Abdominal ultrasonography allows evaluation of the urinary system and measurement of residual urine in the bladder along with the details of the upper urinary tract. The severity of bladder distension can be assessed. Details such as bladder morphology, presence of a bladder tumor or calculi can also be obtained. Transperineal and transvaginal ultrasound are beneficial in assessing the pelvic floor and urethra.

The presence of residual urine greater than 50 mL or 20% of the prevoid urine volume is not normal. The interpretation and management will depend on the clinical situation and urodynamic data available.

Urodynamic Study

This helps to study the bladder capacity, sensation, compliance and bladder contractility along with urethral function. Urodynamic study has to be considered after obtaining a detailed history of patient symptoms, examination and frequency-volume chart. The filling phase in the study can identify a lower or upper motor neuron lesion. The voiding phase will show any disorder of bladder emptying **(Figs. 3 and 4)**.

Urodynamic study is commonly considered in the following conditions:
- Before surgery for stress incontinence
- Urethral obstruction
- Voiding dysfunction
- Overactive bladder
- Neurological disorders
- With history of a prior surgical procedure
- Medicolegal issues

Changes that may be noted in cases of voiding difficulty and history of retention are: delayed first sensation, increased bladder capacity, pressure rise during filling, compliance usually normal, maximum voiding pressure will be raised (absent in a decompensated bladder), isometric pressure reduced or absent (poor detrusor reserve) and significant residual urine. Pressure measurement during voiding can identify a poorly contracting bladder and straining during voiding. Detrusor pressure more than 60 cmH$_2$O and peak flow rate less than 15 mL/s is accepted as obstruction in women.

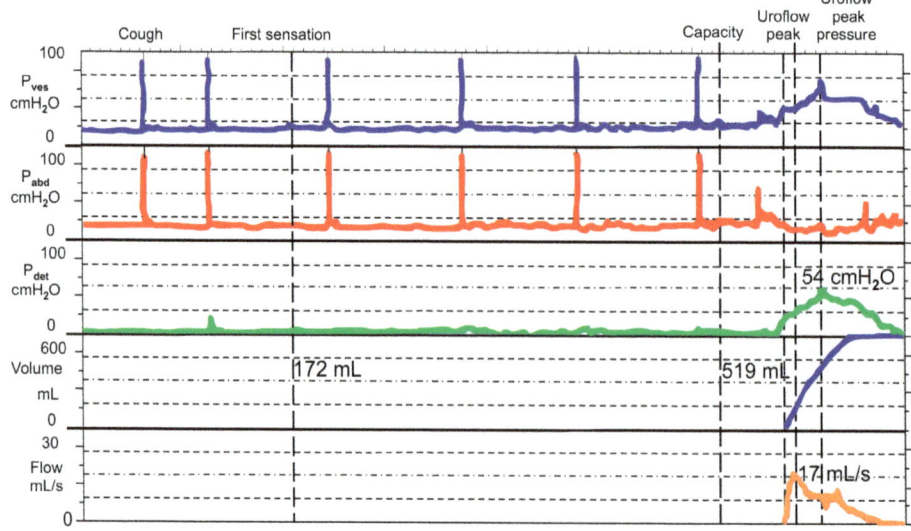

Fig. 3: A normal voiding pattern with normal pressure and flow rate.

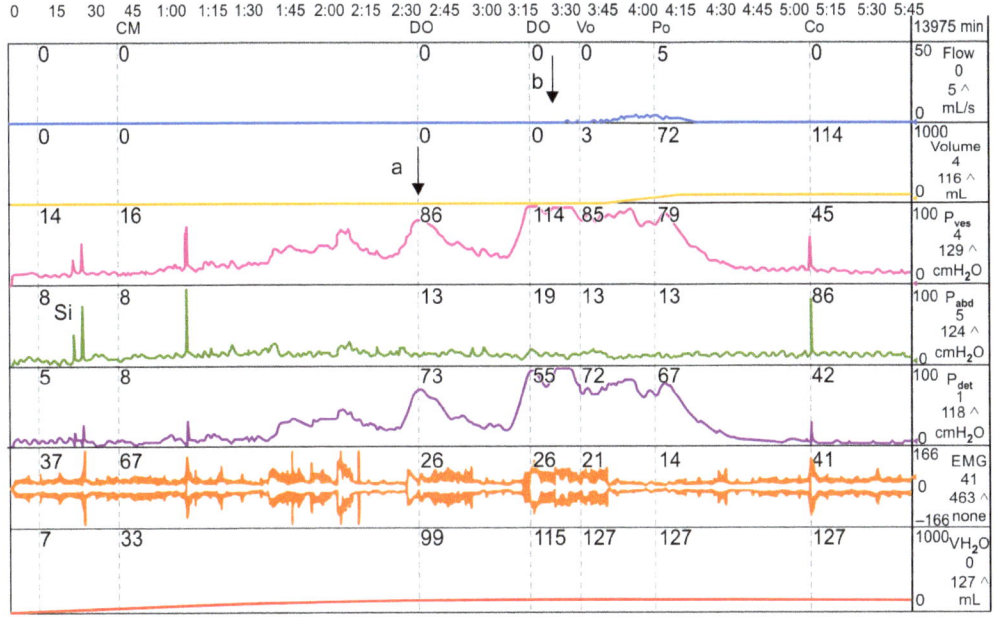

Fig. 4: Urodynamics showing bladder outlet obstruction.

Electromyography

Electromyography (EMG) is used to demonstrate the characteristic decelerating bursts and complex repetitive discharges due to ephaptic transmission which is seen in Fowler's syndrome (urethral sphincter hypertrophy) **(Fig. 5)**.

Cystoscopy

Cystoscopy will allow visualization of the urethra and bladder which will help in identifying urethral and intravesical pathology such as urethral stenosis, bladder calculi, bladder tumor and bladder changes such as trabeculation, sacculation and diverticula.

Other Investigations

A voiding cystourethrogram (VCUG) is useful for diagnosing conditions such as urethral stenosis, vesicoureteric reflux (VUR) and urethral diverticulum.

Computed tomography (CT) and magnetic resonance imaging (MRI): These studies have limited usage in the evaluation of obstructive LUTS. Occasionally or incidentally, where the urinary obstruction is caused by some form of tumor arising from the lower urinary tract or from the pelvic organs causing compression and obstruction, this investigation may be beneficial.

TREATMENT

Early recognition of LUTS may avoid long-term voiding difficulties. Post-continence surgeries, postoperative urinary retention usually resolves spontaneously. However, when urinary retention occurs post radical gynecological surgery, only half of the patients are able to spontaneously resume voiding. Also, difficulty in resumption of spontaneous voiding is seen after epidural anesthesia. In these situations, pre-emptive bladder drainage and emptying can be done. Precise treatment must be dictated by the exact cause in the individual case.

If a catheter is required to be placed for a short duration, a Foley urethral catheter will

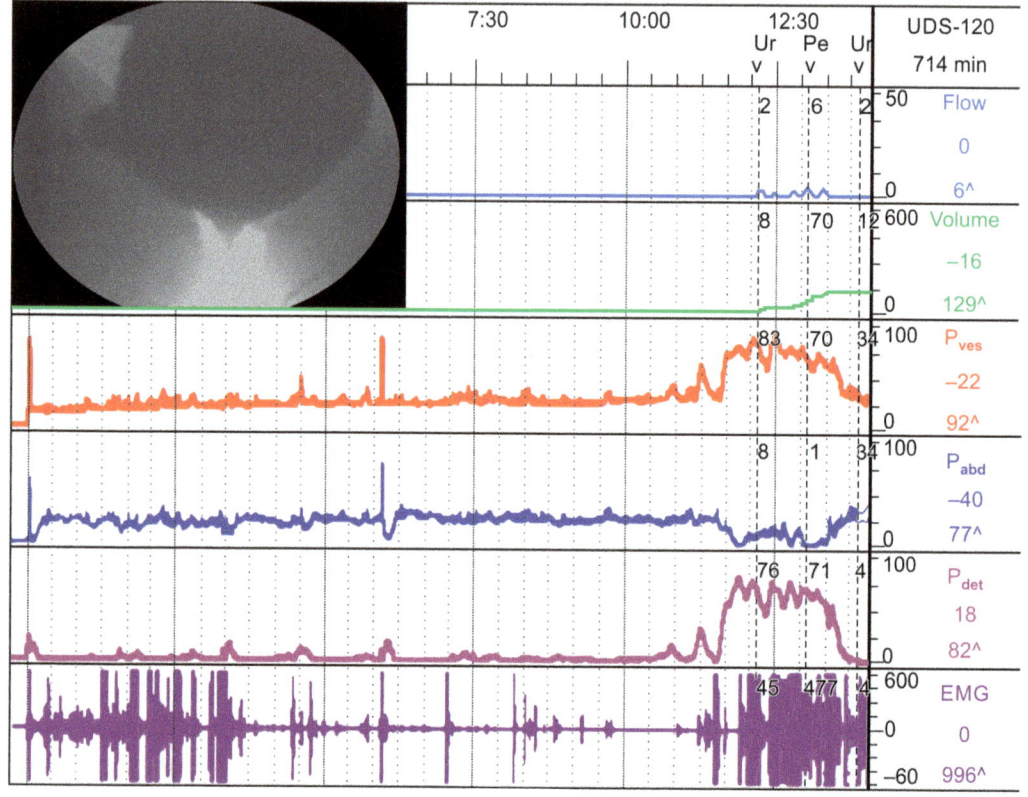

Fig. 5: Urodynamics showing voiding phase dysfunction possibly Fowler's syndrome.
(EMG: electromyography; UDS: urodynamic study)

suffice (e.g., after epidural anesthesia). Where longer term problems may ensue (e.g., after continence surgery), a suprapubic catheter will allow better assessment of voiding and residual volumes and has a lower rate of UTI.

In women with voiding difficulty prior to continence surgery, it is beneficial to teach intermittent self-catheterization. Use of tension free mid-urethral slings has a low but significant incidence of bladder outlet obstruction. The case for routine urethral catheterization for 24 hours after all pelvic surgery remains unresolved.

Clean Intermittent Self-catheterization

Intermittent self-catheterization is a non-sterile practice for urinary drainage **(Fig. 6)**. It is the preferred treatment for lower urinary tract obstruction with chronic urinary retention. The benefit of this is that it allows women to have an independent life with good quality of life and adequate bladder emptying and low chances of UTI.

Intermittent self-catheterization can be sterile or clean. Sterile method is usually preferred for patients with neurogenic bladders to prevent hospital acquired infections. Clean intermittent self-catheterization (CISC) is ideal for everyday use. The patient needs to be reasonably dextrous to do this procedure and can utilize a mirror to do the procedure. Disposable catheters are preferable while reusable catheters are also acceptable with very low risk of infection. The frequency at which CISC needs to be done is patient specific, with the intention to avoid

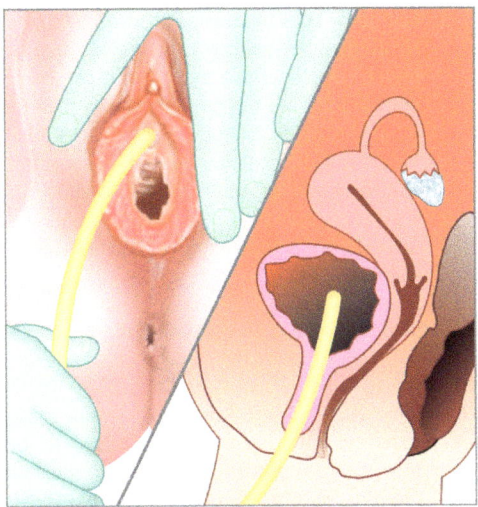

Fig. 6: Technique of clean intermittent self-catheterization.

overfilling and urinary leak. CISC can also be done by a caretaker.

Pharmacotherapy

The female bladder and the urethra are sensitive to the action of estrogens. Atrophic senile urethritis related urethral changes can occur as a result of estrogen deprivation. Systemic or topical hormone replacement therapy (HRT) does have a role in the management of bladder outlet obstruction in females though there is no conclusive evidence.[4] Estrogen and progesterone receptors are present in the vagina, urethra, bladder and pelvic floor.[5] A significant effect of estrogen replacement therapy on urinary incontinence has not been found. The relationship between onset of symptoms and menopause appears to be an important confounder because only symptoms that originated during or after menopause are likely to benefit from hormonal treatment.[6]

Drugs such as cholinergic agents (bethanechol), anticholinesterase (distigmine) and prostaglandins have been used but without much evidence of any clinical benefit. Alpha blockers (Tamsulosin) have been used but they do not have much proven benefit in women. Diazepam used as an anxiolytic may help with postoperative voiding problems. In cases of combined urge incontinence and retention, drugs such as anticholinergic agents (tolterodine) have been used along with CISC with some benefit.

Surgical Treatment

Urethral Dilatation

In urethral stenosis, urethra-cystoscopy and urethral dilatation gives good results. Some favorable long-term outcomes for urethral dilation have been reported. Smith et al. reported a 57% success rate at a mean follow-up of 21 months in seven women after dilation to 30 Fr.[7] Recurrence is noted in few cases which may require repeated dilatations. Self-dilatation by using a female urethral dilator can maintain the urethral passage adequate enough to void comfortably.

Urethrotomy

Urethral strictures are generally amenable to urethrotomy with an Otis Urethrotome. But recurrence rates are high in the long term.

In occasional cases where there is longer narrowing due to stricture of the female urethra, a graft can be placed to achieve good long-term results and reduce the rates of recurrence.[8,9]

Primary bladder neck obstruction in women is rarely seen. Though bladder neck incision as a treatment option in these cases may be considered, there is always a risk of causing urinary incontinence.[10]

Neuromodulation

The S3 nerve root is stimulated through the S3 foramen. It is done in two stages: (1) temporary neurostimulator placement and (2) permanent neurostimulator placement.

In the first stage, percutaneous nerve evaluation is done using a temporary stimulation wire. If this shows any beneficial effect, then a permanent stimulator is implanted. It is useful especially in patients with Fowler's syndrome.

Injection of botulinum toxin into the external urethral sphincter is one of the simpler treatment options in Fowler's syndrome.

Continent urinary diversion with a Mitrofanoff-like stoma can be done in refractory cases of Fowler's syndrome.

REFERENCES

1. Abrams P, Cardozo L, Fall M, Griffiths D, Rosier P, Ulmsten U, et al. The standardisation of terminology in lower urinary tract function: report from the standardisation sub-committee of the International Continence Society. Urology. 2003;61:37-49.
2. Saloniaa A, Zannia G, Nappi RE, Briganti A, Dehò F, Fabbri F, et al. sexual dysfunction is common in women with lower urinary tract symptoms and urinary incontinence: results of a cross-sectional study. Eur Urol. 2004;45(5):642-8.
3. Scarpero HM, Fiske J, Xue X, Nitti VW. American Urological Association Symptom Index for lower urinary tract symptoms in women: correlation with degree of bother and impact on quality of life. Urology. 2003;61:1118-22.
4. Yande S, Joshi M. Bladder outlet obstruction in women. J Midlife Health. 2011;2(1):11-7.
5. Cardozo L. Role of estrogens in the treatment of female urinary incontinence. J Am Geriatr Soc. 1990;38:326-8.
6. Alling L, Lose G, Jørgensen T. Risk factors for lower urinary tract symptoms in women 40 to 60 years of age. Obstet Gynecol. 2000;96(3):446-51.
7. Smith AL, Ferlise VJ, Rovner ES. Female urethral strictures: successful management with long-term clean intermittent catheterization after urethral dilation. BJU Int. 2006;98:96-9.
8. Blaivas JG, Santos JA, Tsui JF, Deibert CM, Rutman MP, Purohit RS, et al. Management of urethral stricture in women. J Urol. 2012;188:1778-82.
9. Osman NI, Chapple CR. Contemporary surgical management of female urethral stricture disease. Curr Opin Urol. 2015;25:341-5.
10. Zhang P, Zhi-Jin W, Ling X, Yong Y, Zhang N, Zhang X. Bladder neck incision for female bladder neck obstruction: long-term outcomes. Urology. 2014;83(4):762-6.

CHAPTER 14: Current Trends in the Management of Recurrent Urinary Tract Infections

Karthik Rao

INTRODUCTION

There have been multiple definitions of recurrent urinary tract infection (rUTI). Most of the urological guidelines agree that two episodes of culture proven UTI within 6 months or three episodes in a year qualifies for rUTI.[1-3] It requires that each episode is a separate infection with complete resolution of symptoms in between.

However, in patients with uncomplicated cystitis who recur within 2 weeks after symptom resolution or have bacterial persistence without resolution of symptoms should be classified as having a complicated UTI requiring further evaluation.

Recurrent urinary tract infections are considered as *relapse* if the recurrence occurs within 2 weeks of completion of treatment with the same organism. rUTIs occurring more than 2 weeks after treatment are considered *reinfections* irrespective of the organism being the same or different.[1-3]

Recurrent urinary tract infections include infections of both the lower urinary tract that manifests as cystitis and upper urinary tract that presents as pyelonephritis.

In young women, acute onset dysuria invariably indicates UTI whereas in older postmenopausal ladies, UTI presentation is more complicated such as increased frequency of urination, urgency associated with or without incontinence, nocturia, generalized fatigue and so on.

RISK FACTORS FOR URINARY TRACT INFECTION

Risk factors are broadly classified into factors that **(Table 1)**:
- *Reduce flow of urine*: Bladder outlet obstruction such as in distal urethral stenosis, neurogenic bladder, voiding dysfunction.
- *Promote colonization of bacteria*: Sexual activity, estrogen depletion, spermicidal creams.
- *Facilitate ascent of organisms*: Catheterization, fecal or urinary incontinence, and significant residual urine.

Biological factors or genetic factors also play a role in recurrent cystitis with increased susceptibility of the vaginal epithelium to get colonized by the uropathogen. Nonsecretors of

TABLE 1: Risk factors as per age group.[4-6]

Young women in the premenopausal age group	Postmenopausal older women
History of UTI in childhood at or before 15 years of age	History of UTI before menopause
Sexual intercourse	Atrophic vaginitis
Multiple partners	Presence of cystocele and significant post-void residual urine
Use of spermicidal creams or lubricants	Urinary catheterization
Instrumentation	Bed ridden patients

ABH blood group antigens have an increased propensity for recurrent UTI as the uroepithelial cells show significant binding capacity to uropathogenic *Escherichia coli*.

Complicated UTI is an infection wherein the patient has factors that put her at a higher risk of contracting a UTI. Factors could be anatomic or a functional abnormality of the urinary tract such as stone disease, bladder diverticulum or neurogenic bladder. Infections in an already immune compromised host or infection with multidrug-resistant bacteria.

EVALUATION

Detailed History

- Lower urinary tract symptoms (LUTS) such as dysuria, frequency, urgency, nocturia, incontinence
- Hematuria
- Fecaluria or pneumaturia
- Bowel symptoms such as constipation or diarrhea, fecal incontinence
- Flank pain
- Vaginal discharge with lower backache
- Menstrual history and use of tampons
- Sexual history including the postcoital status and spermicides or contraceptive used
- Recent use of antibiotics for any condition and any allergies
- Recent instrumentation or catheterization
- History elucidating the risk factors for a complicated UTI

Physical Examination

It includes an abdominal and a detailed pelvic examination. Note to be made regarding prolapse if present, mentioning the compartment and degree. Examination specific to infections in the vagina or inflammatory conditions such as atrophic vaginitis needs to be done. Stress urinary incontinence should be elucidated and mentioned if present.

Urine Analysis and Culture

Sample collection:
- Midstream clean catch urine specimen.
- Catheter specimen collection is more complex. Replace the old catheter to a new one and collect the sample from the freshly inserted catheter. Few catheters come with sampling ports that can be cleaned and urine aspirated through a syringe.
- Suprapubic aspiration of urine following sterile procedures can be done in children and patients with neurogenic bladder.

Urine analysis indicates infection if a chemical dipstick test indicated the presence of leukocyte esterase or nitrite positivity.

Urine culture—diagnostic criteria: >10^5 colony forming units (CFU) in asymptomatic patients and >10^2 CFU in symptomatic patients are considered as positive cultures and uniformly used in majority of studies.[2-4]

Upper Tract Imaging and Cystoscopy

These are not routinely recommended. These procedures are reserved for patients with suspicion of complicated UTI. Symptoms persisting, early recurrence of infection, known cases of urinary tract stone disease, hematuria, and fever with flank pain with suspicion of pyelonephritis.

DIFFERENTIAL DIAGNOSIS

- Bladder neoplasm
- Skene's gland abscess
- Urinary fistulae
- Urethral diverticulum
- Bladder stones

MANAGEMENT[1-4,7]

Treatment of the Acute Episode

Uncomplicated Cystitis

- Oral fosfomycin 3 g single dose
- Trimethoprim-Sulfamethoxazole (TMP-SMX) DS BD for 3 days
- Nitrofurantoin 100 mg BD for 5 days
- Ciprofloxacin 250 mg BD for 3 days

Complicated Cystitis

- Culture specific antibiotic
- Empirical treatment to be started based on previous culture report or antibiogram
- Patients fit for oral antibiotic usage:
  - Ciprofloxacin 500 mg BD for 7 days
  - TMP-SMX DS BD for 14 days

Prophylaxis Management

Behavioral Modification

- Increased fluid intake, modification of contraception methods, postcoital voiding, proper hygiene.
- Use of spermicides, barrier contraceptives and multiple sexual partners have been recognized as significant risk factors for rUTI.

Non-antimicrobial Prophylaxis

- Vaginal estrogen cream application, probiotic usage, cranberry extract, D-Mannose.
- Vaginal application of estrogen helps in bypassing the hepatic first pass mechanism thereby decreasing the dose required to achieve therapeutic effect in comparison to systemic intake of estrogens. Estrogens have shown to improve the local immunity of the vaginal epithelium by decreasing the local pH and inducing the maturation of the urothelial cells.[8]
- D-Mannose is a sugar that is eliminated by the kidneys in urine. It binds to uropathogens such as *Escherichia coli* and prevents its adherence to the uroepithelium.[9]

Antimicrobial Prophylaxis[2,3,7,9]

Continuous Antibiotic Prophylaxis

The ideal schedule of medication for continuous prophylaxis is still ambiguous. It ranges from once a day to alternate days to weekly once prophylaxis. The weekly regimens have shown to have a better safety profile and decreased incidence of bacterial resistance.

- TMP-SMX DS once daily
- Nitrofurantoin 50/100 mg once a day
- Cephalexin 250/500 mg once a day
- Fosfomycin 3 g once in 10 days

Postcoital Prophylaxis

Single dose of Nitrofurantoin 100 mg, TMP-SMX DS or cephalexin 250 mg

Persistent infections are due to stones, bladder diverticulum have to be treated through appropriate surgical measures.

Urinary tract infection in pregnancy is associated with adverse maternal and fetal outcomes. A Cochrane review in 2015[10] of interventions to prevent recurrent urinary tract infections in pregnancy did not find a significant difference between daily dose of Nitrofurantoin with close clinical surveillance and close clinical surveillance alone. Further studies are required to compare the non-pharmacological and pharmacological benefits of prophylaxis in pregnancy.

REFERENCES

1. Wein AJ, Kavoussi LR, Partin AW, Peters CA. Campbell-Walsh Urology, 11th edition. Philadelphia: Elsevier Inc.; 2016. pp. 237-74.
2. Anger J, Lee U, Ackerman L, Chou R, Chughtai B, Clemens Q, et al. Recurrent Uncomplicated Urinary Tract Infections in Women: AUA/CUA/SUFU Guideline. Linthicum, MD: American Urological Association Education and Research, Inc.; 2019.

3. Bonkat G, Pickard R, Bartoletti R, Cai T, Bruyere F, Geerlings SE, et al. EAU guidelines on Urological Infections. Arnhem, Netherlands: European Association of Urology; 2018.
4. Durwood EN. Complicated urinary tract infections. Urol Clin N Am. 2008;35:13-22.
5. Lindsay EN. Uncomplicated urinary tract infection in adults including uncomplicated pyelonephritis. Urol Clin N Am. 2008;35:1-12.
6. Jhang JF, Kuo HC. Recent advances in recurrent urinary tract infection from pathogenesis and biomarkers to prevention. Tzu Chi Med J. 2017;29:131-7.
7. Barber AE, Norton JP, Spivak AM, Mulvey MA. Urinary tract infections: current and emerging management strategies. Clin Infect Dis. 2013;57:719-24.
8. Krause M, Wheeler TL, Snyder TE, Richter HE. Local effects of vaginally administered Estrogen therapy: a review. J Pelvic Med Surg. 2009;15(3):105-14.
9. Hickling DR, Nitti VW. Management of recurrent urinary tract infection in healthy adult women. Rev Urol. 2013;15(2):41-8.
10. Schneeberger C, Geerlings SE, Middleton P, Crowthe AC. Interventions for preventing recurrent urinary tract infection during pregnancy. Cochrane Database of Systemic Reviews; 2015. [online] Available from: https://doi.org/10.1002/14651858.CD009279.pub3.

CHAPTER 15

Urinary Tract Calculi in Pregnancy

Mohan Balaiah Aswathaiya

INTRODUCTION

Symptomatic urinary calculi in pregnancy present a unique challenge to the obstetrician and urologist. This is due to ambiguity in diagnosis, risk of radiation exposure, need for a well-equipped center and multidisciplinary involvement in management.

EPIDEMIOLOGY

Urinary stone disease affects 8/1,000 pregnancies and is more common in white women.[1] Multiparous women are more likely affected.[2] Right and left side are equally affected although gestational hydronephrosis is more common on the right side.[3] Apart from the morbidity due to ureteric colic pain, urinary tract infection and urinary tract obstruction, there is increased risk of spontaneous abortions, preterm delivery, preeclampsia and premature rupture of membranes.[1,3] However, there is no adverse impact on the birth outcomes.[3] Although incidence of urolithiasis is increasing in non-pregnant women in the last two decades, there is no such trend seen in pregnant women.[4] The reasons for such observation is presently unknown.

PATHOPHYSIOLOGY

Although certain physiological changes during pregnancy favor stone formation, the overall risk of stone formation is same as in non-pregnant state due to concomitant increase in stone inhibiting factors[5] **(Table 1)**. Hence, pregnancy itself does not increase risk of stone formation. However, a combination of gestational hypercalciuria and increased urinary pH favors formation of calcium phosphate stone which is the predominant type of stone seen in pregnancy.[6]

EVALUATION

Majority of patients present with acute onset flank pain accompanied by macroscopic or microscopic hematuria. There might be other associated symptoms of nausea, vomiting, dysuria, frequency and urgency.

Laboratory evaluation includes complete blood count, renal function test, urine routine and urine culture. Unique to pregnancy,

TABLE 1: Effect of physiological changes in pregnancy on urinary stone formation.[5-9]

Favor stone formation	Inhibit stone formation
Gestational hydronephrosis	Hypercitraturia and hypermagnesuria (increased GFR)
Hypercalciuria due to increased filtered load of calcium, suppression of parathyroid hormone and placental production of 1,25-dihydroxycholecalciferol	Increased urinary excretion of stone inhibitors such as glycoproteins, uromodulin and nephrocalcin (increased GFR)
Hyperuricosuria due to increased filtered load of uric acid	Increased urine output
Increased urinary pH along with hypercalciuria favors calcium phosphate stone	Increased urinary pH prevents uric acid and calcium oxalate stone

(GFR: glomerular filtration rate)

presence of pus cells in urine routine examination itself does not indicate urine infection. Hence, urine culture should be done to prove or rule out infection.[10]

The physiologic increase in glomerular filtration rate during pregnancy normally results in a decrease in concentration of serum creatinine to a range of 0.4–0.8 mg/dL. Hence, a serum creatinine of 1.0 mg/dL, although normal in a non-pregnant individual, reflects renal impairment in a pregnant woman.[11]

DIAGNOSIS

Diagnosis of urolithiasis involves visualization of stone on an imaging study. Transabdominal is recommended as the first line diagnostic test, magnetic resonance imaging (MRI) without contrast is the second-line test, and low dose non-contrast computed tomography (NCCT) is the last resort test to diagnose urinary stones during pregnancy.[12]

Ultrasound of abdomen and pelvis is the first diagnostic test due to absence of radiation exposure and wide availability. Stones appear as an echogenic focus with posterior acoustic shadow with or without proximal hydroureteronephrosis. USG has sensitivity of 34% and high specificity of 86%.[13] The diagnostic capability of USG can be increased with additional techniques such as Doppler study of ureteral jets,[14] renal resistive index[15] and use of transvaginal ultrasound.[16] However, ultrasound is nondiagnostic in many patients **(Figs. 1A to D)**.

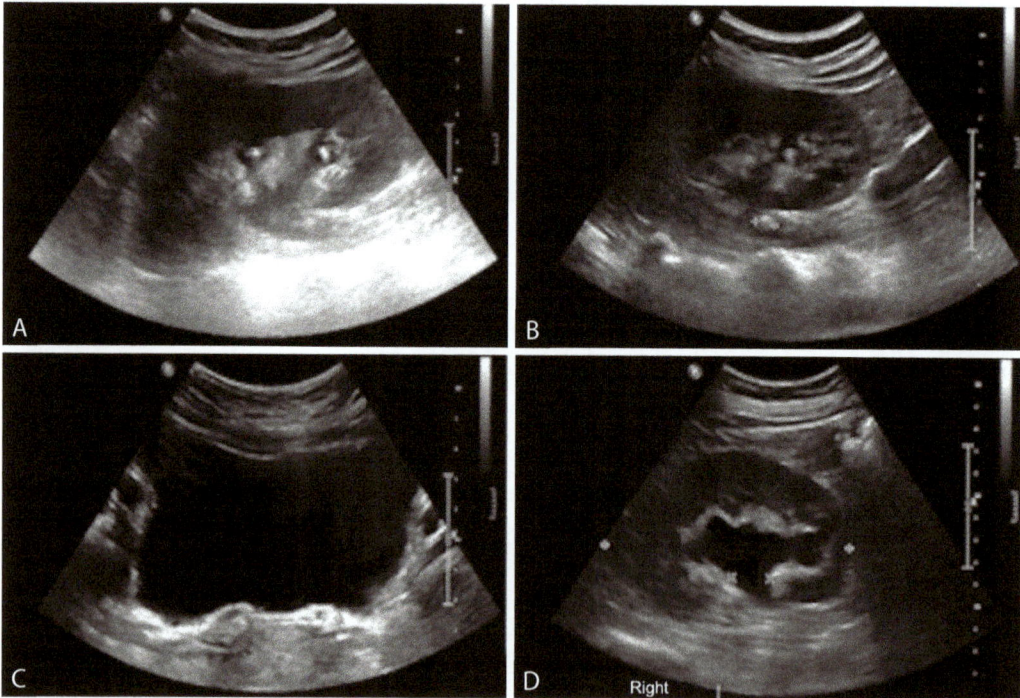

Figs. 1A to D: Diagnosis by transabdominal ultrasonography during pregnancy. (A) Two kidney stones; (B) A proximal ureteral calculus at the ureteropelvic junction; (C) A distal ureteral calculus at the ureterovesical junction; (D) Hydronephrosis without definite echogenicity of ureteral calculi in ultrasonography.[17]
Source: Choi C, Yu Y, Park D. Ureteral stent insertion in the management of renal colic during pregnancy. Chonnam Med J. 2016;52:123-7.

Magnetic resonance imaging is the second line imaging study in case ultrasound is nondiagnostic. MRI is helpful to differentiate between physiological and pathological hydronephrosis. The typical findings of pathologic obstruction include visualization of stone as a filling defect at a point of ureteral constriction, renal edema or perirenal extravasation, and the "double-kink" sign where constriction is present at the pelvic brim and ureterovesical junction **(Fig. 2)**.[18] 1.5 T MRI is currently recommended in pregnancy. There is no radiation risk. Gadolinium is not recommended in pregnancy due to toxic effects on the fetus. However, cost, availability and claustrophobia limit its widespread use. T2-weighted half-Fourier acquisition single-shot turbo spin-echo (HASTE) protocol, has emerged as a promising option in pregnancy.[19]

Low-dose NCCT scan protocols have been developed to reduce radiation exposure while maintaining the high sensitivity and specificity. White et al. examining low-dose CT scans in pregnancy confirmed very low radiation exposure of 7.1 mGy[20] and demonstrated the highest positive predictive value (96%) of all imaging modalities in pregnancy for detection of urolithiasis.[21] The incidence of negative ureteroscopy (URS) (no stone) was least (4.5%) when preoperative imaging done was low-dose CT, highest (28%) when ultrasound alone was done and 20% when MRI was done.[22]

MANAGEMENT

A multidisciplinary approach with involvement of a urologist, obstetrician, radiologist, neonatologist, and possibly an anesthesiologist is highly recommended.

Almost half (48%) of pregnant women with symptomatic urinary stones will pass their stone spontaneously.[23] If the stone does not pass during pregnancy, then approximately 50% of them are passed spontaneously within first month of postpartum.[24] Hence, conservative treatment is the first line of management unless there is clear indication for intervention such as sepsis, anuria, acute kidney injury or infection. URS can be safely done if conservative treatment fails. Temporary treatments in the form of ureteral stent or nephrostomy tube placement are the other alternatives. An algorithm to guide management of pregnant women with urolithiasis has been formulated by Semins and Matlaga **(Flowchart 1)**.[19]

Expectant Management

Conservative management involves aggressive hydration (oral/intravenous), adequate pain control, antiemetic measures, medical expulsive therapy (MET), serial monitoring of symptoms, renal function test and periodic ultrasound to confirm stone passage.

Pain management is challenging in pregnancy. Nonsteroidal anti-inflammatory drugs (NSAIDs) are contraindicated in pregnancy due to risk of premature closure of patent

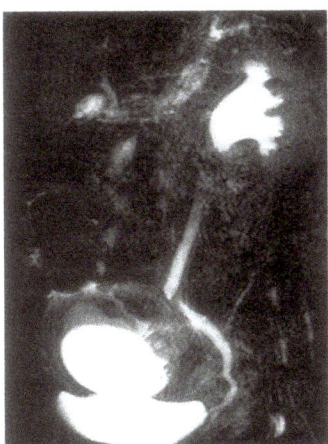

Fig. 2: The "double-kink" sign where physiologic constriction is present at the pelvic brim and stone obstruction at the ureterovesical junction.[19]
Source: Spencer JA, Chahal R, Kelly A, Taylor K, Eardley I, Lloyd SN. Evaluation of painful hydronephrosis in pregnancy: magnetic resonance urographic patterns in physiological dilatation versus calculus obstruction. J Urol. 2004;171(1):256-60.

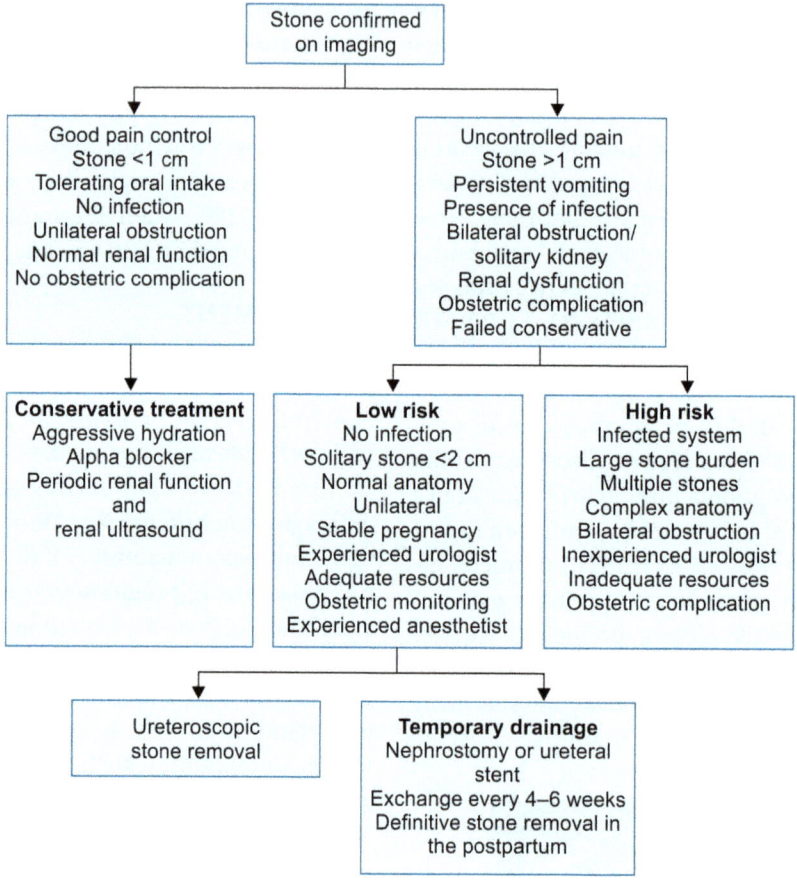

Flowchart 1: Algorithm to guide management of urolithiasis in pregnancy (Semins and Matlaga).[19]

ductus arteriosus and fatal pulmonary hypertension.[25] Paracetamol and antispasmodics are the mainstay of pain management.[26] Continuous segmental epidural block (T11 and L2) has been found to be an effective analgesic strategy and also improve spontaneous passage of the calculi.[27] In an interesting trial, Xue et al. reported that intracutaneous injection of sterile water was significantly superior to oral paracetamol for pain management.[28]

Another strategy to improve spontaneous stone passage is MET. Alpha blocker (Tamsulosin) or calcium channel blocker (Nifedipine) is recommended in the adult population for uncomplicated unilateral distal ureteral stones measuring less than 10 mm. These medications are Category B in pregnancy and thought to be safe with no harmful effects demonstrated in humans.[29] In a recent retrospective study, use of Tamsulosin as MET in pregnancy did not affect maternal or fetal outcomes and improved stone passage rate by 24%.[30] American Urology Association Guidelines (2016) recommend that should MET be considered for the pregnant patient, the patient should be counseled that MET has not been adequately investigated in the pregnant population, and the pharmacologic agents are being used for an "off-label" purpose.[31]

Active Intervention

Urological intervention is required in cases of failed conservative treatment, intractable pain/vomiting, large stone burden (>1 cm), presence of urine infection, severe hydronephrosis, renal dysfunction, solitary kidney, bilateral ureteric obstruction and obstetric complications.[19] Ureteral stent placement or percutaneous nephrostomy tube placement are effective intervention strategy for quick relief of symptoms.[32] They can be performed under local anesthesia or sedation with ultrasound guidance. However, many patients do not tolerate them well, need multiple exchanges (every 4-6 weeks) due to risk of rapid encrustation during pregnancy.[33]

With advancement in technology and techniques, definitive stone removal with URS can be safely and effectively performed during pregnancy. Obstetric complications (preterm labor) at time of surgical intervention are rare (4%).[22] A meta-analysis has shown surgical complications of URS in pregnant women to be similar to those in nonpregnant patients.[34] URS has been found to be cost-effective compared to stenting or nephrostomy in pregnancy.[35] However, the relative benefit of URS decreases in the third trimester so temporary drainage procedures may be reasonable and justified for patients presenting late in pregnancy.[35] URS should be performed during second trimester by an experienced urologist in a center well-equipped to manage obstetric and neonatal emergencies.[34]

INTERVENTIONS CONTRAINDICATED IN PREGNANCY

Shock wave lithotripsy (SWL) is an excellent noninvasive treatment for urolithiasis in a nonpregnant state. However, it is absolutely contraindicated in pregnancy based on animal studies showing potential for fetal loss from shock wave injury.[36]

Percutaneous nephrolithotomy is the treatment of choice for renal stones > 2 cm.[12] Generally, the procedure involves prolonged anesthesia time, need for prone position and significant intraoperative radiation exposure due to fluoroscopy. Hence, it is generally avoided in pregnancy. Pregnant women with large stone burdens (>2 cm) are best managed with ureteral stent or nephrostomy tube during pregnancy and percutaneous nephrolithotomy done in the postpartum period.

REFERENCES

1. Sohlberg EM, Brubaker WD, Zhang CA, Anderegg LDL, Dallas KB, Song S, et al. Urinary stone disease in pregnancy: a claims based analysis of 1.4 million patients. 2020;203(5):957-61.
2. Rodriguez PN, Klein AS. Management of urolithiasis during pregnancy. Surg Gynecol Obstet. 1988;166(2):103-6.
3. Rosenberg E, Sergienko R, Abu-Ghanem S, Wiznitzer A, Romanowsky I, Neulander EZ, et al. Nephrolithiasis during pregnancy: characteristics, complications, and pregnancy outcome. World J Urol. 2011;29(6):743-7.
4. Riley JM, Dudley AG, Semins MJ. Nephrolithiasis and pregnancy: has the incidence been rising? J Endourol. 2014;28:383-6.
5. Biyani CS, Joyce AD. Urolithiasis in pregnancy. I: pathophysiology, fetal considerations and diagnosis. BJU Int. 2002;89(8):811-8.
6. Ross AE, Handa S, Lingeman JE, Matlaga BR. Kidney stones during pregnancy: an investigation into stone composition. Urol Res. 2008;36(2):99-102.
7. Meria P, Hadjadj H, Jungers P, Daudon M. Stone formation and pregnancy: pathophysiological insights gained from morphoconstitutional stone analysis. J Urol. 2010;183:1412-6.
8. Smith CL, Kristensen C, Davis M, Abraham PA. An evaluation of the physicochemical risk for renal stone disease during pregnancy. Clin Nephrol. 2001;55:205-11.
9. Resim S, Ekerbicer HC, Kiran G, Kilinc M. Are changes in urinary parameters during pregnancy clinically significant? Urol Res. 2006;34:244-8.
10. Parulkar BG, Hopkins TB, Wollin ML, Howard PJ Jr, Lal A. Renal colic during pregnancy: a case for conservative treatment. J Urol. 1998;159:365-8.

11. Fischer MJ. Chronic kidney disease and pregnancy: maternal and fetal outcomes. Adv Chronic Kidney Dis. 2007;14:132-45.
12. Turk C, Skolaris A, Neisius A, Petrik A, Seitz C, Thomas K. EAU Guidelines on Urolithiasis. Arnhem, Netherlands: European Association of Urology; 2019.
13. Stothers L, Lee LM. Renal colic in pregnancy. J Urol. 1992;148:1383-7.
14. Deyoe LA, Cronan JJ, Breslaw BH, Ridlen MS. New techniques of ultrasound and color Doppler in the prospective evaluation of acute renal obstruction. Do they replace the intravenous urogram? Abdom Imaging. 1995;20(1):58-63.
15. Onur MR, Cubuk M, Andic C, Kartal M, Arslan G. Role of resistive index in renal colic. Urol Res. 2007;35:307-12.
16. Laing FC, Benson CB, DiSalvo DN, Brown DL, Frates MC, Loughlin KR. Distal ureteral calculi: detection with vaginal US. Radiology. 1994;192:545-8.
17. Choi C, Yu Y, Park D. Ureteral stent insertion in the management of renal colic during pregnancy. Chonnam Med J. 2016;52:123-7.
18. Spencer JA, Chahal R, Kelly A, Taylor K, Eardley I, Lloyd SN. Evaluation of painful hydronephrosis in pregnancy: magnetic resonance urographic patterns in physiological dilatation versus calculous obstruction. J Urol. 2004;171:256-60.
19. Semins JM, Matlaga BR. Management of urolithiasis in pregnancy. Int J Womens Health. 2013;5:599-604.
20. White WM, Zite NB, Gash J, Waters WB, Thompson W, Klain FA. Low-dose computed tomography for the evaluation of flank pain in the pregnant population. J Endourol. 2007;21:1255-60.
21. White WM, Johnson EB, Zite NB, Beddies J, Krambeck AE, Hyams E, et al. Predictive value of current imaging modalities for the detection of urolithiasis during pregnancy: a multi-center, longitudinal study. J Urol. 2013;189:931-4.
22. Johnson EB, Krambeck AE, White WM, Hyams E, Beddies J, Marien T, et al. Obstetric complications of ureteroscopy during pregnancy. J Urol. 2012;188:151-4.
23. Burgess KL, Gettman MT, Rangel LJ, Krambeck AE. Diagnosis of urolithiasis and rate of spontaneous passage during pregnancy. J Urol. 2011;186:2280-4.
24. Razvi H, Bensalah K, Peyronnet B, Gross A, Krambeck A, Smith A, et al. Stones in special situations. In: Denstedt J, Rosette J (Eds.). Stone disease. Montreal: Societe Internationale d'Urologie (SIU); 2014. pp. 409-501.
25. Burdan F, Starosławska E, Szumiło J. Prenatal tolerability of acetaminophen and other over-the-counter non-selective 93 cyclooxygenase inhibitors. Pharmacol Rep. 2012;64:521-7.
26. Guichard G, Fromajoux C, Cellarier D, Loock E, Chabannes S, Bernardini R, et al. Prise en charge de la colique néphrétique chez la femme enceinte: à propos de 48 cas [Management of renal colic in pregnant women, based on a series of 48 cases]. Prog Urol. 2008;18(1):29-34.
27. Maikranz P, Coe FL, Parks J, Lindheimer MD. Nephrolithiasis in pregnancy. Am J Kidney Dis. 1987;9:354-8.
28. Xue P, Tu C, Wang K, Wang X, Fang Y. Intracutaneous sterile water injection versus oral paracetamol for renal colic during pregnancy: a randomized controlled trial. Int Urol Nephrol. 2013;45(2):321-5.
29. Weber-Schoendorfer C, Hannemann D, Meister R, Elefant E, Cuppers-Maarschalkerweerd B, Arnon J, et al. The safety of calcium channel blockers during pregnancy: a prospective, multicenter, observational study. Reprod Toxicol. 2008;26:24-30.
30. Bailey G, Vaughan L, Rose C, Krambeck A. Perinatal outcomes with tamsulosin therapy for symptomatic urolithiasis. J Urol. 2016;195:99.
31. Assimos D, Krambeck A, Miller N, Monga M, Murad MH, Nelson CP, et al. Surgical management of Stone: AUA/Endourology Society Guideline; 2016.
32. Mokhmalji H, Braun PM, Martinez Portillo FJ, Siegsmund M, Alken P, Köhrmann KU, et al. Percutaneous nephrostomy versus ureteral stents for diversion of hydronephrosis caused by stones: a prospective, randomized clinical trial. J Urol. 2001;165:1088-92.
33. Ngai HY, Salih HQ, Albeer A, Aghaways I, Buchholz N. Double-J ureteric stenting in pregnancy: a single-centre experience from Iraq. Arab J Urol. 2013;11:148.
34. Semins MJ, Trock BJ, Matlaga BR. The safety of ureteroscopy during pregnancy: a systematic review and meta-analysis. J Urol. 2009;181:139-43.
35. Clennon EK, Duty DB, Caughey AB. Cost-effectiveness of urolithiasis management in pregnancy. Urol Pract. 2019;6:337-44.
36. Ohmori K, Matsuda T, Horii Y, Yoshida O. Effects of shock waves on the mouse foetus. J Urol. 1994;151:255.

16 Basics of Cystoscopy

Ramesh Hanumegowda

INTRODUCTION

Cystoscopy is the visualization of bladder and urethra through an endoscope. Although it is a primary urological tool, it has wide application in gynecological practice as well. It is particularly useful in the evaluation of lower urinary tract injury in gynecological surgeries as the female genital tract and urinary tract are closely related anatomically and embryologically.[1]

Philipp Bozzini was the first to introduce cystoscopy in 1806, later in 1877 Max Nitze developed a cystoscope with good illumination using optical lenses.[2] The improvement of light transmission while simultaneously reducing size of the scope was achieved in 1979 by Harold Hopkins by adding glass rods with only short gaps of air in between. Later the advent of fiberoptics made development of flexible cystoscopes possible.[3]

Indications for cystoscopy, basic understanding of the equipment and systematic approach to perform the procedure are discussed in this chapter.

INDICATIONS

- Suspected urinary tract injury during gynecological surgeries, e.g., cystotomy, ureteral injury, intravesical/urethral erosion of mesh or suture.
- Suspected urinary tract involvement by endometriosis or gynecological malignancies
- Suspected urinary tract involvement following lower genital tract trauma
- In the evaluation of postvoid dribbling of urine (cause may be urethral diverticulum)
- Evaluation for leakage of urine per vagina (genitourinary fistula)
- Evaluation of lower urinary tract symptoms such as urgency, frequency, incontinence in the absence of urinary tract infection (UTI)
- Recurrent UTI in the setting of prior pelvic surgery as this could be due to foreign body in urinary tract.
- Also indicated in the evaluation of hematuria, genitourinary tuberculosis
- During sling procedures for incontinence, cystoscopy is an essential too as it helps for proper tensioning of sling and to rule out the intravesical or intraurethral involvement by sutures or mesh.
- Instillation of therapeutic agents such as intravesical botulinum toxin for detrusor overactivity or periurethral bulking agents
- Evaluation of bladder diverticula, bladder stones
- Visual urethral dilatation

CONTRAINDICATIONS

- Active urinary tract infection
- Complete urethral obstruction

PREOPERATIVE PREPARATION

Informed consent: Patient should be explained about the nature of the procedure and the associated complications in understandable language.

Following risks to be explained before the procedure:

Common Risks
Immediately after cystoscopy, transient mild burning or bleeding on voiding might be encountered.

Occasional Risks
Bladder infection requiring antibiotics.

Rare Risks
- Delayed bleeding requiring clot removal or further surgery
- Urethral injury leading to delayed stricture formation
- Very rarely, bladder perforation requiring temporary catheter or open surgical repair.

PREOPERATIVE EVALUATION
Cystoscopy is a minimally invasive procedure that does not warrant detailed evaluation in low risk women who are undergoing diagnostic cystoscopy only. However, in women who have symptomatic UTI, pregnant women, and in patients who require therapeutic manipulation, it would be prudent to screen them for infection and treat them with antibiotics. In addition, examination of abdomen and pelvis is to be done with particular attention to condition and position of urethral meatus.

PROPHYLACTIC ANTIBIOTICS
For a routine diagnostic cystoscopy in the absence of risk factors, prophylactic antibiotics are not recommended as per the American Urological Association (AUA) Best Practice recommendations (**Box 1 and Table 1**).

In high-risk patients, single intravenous dose of prophylactic antibiotic can be given within 60 minutes before the procedure. If a fluoroquinolone is used, the infusion can be started even 120 minutes prior to the procedure in order to achieve adequate tissue levels at the time of procedure and also to minimize the possibility of a drug reaction close to the time of induction of anesthesia.

Operative setting: Cystoscopy for gynecologic conditions may be performed in an office setting or in the operating room.

Anesthesia
Local application of lignocaine gel: Most women will tolerate the office cystoscopy. The prefilled 2% lignocaine syringe is inserted into the mid-urethra. The gel is slowly injected and the procedure can be started after 5–15 minutes.

Sedation or regional or general anesthesia for this procedure may be used based upon the preference of patient, surgeon or the nature of surgery.

TABLE 1: Antimicrobial prophylaxis.[5]

Nature of operation	Common pathogens	Recommended antimicrobials
Cystoscopy alone	Enteric gram-negative bacilli, enterococci	High-risk only: ciprofloxacin or Trimethoprim-sulfamethoxazole
Cystoscopy with manipulation or upper tract instrumentation	Enteric gram-negative bacilli, enterococci	Ciprofloxacin or Trimethoprim-sulfamethoxazole

BOX 1: Policy statement.[4]

Patient risk factors requiring antibiotic prophylaxis
- Advanced age
- Anatomic anomalies of the urinary tract
- Poor nutritional status
- Smoking
- Chronic corticosteroid use
- Immunodeficiency
- Externalized catheters
- Distant coexistent infection
- Prolonged hospitalization

INSTRUMENTS

Types of Cystoscopes
1. Rigid cystoscope
2. Flexible cystoscope

Rigid Cystoscope

Rigid cystoscope is routinely used for cystoscopy unless special circumstances require the use of flexible cystoscope, e.g., when a patient cannot be placed in dorsal lithotomy position.

Parts of Rigid Cystoscope
- Cystoscope sheath
- Bridge
- Telescope
- Light source with cable

Cystoscope sheath: All cystoscopes are made of stainless steel alloy, calibrated in French (F) which is the outer diameter of the instrument. 1 mm is equal to 3 F, all sheaths are 22 cm in length regardless of the size **(Table 2)**.

Female cystoscope sheath: 17 F sheath is also called female cystoscope sheath because it has a shorter beak length which helps in distension of short female urethra, whereas the other sheaths has longer beak length which cause leakage of irrigating fluid leading to nondistension of urethra and poor vision **(Fig. 1)**. This problem can also be circumvented by the use of Nickel adapters **(Fig. 2)**.

The adapter should be passed against the urethral orifice after the insertion of the cystoscope to avoid leakage of irrigating fluid and the resultant collapse of the urethra.[6]

Sheath has inlet and outlet vent to allow ingress and egress of irrigating fluid. Numbering on the sheath denotes the size of the working instrument which can be passed.

Bridge: All adult bridges are universal and can fit into all sizes of sheaths, length is 6 cm. Bridge has telescope channel and accessory channel for instruments, and the bridge is detachable which helps in emptying the bladder efficiently **(Fig. 3)**.

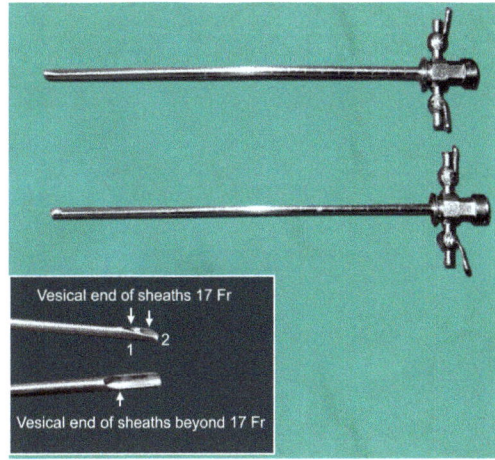

Fig. 1: Cystoscope sheaths. Note the 17 Fr sheath has shorter beak length.

TABLE 2: Standard Karl Storz sheath sizes with color code.*

Sheath size	Color code
17 F	Yellow
19 F	Green
20 F	Red
22 F	Blue
25 F	White

*For diagnostic cystoscopy the lowest diameter sheath is used.

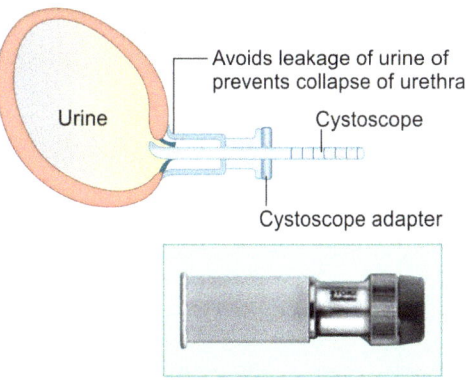

Fig. 2: Cystoscope adapter used during the procedure.

Telescope: Telescopes are classified depending on the viewing angle. The degree indicates the deflection of the lens **(Fig. 4 and Table 3)**.[6] It has a light pillar which connects to the light cable and an eye piece.

Flexible Cystoscope

Advantage is procedure can be done in a supine position with comfort to patient, useful in manipulation across difficult curves, easy visualization of the entire bladder and gives access to the laterally positioned ureteral orifices **(Fig. 5)**.

Irrigating fluid: Fluid is instilled to distend the bladder and improve visualization, we use either normal saline or distilled water as irrigating fluid. If monopolar cautery is required to be used, it is necessary to use nonconductive solutions (e.g., water, glycine) to avoid dispersing the electrical current. Use of any irrigating fluid for operative purposes requires monitoring of fluid

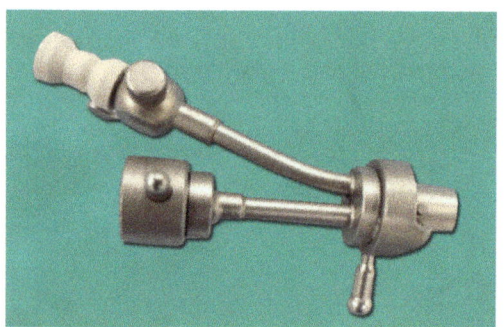

Fig. 3: Bridge with single side channel, straight channel is for telescope.

TABLE 3: Different telescope lenses.

Degree	Features
0°	Straight forward telescope is focused to view straight ahead, is usually used for urethroscopy
30°	Forward oblique telescope best visualizes the base and anterolateral wall of the bladder and is the best choice if a ureteral procedure is performed (e.g., stent placement), it is the most commonly used telescope
70°	Lateral telescope to view the dome of bladder
120°	Retrospective telescope to visualize anterior bladder neck from inside

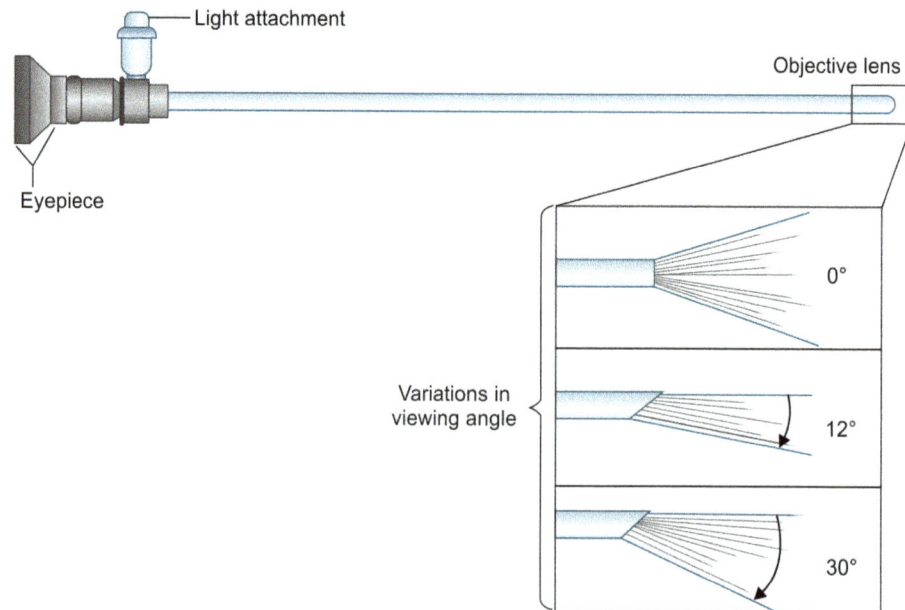

Fig. 4: Telescope with different viewing angles.

INSTRUMENTS

Types of Cystoscopes
1. Rigid cystoscope
2. Flexible cystoscope

Rigid Cystoscope

Rigid cystoscope is routinely used for cystoscopy unless special circumstances require the use of flexible cystoscope, e.g., when a patient cannot be placed in dorsal lithotomy position.

Parts of Rigid Cystoscope
- Cystoscope sheath
- Bridge
- Telescope
- Light source with cable

Cystoscope sheath: All cystoscopes are made of stainless steel alloy, calibrated in French (F) which is the outer diameter of the instrument. 1 mm is equal to 3 F, all sheaths are 22 cm in length regardless of the size **(Table 2)**.

Female cystoscope sheath: 17 F sheath is also called female cystoscope sheath because it has a shorter beak length which helps in distension of short female urethra, whereas the other sheaths has longer beak length which cause leakage of irrigating fluid leading to nondistension of urethra and poor vision **(Fig. 1)**. This problem can also be circumvented by the use of Nickel adapters **(Fig. 2)**.

The adapter should be passed against the urethral orifice after the insertion of the cystoscope to avoid leakage of irrigating fluid and the resultant collapse of the urethra.[6]

Sheath has inlet and outlet vent to allow ingress and egress of irrigating fluid. Numbering on the sheath denotes the size of the working instrument which can be passed.

Bridge: All adult bridges are universal and can fit into all sizes of sheaths, length is 6 cm. Bridge has telescope channel and accessory channel for instruments, and the bridge is detachable which helps in emptying the bladder efficiently **(Fig. 3)**.

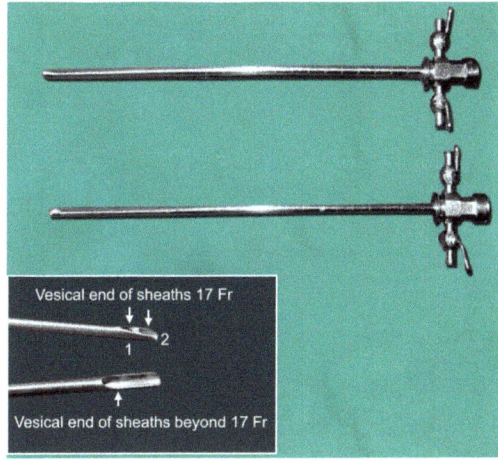

Fig. 1: Cystoscope sheaths. Note the 17 Fr sheath has shorter beak length.

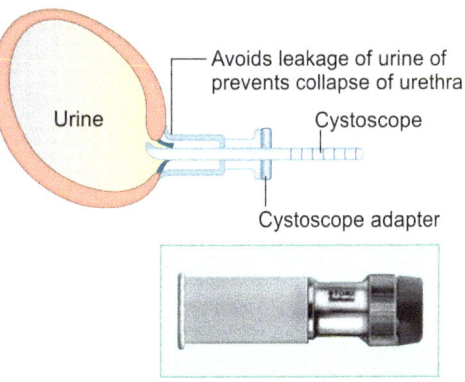

Fig. 2: Cystoscope adapter used during the procedure.

TABLE 2: Standard Karl Storz sheath sizes with color code.*	
Sheath size	**Color code**
17 F	Yellow
19 F	Green
20 F	Red
22 F	Blue
25 F	White

*For diagnostic cystoscopy the lowest diameter sheath is used.

Telescope: Telescopes are classified depending on the viewing angle. The degree indicates the deflection of the lens **(Fig. 4 and Table 3)**.[6] It has a light pillar which connects to the light cable and an eye piece.

Flexible Cystoscope

Advantage is procedure can be done in a supine position with comfort to patient, useful in manipulation across difficult curves, easy visualization of the entire bladder and gives access to the laterally positioned ureteral orifices **(Fig. 5)**.

Irrigating fluid: Fluid is instilled to distend the bladder and improve visualization, we use either normal saline or distilled water as irrigating fluid. If monopolar cautery is required to be used, it is necessary to use nonconductive solutions (e.g., water, glycine) to avoid dispersing the electrical current. Use of any irrigating fluid for operative purposes requires monitoring of fluid

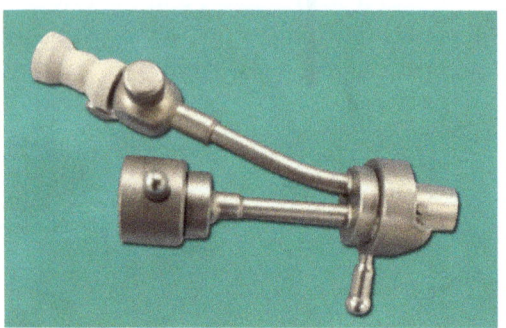

Fig. 3: Bridge with single side channel, straight channel is for telescope.

TABLE 3: Different telescope lenses.

Degree	Features
0°	Straight forward telescope is focused to view straight ahead, is usually used for urethroscopy
30°	Forward oblique telescope best visualizes the base and anterolateral wall of the bladder and is the best choice if a ureteral procedure is performed (e.g., stent placement), it is the most commonly used telescope
70°	Lateral telescope to view the dome of bladder
120°	Retrospective telescope to visualize anterior bladder neck from inside

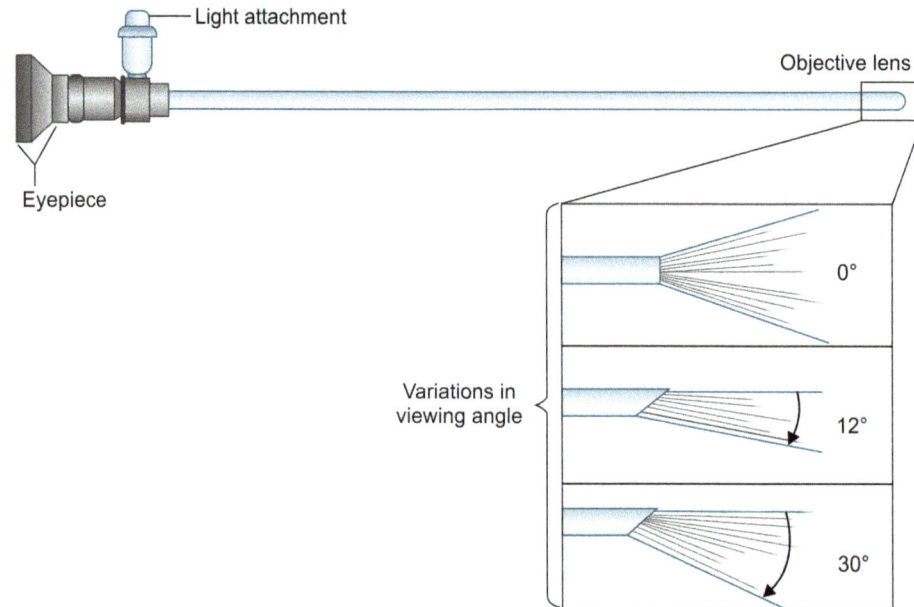

Fig. 4: Telescope with different viewing angles.

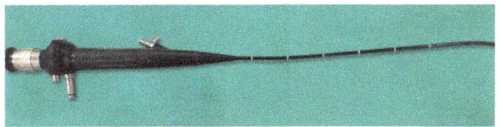

Fig. 5: Flexible cystourethroscope.

absorption to avoid volume overload and possible hyponatremia.

HOW TO PERFORM A RIGID CYSTOSCOPY?

With the patient in dorsal lithotomy position, the perineum including urethral meatus is cleaned with a sterile solution (e.g., iodine) and surgical drapes are placed. A sterile lubricant is placed on the cystoscope sheath and the fluid inflow is opened. The cystoscope is passed with irrigation turned on to prevent excess bubbles in the bladder.

The cystoscopic lens and sheath are inserted into the urethra with the scope directed toward the ceiling as the normal angle is slightly upward under the pubic bone. For women with pelvic organ prolapse, it is helpful to reduce the prolapse prior to performing cystoscopy.

Bladder is filled adequately to visualize the bladder, but care needs to be taken not to over distend the bladder to prevent urothelium distortion which may hide the subtle changes. It is particularly important not to overdistend especially if we are taking biopsies, as the thin stretched bladder wall will predispose to bladder perforation.

Examination of Urethra

The urethral meatus is examined: look for stenosis, mucosal prolapse.

The urethral mucosa is then examined for erythema, pallor, exudate, polyps, condylomata or diverticula. The presence of an exudate suggests the presence of a diverticulum, although this is rarely visualized during urethroscopy. Also the surgeon can use a 0° lens to attempt to visualize a diverticular ostium which may not be seen always.

Bladder neck (urethrovesical junction) is also visualized for its patency or presence of any lesions.

Examination of Bladder

Initially look at the bladder base. For this, the hand holding the cystoscope is gently moved upward which moves the tip of the scope toward the bladder base. The scope is slowly withdrawn in midline to see the interureteric bar, at this time, the scope is moved laterally to look for the ureteric orifices. Typically 30° or 70° lenses are used in bladder visualization.

The air bubble in the bladder is visualized in the anterior dome of the bladder, which is oriented at the superior aspect for better orientation during rest of the procedure.

Systematic examination of the bladder is done to look for trigone, ureteral orifices, posterior wall, lateral walls, anterior wall with dome. Biopsy can be taken from suspicious areas. Gentle pressing of the suprapubic area with one hand when the bladder is partially full, best visualizes the dome and anterior wall of the bladder.

CYSTOSCOPY IN SPECIFIC CONDITIONS

Identifying bladder injury: During abdominal hysterectomy, there is a 0.5–1% chance of bladder injury.[7] Cystoscopic visualization of perivesical fat, bleeding, if the rent is large intestine can be seen and loss of bladder distension are the signs of bladder perforation. Any bleeding site should be cauterized and the bladder should be reinspected. Most cystotomies at the time of hysterectomy are located in the bladder base just above the trigone.

Inadvertently placed sutures are to be removed and appropriate repair is done. Cystoscopy can miss small injuries approximately 1 in 1,000 cytoscopies.

Ureteral injury: Ureteral orifices are carefully observed for 5–10 minutes to look for the normal efflux of urine jet. Inability to see the urine jets even after 5–10 minutes, blood coming from the orifice are suggestive of possible ureteral injury. Appropriate action to be taken for further evaluation and management such as ureteroscopy and intravenous urography.

For better visualization of urine jet, coloring agents such as intravenous sodium fluorescein or indigo carmine or oral agents such as phenazopyridine can be used.

Vesicovaginal fistula: When the fistulae are immature, they may appear as areas of localized bullous edema without distinct ostia. A mature fistula may have smooth margins with variable sized ostia. In case of small VVF, it may be difficult to identify the exact tract, and in these cases a guidewire is passed through the suspected ostia, retrieval of guidewire in the vagina confirms the presence of the fistulous tract.

Points to note during cystoscopy: Location, number and with note being made of location of ureteral orifices in relation to distance from fistula **(Fig. 6)**.

When there is a history of prior malignancy or radiation, a biopsy of the fistula needs to be done to rule out recurrence of malignancy.

For urethrovaginal fistula, scope with short beak should be used to see the urethra adequately.

Bladder lesions: Biopsy of the suspected lesions to be done using biopsy forceps.

Bladder diverticula: Diverticula are herniation of the bladder mucosa through muscularis propria of the bladder, which can lead to recurrent UTI, stone formation and malignancy. The bladder diverticulum should be thoroughly inspected for calculi or any

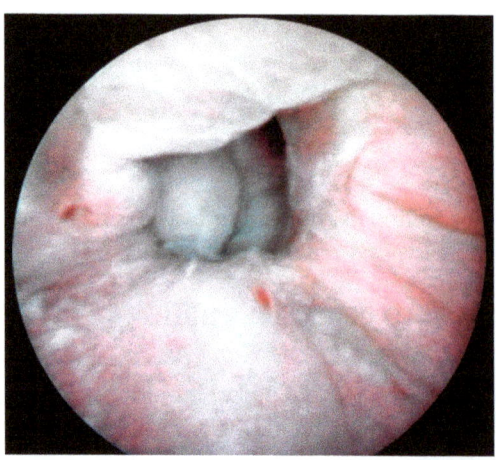

Fig. 6: Endoscopic view of vesicovaginal fistula (VVF). The fistula as seen from the bladder side. This VVF is large enough to allow one to see directly into the vagina from the bladder.[8]

changes in the mucosa. To do this thoroughly, a flexible cystoscope would be ideal. In case of any abnormalities noted in urothelium, a biopsy is taken very carefully so as to avoid perforation in an already thin mucosal diverticulum. The size and location of the diverticula in relation to the ureteric orifices and the urethra is noted.

Use of cystoscopy in anti-incontinence sling surgeries: Here, cystoscopy is performed to exclude the needle penetration of the bladder or urethra. This is ideally performed with a 70° lens. If perforation is noted, the needle is withdrawn and reinserted with caution, to avoid further injury. Cystoscopy is also useful in assessing adequate tensioning during the surgery.

COMPLICATIONS

Complications following diagnostic cystoscopy are rare.

Infection: Incidence of symptomatic UTI is 2–5%, a urine culture should be sent and infection is treated appropriately.

Bleeding: Minimal bleeding is common and it will stop spontaneously. Bleeding which requires intervention is extremely rare.

Injury to urethra and bladder: Minor mucosal abrasions may be seen frequently, perforations requiring catheter placement or repair are very rare.

Complications associated with anesthesia and positions of patient are also rare.

POSTOPERATIVE CARE

Patients may experience mild dysuria, frequency, urgency and small amounts of bleeding that should clear within 10–12 hours. Persistent bleeding or symptoms require immediate attention. Patients can resume their routine work as soon as the anesthesia effect wears off.

REFERENCES

1. Weinberger MW. Cystourethroscopy for the practicing gynaecologist. Clin Obstet Gynecol. 1998;41:764-6.
2. Ramai D, Zakhia K, Etienne D, Reddy M. Philipp Bozzini (1773–1809): The earliest description of endoscopy. J Med Biogr. 2018;26(2):137-41.
3. Duffey B, Monga M. Principles of endoscopy. In: Wein AJ, Kavoussi LR, Novick AC, Partin AW, Peters CA. Campbell-Walsh Urology, 10th edition. Philadelphia: Saunders-Elsevier; 2012. pp. 192-4.
4. Cruse PJ. Surgical wound infection. In: Wonsiewicz MJ (Ed). Infectious Diseases. Philadelphia: WB Saunders Co.; 1992. p. 758.
5. Wolf JS Jr, Bennett CJ, Dmochowski RR, et al. Best practice policy statement on urologic surgery antimicrobial prophylaxis. J Urol. 2008;179:1379-90.
6. Sabnis RB. Urology instrumentation: A comprehensive guide (Instruments pictures). New Delhi: Jaypee Brothers Medical Publishers; 2016.
7. Keettel WC, Sehring FG, deProsse CA, Scott JR. Surgical management of urethrovaginal and vesicovaginal fistulas. Am J Obstet Gynecol. 1978;131:425-31.
8. Rovner ES. Bladder and Female Urethral Diverticula. In: Wein AJ, Kavoussi LR, Novick AC, Partin AW, Peters CA. Campbell Walsh Urology, 10th edition. Philadelphia: Saunders-Elsevier; 2012. p. 2266.

17: Urinary Tract Injuries in Difficult Gynecologic Surgeries: Tips and Tricks to Anticipate and Avoid

Manjula Anagani, Prabha Agrawal

INTRODUCTION

While operating on either the reproductive or the urinary tract in women, the potential of injuring the other should always be considered, owing to the close association between the two, both anatomically and embryologically. A careful dissection and the precise knowledge of the urinary tract structures within the operating field, form the basis of the fundamental and preliminary approach to prevention. This elementary approach holds true to prevent injuries that involve the ureter, which typically go unrecognized and are potentially life-threatening or result in long-term sequelae. Most of the bladder injuries on the other hand are recognized and treated early and have lesser potential for major complications.

INCIDENCE

The several reasons for widely reported differences in the incidence of urological injuries include the experience of the surgeon, the pelvic anatomy whether normal or distorted, the type of the operation and its complexity. Rate of urinary tract injury in females with pelvic surgery varies from 0.3 to 1%.[1] Bladder injury is approximately three times more common than ureteral injury.[1] Overall the incidence of all major complications associated with laparoscopic surgery have declined over time except for ureteric injuries which has stayed constant at approximately 1%.[2] Altgassen et al. found that the complication rate were nearly half for experienced surgeons as compared with the less experienced ones.[3]

RELEVANT ANATOMY

Ureters are 25–30 cm long retroperitoneal structures extending from the renal pelvis to the urinary bladder. The ureter is crossed anteriorly by ovarian vessels as it enters the pelvis and at the mid-plane of the pelvis it is crossed anteriorly by the uterine artery. Here it tunnels into the cardinal ligament and enters into the trigone of the bladder approximately 1.5–2.0 cm lateral to the cervix at the level of internal os.[4]

Ureters have a unique blood supply, the knowledge of which is important to prevent ischemic injury to the ureter. They derive blood supply from small vessels approaching from medial in abdomen and approaching from lateral in pelvis.[4] Hence, to expose the ureter peritoneal incision should be made laterally to the ureter in the abdomen and medially in the pelvis.[4]

MECHANISM AND SITE OF INJURY

Ureteric injury may be due to in advertant ligation, angulation, transaction, laceration, crush, ischemia or resection.[4] The most common form of injury is inadvertent ligation followed by ureteral kinking and obstruction.[6] Iatrogenic injuries most commonly affect the distal third of the ureter, accounting for 91% of injuries.[5]

Conditions which displace cervix laterally predisposing lower ureter to injury:
- Any mass or abscess in the broad ligament
- Gravid uterus

Conditions which encase ureter closer to reproductive tract by fibrosis/retraction:
- Endometriosis
- Active infection, pelvic inflammatory disease
- Advanced cervical or ovarian neoplasms
- Radiation therapy

Other conditions which predispose to ureteric injury: The others listed:

The most common sites of intraoperative ureteric injuries during gynecological surgeries are at the pelvic brim, over the iliac arteries, within the cardinal ligament and at the anterolateral fornix of the vagina.

Hurd et al. in their study showed that the distance of ureter from the cervix was on an average 2.3 ± 0.8 cm.[6] In 52 women with apparently normal pelvic anatomy, analysis of CT images showed that in 12% of the patients the distance of ureter from the cervix was less than 0.5 cm. Additionally it was found that the higher the body mass index, the nearer the ureter was to the cervix.[7]

Maximum risk for ureteral injury in abdominal hysterectomy is during uterine arteries ligation, followed by ligation of ovarian vessels in infundibulopelvic ligament whereas in vaginal hysterectomy, the risk is during ligation of the cardinal ligaments. A high incision on the cervix can incorporate ureters in it. Radical hysterectomy can skeletonize ureter resulting in avascular necrosis and injury to the pelvic nerves can affect lower urinary tract dysfunction.[8]

Ureteral injuries during laparoscopic endometriosis surgery or laparoscopic-assisted vaginal hysterectomy (LAVH) occur mostly near the cardinal and uterosacral ligaments and are either due to thermal-electrocautery or sharp dissection.[9]

RISK FACTORS

More than 75% of ureteral injuries occur during gynecologic procedures that surgeons describe as routine and uncomplicated with normal pelvic anatomy.[9]

Few predisposing factors for urological injuries are:
- Uterus ≥ 12 weeks gestation size
- Ovarian cysts ≥ 4 cm size
- Tubo-ovarian mass/abscess
- Cervical fibroids, broad ligament fibroids
- Any mass or abscess in the broad ligament
- Pregnant uterus
  These masses predispose lower ureter to injury by lateral displacement of the cervix.
- Endometriosis
- Active infection, pelvic inflammatory disease
- Prior intra-abdominal surgery, pelvic adhesions
- Advanced state of malignancy, cervical cancer, ovarian neoplasms
- Radiation therapy
  These conditions can cause fibrosis, retract, and encase the ureter toward the gynecologic tract. Prior irradiation can compromise ureteric blood supply and increase the risk of ureter injury.
- Anatomical anomalies of the urinary tract, such as ectopic ureter, ectopic kidney, ureteral duplication or a wide ureter can displace the ureter into an abnormal location.
- Obesity (high BMI)
- Certain procedures such as anterior vaginal wall surgery, neovaginoplasty, severe genital organ prolapse repair, post hysterectomy ovariectomy.
- During surgery, hemorrhage is a clear risk factor for ureteric injury.
- Surgical experience is an important factor in causation, intraoperative diagnosis, and early treatment of urinary tract injury.

PREOPERATIVE EVALUATION

It includes the following:
- *Informed consent:* Preoperative counseling and consent required for patients with high risk factors for urological injury.
- *Imaging studies:* Preoperative ultrasonography, MRI, and intravenous pyelography (IVP) may help the surgeon to plan surgery whenever there is suspicion of distorted anatomy. Though cost-effectiveness of IVP in all patients is not established.[10]
- *Preoperative stent insertion:* It is recommended in patients with suspicion of pelvic adhesions or history of previous pelvic surgery.[10] Preoperative stenting helps surgeon to palpate ureters and prevent injury but in majority of cases, ureters are identified easily, making the procedure unnecessary.

However, stent placement helps in intraoperative diagnosis of ureteral injury if it happens.[9] A stented ureter becomes rigid and is difficult to lateralize and may lead to more injuries and the practice is not evidence-based. It is reported that cost-effectiveness was lower than expected[10] **(Figs. 1 and 2)**.

INTRAOPERATIVE PREVENTIVE MEASURES

These include proper examination of the disease, enough exposure, planned operative approach, restoration of anatomy and early urological assistance when required. Operating close to the pathology and avoiding blind clamping or suturing of blood vessels is important. Sudden hemorrhage should be handled by applying pressure, visualization of bleeding vessels followed by precise suturing.

Safety Measures to Prevent Laparoscopic Electrosurgical Complications

Up to one-fourth of ureteric injuries may be related to energy source usage during surgery, hence it is important to adhere to rules of safe electrosurgery.[7] Inadvertent tissue contact, insulation failure, direct coupling, and capacitive coupling may lead to injuries at a site distant to the surgeon's view, are difficult to identify intraoperatively and present several days later.

The important safety measures are:
- Careful inspection of insulation before use
- Newer technology such as tissue response generators and active electrode monitoring help in decreasing concerns about insulation failure and capacitive coupling.
- Usage of lowest possible effective power setting with low-voltage waveform for monopolar current.
- Bipolar utilizes high current concentration and low voltages leading to damage

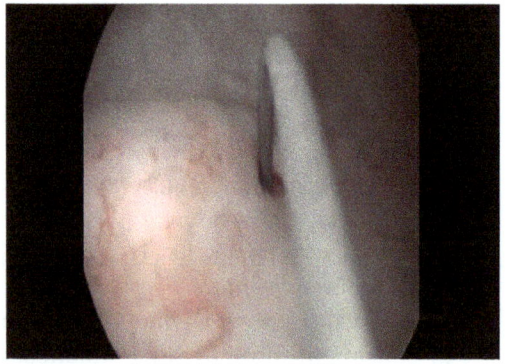

Fig. 1: Cystoscopic-guided ureteric catheterization.

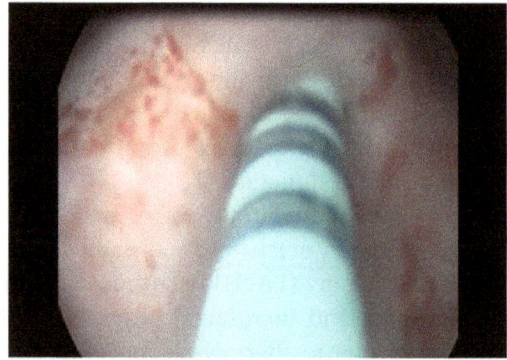

Fig. 2: Cystoscopic-guided ureteral stenting.

beyond the electrode contact. Current settings in bipolar should be much less than with monopolar.
- Use brief intermittent activation/pulse technique as tissue desiccates, resistance increases and the current seeks an alternate pathway. Pulsing of the energy on and off every few seconds allows the tissues to cool and prevents lateral thermal damage.
- Put cool irrigant liquid after use of energy sources.
- Energy source should never be activated in close proximity or in direct contact with another instrument. Both the heel and the tips of the bipolar forceps should be under vision when activating.
- Resistance of biologic tissues varies depending upon the water content. Water content varies by tissue type, organ system, age, illness, inflammation, and fever. As water content decreases rate of temperature rise increases leading to lateral thermal damage.
- Compression of tissue in bipolar forceps decreases water content thereby decreasing sealing time and less use of energy sources.
- Ultrasonic scalpel blade vibration produces a transient low-pressure area at the blade tip due to which fluid within the cells vaporizes and subsequently rupture. Vapor between tissue planes expands and aids in plane dissection near bladder hence advisable in previous cesarean adhesions.
- Fallopian tubes should be pulled medially, away from pelvic side walls before coagulation.
- Avoid electrocoagulation on uterosacral ligaments bleeders, rather secure it with clips or sutures. Same applies for uterine vessels and cardinal ligaments during LAVH.

SURGICAL TECHNIQUE TO AVOID BLADDER INJURY

Interureteric bar is the most common site of injury and occurs mostly during dissection of the bladder from the cervix **(Fig. 3)**.[7] Adequate development of vesicovaginal space, meticulous and sharp dissection in presence of adhesions and being intrafascial in approach helps.

During laparoscopic gynecological surgery urinary bladder is at risk of injury due to its close association with the operating field and while suprapubic insertion of the Veress needle/trocar. In cases like deep infiltrating endometriosis the bladder can be directly involved and may get injured.

Prevention

Bladder catheterization before pneumoperitoneum creation and trocar insertion is recommended to avoid injury to distended bladder.[4] An empty bladder is of lesser size and cannot be penetrated as easily as a distended one. The Royal College of Obstetricians and Gynaecologists advises against suprapubic insertion of the Veress needle due to high failure rate and more risk of injury.[11] In addition, insertion of secondary trocars should be performed under vision.

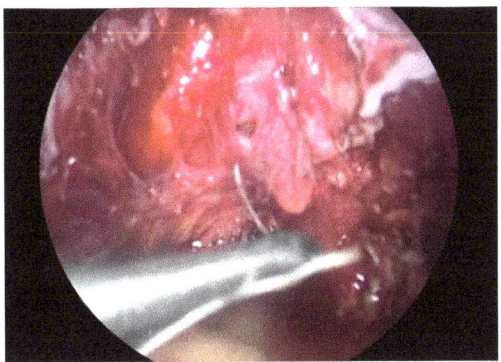

Fig. 3: Laparoscopy showing rent in dome of urinary bladder.

Preferably vault suturing to be done laparoscopically during total laparoscopic hysterectomy and vaginally in LAVH.[7]

Recognition

Direct recognition of bladder injury is by:
- Rent/cystotomy or urinary leak from bladder **(Fig. 4)**
- Visualization of Foley bulb in abdomen **(Fig. 5)**
- Hematuria
- Pneumaturia—carbon dioxide gas leaking through the bladder defect into the uro bag distends it.
- Suprapubic bruising
- Abdominal wall/pelvic mass
- Urine drainage from accessory trocar site

The investigations which can be performed on table to recognize bladder injury include:
- Cystosufflation with 200–300 mL of methylene blue or indigo carmine through the Foley catheter delineates the bladder edges and help recognize the extent and site of the injury. Carbon dioxide cystosufflation can be used as an alternative.[7]
- In cases where the bladder injury opens into the retropubic space of Retzius, the dye may not be seen leaking intra-abdominally. In all cases of suspected bladder injury, intraoperative cystoscopy is recommended. Few authors suggest routine cystoscopy after major gynecologic surgery but unanimous consent is not there[7] **(Fig. 6)**.
- Perioperatively, ultrasound examination can help in measuring bladder volumes and pelvic or abdominal fluid but it lacks the ability to identify a specific source of leak, hence, not recommended to diagnose bladder injury.[5]
- CT cystography is now the gold standard diagnostic tool for intraoperative suspected iatrogenic bladder injury.[5]
- *Intentional cystotomy:* A 5 mm laparoscope inserted through the bladder injury can help in inspecting the bladder mucosa, trigone and ureteral orifices.[7]

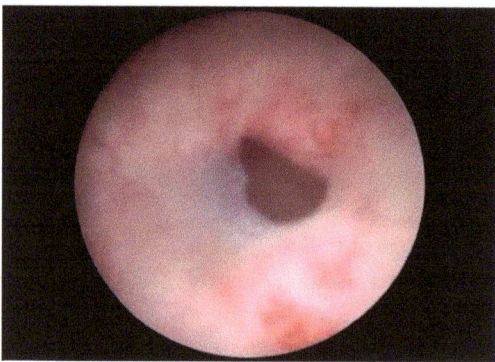

Fig. 4: Cystoscopy showing rent in dome of urinary bladder.

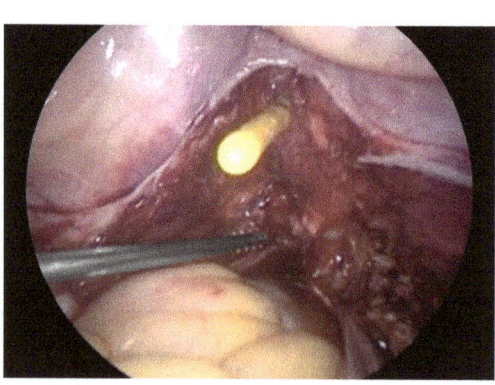

Fig. 5: Laparoscopy showing intraperitoneal Foley catheter.

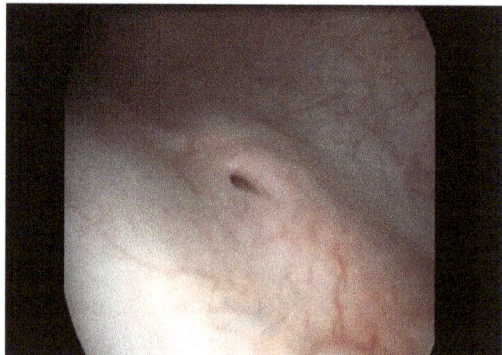

Fig. 6: Cystoscopy showing normal fish mouth opening of ureteral orifice.

SURGICAL TECHNIQUE TO AVOID URETERIC INJURY

The leading cause of iatrogenic ureteric injury has now shifted from urologic to gynecologic surgeries due to increasing number of minimally invasive gynecological laparoscopic procedures. In fact, an estimated 75% of all ureteric injuries are iatrogenic.[5]

Prevention of Injury

- Identification of ureteric peristalsis and following its course before dissection is the safest way to prevent ureteric injury. Ureter typically elicits peristalsis on gentle stroking and has a characteristic snap on palpation which helps in distinguishing it from other vascular structures.
- Operating close to the pathology and careful mobilization from the operative site helps.
- On opening, the anterior leaf of the broad ligament ureter can be exposed. It is then gently pushed laterally and downward with posterior leaf of broad ligament thus keeping it away from the cervix. Take small bites of parametrial and paracervical tissue and avoid double clamping of uterosacral ligaments to prevent injury.
- During active bleeding hemostasis must be secured by gently pulling uterines medially and then doing coagulation.
- Doing resection of adnexa at the end of hysterectomy helps in pulling adnexa medially to achieve an adequate space between ovarian vessels and ureter.
- Carefully preserving the mesentery of ureter by preserving its attachment medially and gentle dissection of ureter from peritoneal wall is recommended.
- Doing vaginal oophorectomy cautiously.

Recognition

- Any intraoperative suspicion of ureteric injury should be followed by prompt recognition along with assessment of severity and nature of the injury.
- Intravenous administration of 10 mL of indigo carmine or methylene blue with 20 mg of furosemide leads to extravasation of blue dye indicating ureteric discontinuity. On cystoscopy, failure to visualize the passage of blue urine even after 15 minutes, suggests unilateral/bilateral ureteric obstruction **(Fig. 7)**.
- Complete transection or occlusion can be ruled out by passing a ureteric catheter in a retrograde fashion to the renal pelvis.
- Cystoscopy is cost-effective, hence, should be considered as routine in complex cases wherein it allows early diagnosis and repair of bladder/ureteric injury. Cystoscopy rules out immediate obstruction by direct visualization of the ureteric orifices and ureteric jets, but not other types of injuries. The detection rate of ureteric injury is 6.2 in 1,000 with and 1.6 in 1,000 without cystoscopy.[1] As an alternative 10% sodium fluorescein given intravenously results in good visualization

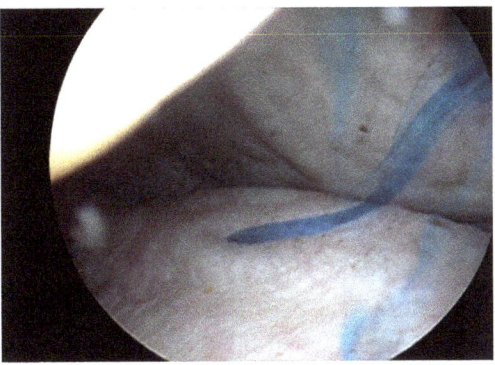

Fig. 7: Cystoscopy showing blue dye jetting from ureter.[13]

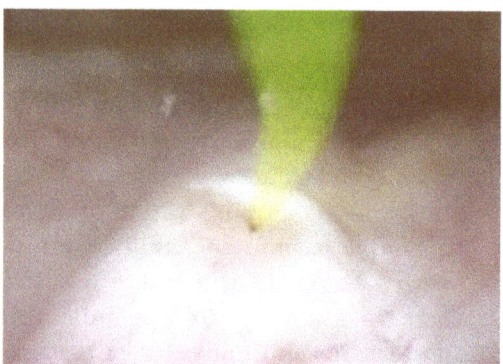

Fig. 8: Cystoscopy showing sodium fluorescein giving a brilliant yellow ureteric jet.[14]

of brilliant yellow ureteric jet minutes after injection **(Fig. 8)**.[12]
- Gold standard for recognizing extravasation of dye or stricture is cystoscopy with bilateral retrograde pyelography and a normal retrograde pyelogram precludes the need for further ureteroscopy.[5]
- Ureteroscopy allows direct inspection of the ureters if retrograde pyelography is inconclusive.
- Alternatively, an on-table intravenous pyelogram can be done followed by an abdominal X-ray 10 minutes later to look for extravasation of contrast.
- Ureterolysis: In complex cases with dense pathology, dissection and exposure of ureter is required, but to be performed only by surgeons with appropriate laparoscopic expertise.
- Ureteric stenting (including lighted stents) reserved for cases when routine methods of ureteric identification have failed and with severely distorted pelvic anatomy.[7]
- Signs of ureteric devascularization such as discoloration, absence of capillary refill, or lack of a bleeding edge should be checked. Use of intravenous fluorescein and Wood's lamp has been suggested to assess the blood supply of ureter.[9]

CONCLUSION

Most common cause of iatrogenic ureteric injury is pelvic surgery. There are no identifiable risk factors in majority of such patients. The cognizance of pelvic anatomy, precise understanding of the ureteric location and the sites where it is most susceptible to injury, thorough training and technique, the consciousness of possible urological injury and appropriate preventive measures, helps the gynecologists to not be frightened and pushed to inactivity in such an event of injury. Urological injury, when discovered intraoperatively, can be corrected, substantially minimizing risk of long-term sequelae.

REFERENCES

1. UpToDate. Urinary tract injury in gynecologic surgery: epidemiology and prevention. [online] Available from: https://www.uptodate.com/contents/urinary-tract-injury-in-gynecologic-surgery-epidemiology-and-prevention [Last accessed on April, 2021].
2. Purandare CN. Urological injuries in gynecology. J Obstet Gynecol India. 2007;57(3):203-20.
3. Altgassen C, Michels W, Schneider A. Learning laparoscopic-assisted hysterectomy. Obstet Gynecol. 2004;104:308-13.
4. Leanza V, Di Prima AF, Leanza G, Teodoro MC, Carbonaro A, D'Agati A, et al. How to prevent ureteral injuries during pelvic gynecological procedures. J Appl Med Sci. 2013;2(3):2241-328.
5. Esparaz AM, Pearl JA, Herts BR, LeBlanc J, Kapoor B. Iatrogenic Urinary Tract Injuries: Etiology, Diagnosis, and Management. Semin Intervent Radiol. 2015;32(2):195-208.
6. Hurd WW, Chee SS, Gallagher KL, Ohl DA, Hurteau JA. Location of the ureters in relation to the uterine cervix by computed tomography. Am J Obstet Gynecol. 2001;184:336-9.
7. Minas V, Gul N, Aust T, Doyle M, Rowlands D. Urinary tract injuries in laparoscopic gynaecological surgery; prevention, recognition and management. Obstet Gynecol. 2014;16(1)19-28.
8. Ito E, Saito T Nerve-preserving techniques for radical hysterectomy. Eur J Surg Oncol. 2004;30(10):1137-40.

9. Washington University. Urologic Complications from Surgery. [online] Available from: https://urology.wustl.edu/patient care/reconstructivesurgery/urologic-complications-from-surgery/ [Last accessed on April, 2021].
10. Lee JS, Choe JH, Lee HS, Seo JT. Urologic complications following obstetric and gynecologic surgery. Korean J Urol. 2012;53(11):795-9.
11. RCOG. Preventing Entry-Related Gynaecological Laparoscopic Injuries. Royal College of Obstetricians and Gynaecologists, Greentop Guideline No. 49. London: RCOG; 2008.
12. Doyle PJ, Lipetskaia L, Duecy E, Buchsbaum G, Wood RW. Sodium fluorescein use during intraoperative cystoscopy. Obstet Gynecol. 2015;125(3):548-50.
13. GynSafe. Cystoscopy. [online] Available from: Cystoscopy, http://gynsafe.com/cystoscopy.html [Last accessed on April, 2021].
14. Green Journal. Sodium Fluorescein Use during Intraoperative Cystoscopy. [online video] Available from: www.youtube.com/watch?v=3SilnYqoOVc [Last accessed on April, 2021].

Identification and Management of Ureteric Injuries in Gynecological Surgeries

CHAPTER 18

Sreeharsha Harinatha

INTRODUCTION

Ureteric injuries occur in about 0.2–1% of all gynecological surgeries[1] and can be a source of significant morbidity to the patient especially if detected late. Hence, prompt identification and management of ureteric injuries is of paramount importance.

Predisposing factors for ureteric injuries include malignancy, endometriosis, enlarged uterus, adhesions, pelvic abscess, and intra-operative bleeding.

Mechanism of injury can be suture ligation, avulsion, transection or more commonly due to thermal damage. About one-third of injuries are detected intraoperatively, while the rest two-thirds are detected postoperatively.[2]

Most common site of injury is at the lower one-third of ureter, followed by upper and then middle third.[3] At the lower one-third, ureter is generally injured just lateral to uterine vessels or close to fornices before it enters the bladder.

CLASSIFICATION

According to the American Association for the Surgery of Trauma,[4] ureteric injuries are classified as follows:
- *Grade I hematoma*: Contusion or hematoma without devascularization
- *Grade II laceration*: < 50% transection
- *Grade III laceration*: ≥ 50% transection
- *Grade IV laceration*: Complete transection with <2 cm of devascularization
- *Grade V laceration*: Avulsion with >2 cm of devascularization.

IDENTIFICATION

Intraoperative

Intraoperative identification of ureteric injuries is crucial to minimize morbidity to the patient and hence high index of suspicion is required especially in challenging cases. Surgeon should carefully inspect the ureter with particular attention to the common areas of ureteric injury especially close to the infundibulopelvic and cardinal ligaments. Note should be made of the peristaltic movements of the ureter although it does not necessarily rule out ureteric injury.

Intravenous indigo carmine and methylene blue dye may be utilized to identify the location of ureteric injury in difficult cases.

Keeping a low threshold for Intraoperative cystoscopy and retrograde pyeloureterography is useful in early and accurate detection of ureteric injury. On cystoscopy, urine efflux from bilateral orifices indicates intact ureter, while blood stained urine efflux can signify a partial ureteric injury. Retrograde injection of contrast into the ureter under fluoroscopic guidance can identify the level of ureteric ligation or injury represented by cutoff of contrast or extravasation of contrast, respectively.

Postoperative

More than two-thirds of ureteric injuries are detected postoperatively. These are usually the injuries which are missed intraoperatively but occasionally could be delayed presentation of thermal necrosis of the ureteric wall.

Presentation could be with flank pain, fever, hematuria, oliguria, anuria, abdominal distension with ileus or leakage of urine.

Rarely, some patients may be asymptomatic and present years later. These are the more unfortunate ones as they may present with a nonfunctioning kidney or sometimes with hypertension.

Any delay in recovery postgynecologic surgery should prompt investigation, at the very least with an ultrasound scan and a renal function test.

Any deterioration in renal function or presence of hydronephrosis or urinoma warrants further investigation.

Intravenous urogram or CT urogram is quite sensitive at detecting ureteric injuries. Complete cutoff or nondrainage of contrast into lower ureter signifies ligation of ureter, whereas extravasation of contrast signifies injury to ureteral wall and site of extravasation gives an estimate of the level of ureteric injury with or without fistula **(Fig. 1)**.

Cystoscopy and retrograde pyeloureterography is a very specific investigation to accurately characterize the ureteric injury. It may be utilized when immediate surgery is planned, when CT findings are nonconclusive or as part of the stenting/nephrostomy procedure **(Fig. 2)**.

Traditional swab tests may be utilized when the predominant symptom is urine leakage.

In two swab test, oral Pyridium may be administered and intravesical methylene blue instilled to color the vaginal swab and hence indicate ureteral or bladder injury.

In three swab test, three swabs are placed in the vagina and the bladder is filled with methylene blue. Discoloration of topmost or middle swab signifies vesicovaginal fistula, whereas wetting of the topmost swab without discoloration indicates ureterovaginal fistula. Discoloration of the lowermost swab indicates urethrovaginal fistula.

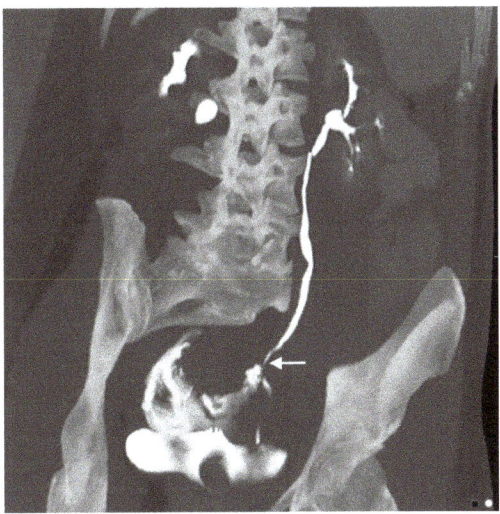

Fig. 1: CT urogram showing lower ureteric injury following abdominal hysterectomy.
Source: Radiopaedia. Ureteric injury. [online] Available from: https://radiopaedia.org/articles/ureteric-injury?lang=ushttps://radiopaedia.org/articles/ureteric-injury?lang=us [Last accessed on April, 2021].

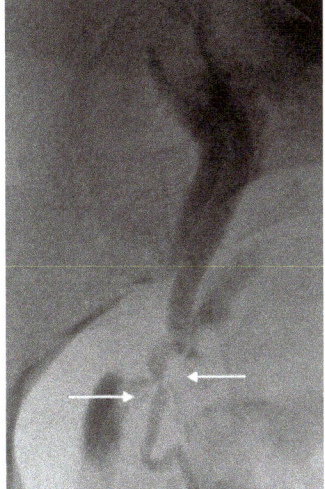

Fig. 2: Retrograde pyeloureterography demonstrating a lower ureteric injury with contrast extravasation.
Source: EPOS. Iatrogenic injury to the urinary tract—A pictorial review of imaging appearances and radiological management. [online] Available from: https://epos.myesr.org/poster/esr/ecr2015/C-2044 [Last accessed on April, 2021].

MANAGEMENT

Management depends upon the timing of presentation, type of surgery performed, patient's general condition and extent of injury.[5] Immediate repair is preferable whenever feasible.

No Action Required

In selected cases with minor ureteric contusions or suture ligated ureters which are removed intraoperatively and continuity is restored and any other injuries ruled out, no further action is required, although it is recommended to keep a low threshold for ureteric stenting in case of any concern.

Percutaneous Nephrostomy

In an unstable patient in whom ureteric injury is recognized or in a patient with extensive hematoma or abscess, in whom delayed repair is planned, percutaneous nephrostomy provides for diversion of urine till the patient is deemed fit for definitive repair. Also in failed ureteric stenting, where immediate repair is not possible, nephrostomy can be planned. Percutaneous nephrostomy can be done under ultrasound or fluoroscopic guidance with local anesthetic infiltration (**Fig. 3**).

Ureteric Stenting

Ureteric stenting with double J stent is by far the most commonly performed procedure for partial or suspected ureteric injuries as well as being a part of the more major reconstructions of the ureter.

All grade 1 and 2 ureteric injuries generally heal well with stenting. Selected grade 3 injuries can also be stented and followed up. Trial of stenting is also advisable in patients with urine leak as in urinoma or ureterovaginal fistula and reviewed after 6 weeks to check the continuity of ureter with retrograde ureterogram or CT urogram.

Ureteroureterostomy

Mid ureteric injuries due to transection or ligation with minimal loss of length are repaired with ureteroureterostomy. Healthy proximal and distal ends are anastomosed with 4-0 absorbable suture (**Fig. 4**). Both ends are spatulated on opposite sides to prevent stenosis. Stent can be removed after 4–6 weeks.

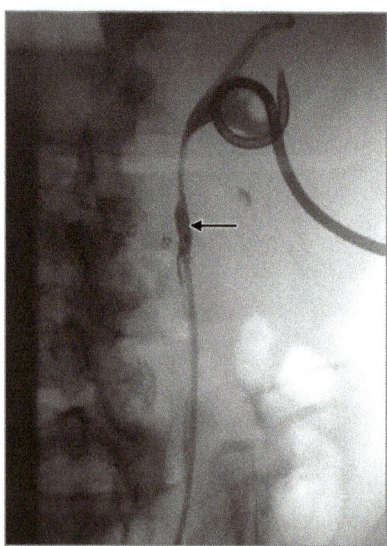

Fig. 3: Percutaneous nephrostomy in a patient with ureteric injury.
Source: Santucci RA, Bartley JM. Urologic trauma guidelines: a 21st century update. Nat Rev Urol. 2010;7:510-9.

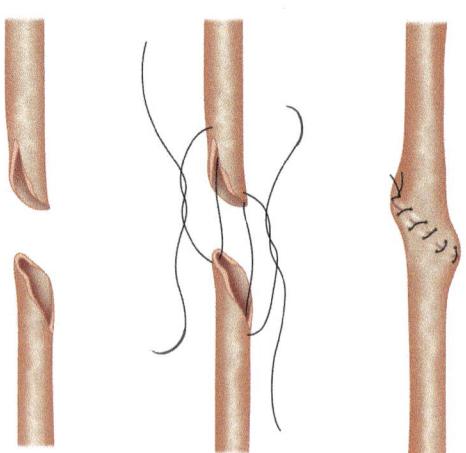

Fig. 4: Ureteroureterostomy.

Ureteroneocystostomy

When the lower ureter is injured and the loss of length is less than 5 cm, ureteroneocystostomy is the ideal procedure to bridge the gap. Ureter is reimplanted in the posterolateral wall of bladder and submucosal tunnel is created to prevent reflux of urine **(Figs. 5 A to D)**. Any tension on the anastomosis will necessitate Psoas hitch of the bladder.

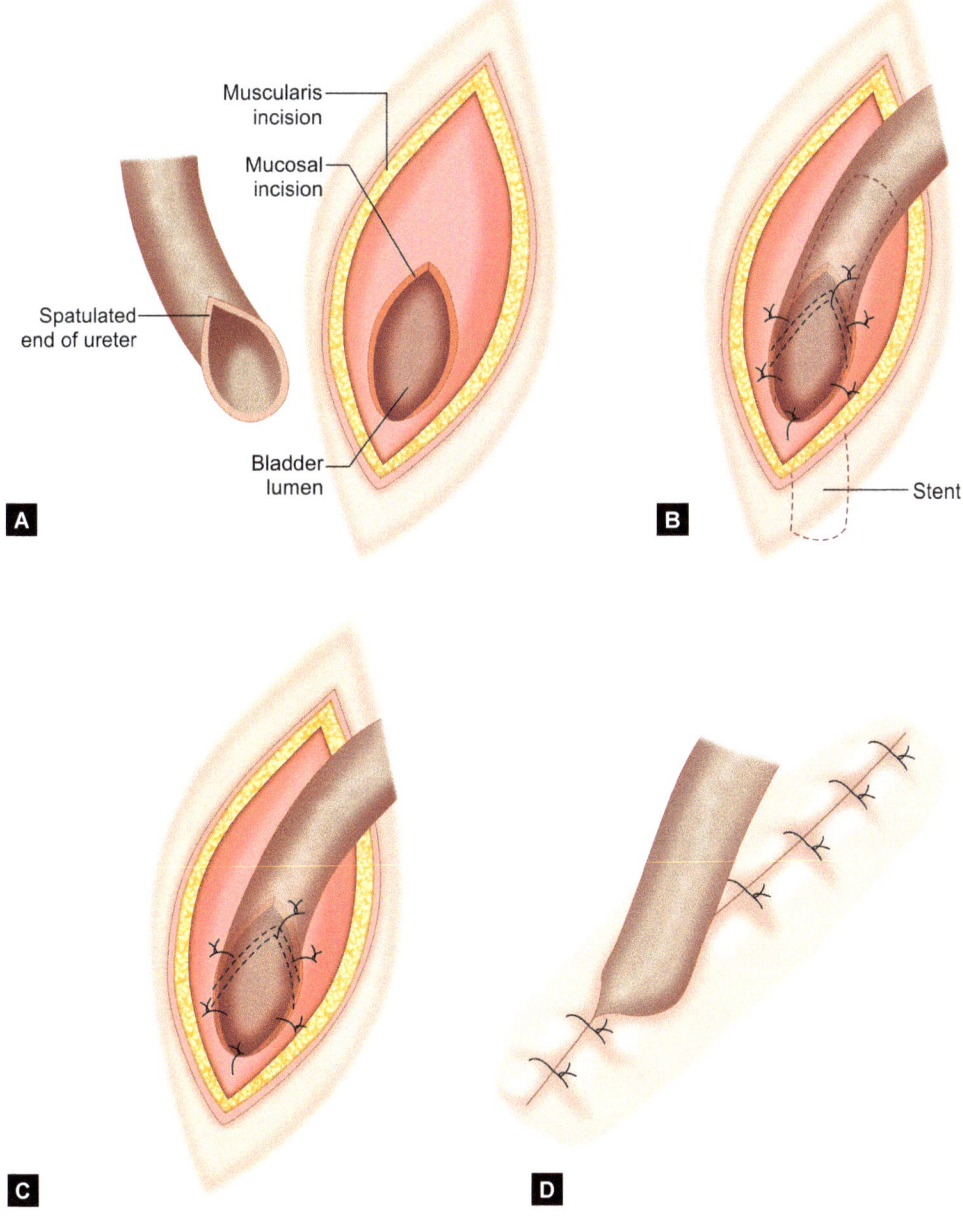

Figs. 5A to D: Ureteral reimplantation technique.

Psoas Hitch

Psoas hitch is utilized when the loss of lower ureteric length is more than 5 cm and ureteroneocystostomy alone is unable to provide a tension free anastomosis **(Fig, 6)**.

Ipsilateral side of the bladder wall is mobilized and hitched to the psoas muscle so as to move the bladder toward the ureter to bridge the gap.

Boari Flap

In mid and lower ureteric injuries with loss of ureteric length unto 15 cm, Boari flap can be utilized with Psoas hitch, to bridge the gap. Spiral flap with a wide base is raised from the bladder wall, tubularized and anastomosed to the proximal ureteric end **(Fig. 7)**.

Transureteroureterostomy

Transureteroureterostomy is infrequently used in mid and lower ureteric injuries as it is technically demanding and exposes the contralateral normal ureter for intervention **(Fig. 8)**. But it can be useful in occasional cases where Boari flap is not possible because of small capacity bladder and ileal interposition is contraindicated. In these cases, posterior peritoneum is incised to expose both the ureters and proximal end of injured ureter is swung across the great vessels to be anastomosed to the normal ureter end-to-side.

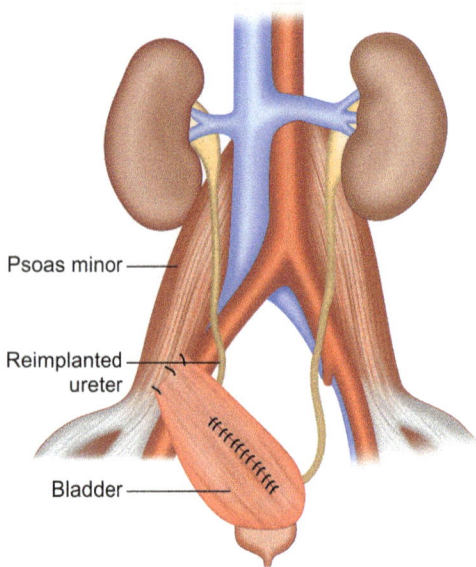

Fig. 6: Ureteroneocystostomy with Psoas Hitch.

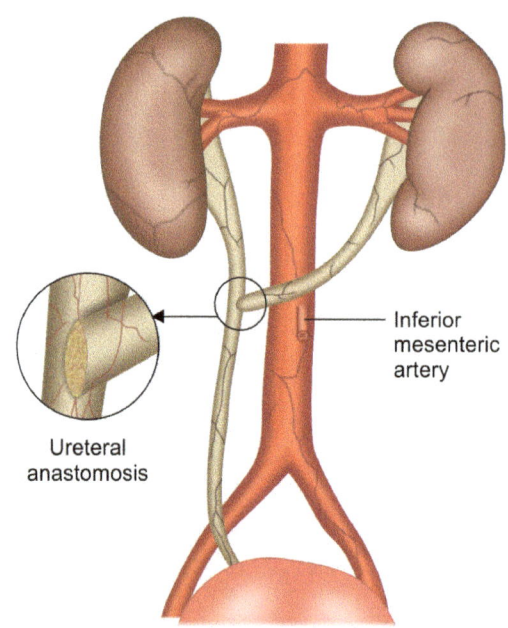

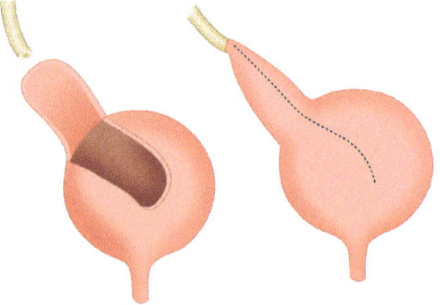

Fig. 7: Boari flap.

Fig. 8: Transureteroureterostomy.
Source: MedScape. Ureteroureterostomy. [online] Available from: https://emedicine.medscape.com/article/1893926-overview [Last accessed on April 2021].

Ureterocalycostomy

When there is injury to the upper ureter like avulsion or transection and proximal ureteric damage precludes end to end anastomosis, ureterocalycostomy can be an option to restore the ureteric drainage **(Fig. 9)**. Here, a small portion of the lower pole is amputated to expose the infundibulum of the lower calyx, which is anastomosed to the distal ureter end-to-end.

Ileal Ureteric Replacement

Ileal ureteric replacement is one of the last resort procedures, when it is not possible to bridge the gap by other techniques. Advantage is that the entire length of ureter can be replaced by isolating the required length of ileum and anastomosing proximally with renal pelvis and distally with the bladder in isoperistaltic fashion **(Fig. 10)**. Disadvantages include mucous plugging and higher incidence of urinary tract infections. Also, patients with compromised renal function should not be advised this procedure due to the high incidence of acidosis.

Renal Autotransplantation

Autotransplantation is also a last resort procedure when other methods are not possible or contraindicated. Example would be a patient with near total loss of ureteric length with compromised renal function and relatively small capacity bladder. Procedure is similar to a regular renal transplant, where renal vessels are anastomosed to iliac vessels and hence technically demanding **(Fig. 11)**. Residual pelvis or ureter can be anastomosed to a bladder opening and continuity restored.

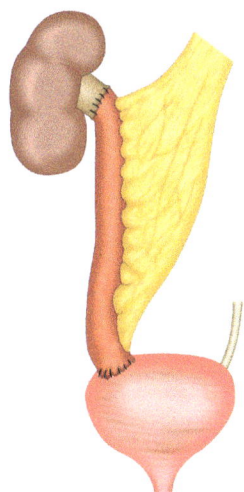

Fig. 10: Ileal ureter.

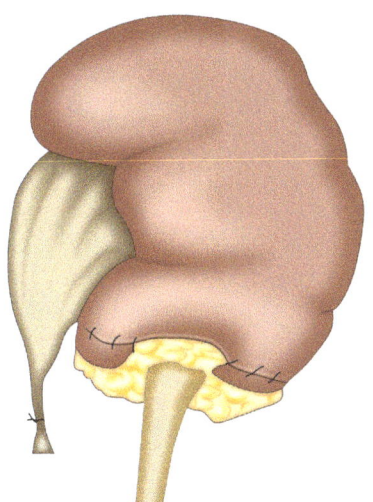

Fig. 9: Ureterocalycostomy.

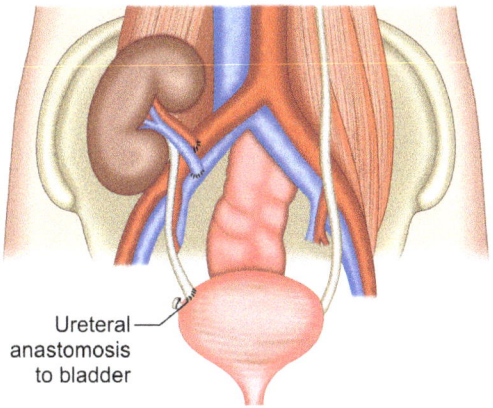

Fig. 11: An autotransplanted kidney.

PREVENTIVE MEASURES

While it is possible to reconstruct and restore nearly any type or extent of ureteric injury, it is imperative on the part of the surgeon to take all measures to avoid injury in the first place. Hence, preventive measures such as meticulous dissection, positive identification of ureter, avoiding blind clamping of vessels, minimal use of cautery with point coagulation and keeping a low threshold for preoperative stenting should be done in all cases to prevent ureteric injury.

REFERENCES

1. Gilmour DT, Dwyer PL, Carey MP. Lower urinary injury during gynecologic surgery and its detection by intraoperative cystoscopy. Obstet Gynecol. 1999;94:883-9.
2. Mann WJ, Arato M, Patsner B, Stone ML. Ureteral injuries in an obstetrics and gynecology training program: etiology and management. Obstet Gynecol 1988;72:82-5.
3. Berkmen F, Peker AE, Alagol H, Ayyildiz A, Arik AI, Basay S. Treatment of iatrogenic ureteral injuries during various operations for malignant conditions. J Exp Clin Cancer Res. 2000;19:441-5.
4. American Association for the Surgery of Trauma. Injuries of ureter. [online] Available from: www.aast.org/injury/t15-20.html#ureter [Last accessed on April, 2021].
5. Mendez LE. Iatrogenic injuries in gynecologic cancer surgery. Surg Clin North Am. 2001; 81:897-923.

CHAPTER 19: Urinary Bladder Injuries during Cesarean Section

Mala Raj, Prashanth K Adiga

INTRODUCTION

Cesarean delivery (CD) is the most common obstetric procedure performed. Bladder injuries are uncommon during cesarean deliveries. With the increased prevalence of cesarean deliveries, the obstetrician needs to be aware of the potential complications, which includes bladder injury. In this chapter, we will discuss incidence, risk factors, identification, management, and prevention of bladder injuries.

INCIDENCE

Bladder injury is defined as any full-thickness injury to the bladder identified by the patient's physician during their course of care, requiring repair. The incidence of bladder injuries during CD ranges from 0.28 to 0.47%.[1,2]

RISK FACTORS

Box 1 shows the risk factors for bladder injury.

Previous Cesarean Delivery

Previous CD is a risk factor for bladder injury. In a study by Phipps et al., there was a fourfold risk of bladder injury in previous CD, compared with primary CD.[1] The chances of bladder injury increase with increasing number of CD: 0.13% first, 0.09% second, 0.28% third, 1.17% fourth, 1.94% fifth, and 4.49% sixth CD.[3]

Previous Abdominal Surgery

Previous abdominal surgery is another risk factor for bladder injury.[1] In a study by Gungorduk et al., using regression analysis of risk factors, previous pelvic surgery had odds ratio of 2.63 (95% confidence interval 1.23–5.61).[4]

Emergency Cesarean Delivery

Emergency CD is a significant risk factor for bladder injury. Studies by Phipps et al., and Rajasekar et al. have suggested that emergency delivery (ED) was a risk factor for bladder injuries. This association could be due to the need of uterine incision without a bladder flap and even when a bladder flap is formed, the emergency to deliver the baby might preclude bladder care.[1,5] There has been conflicting opinion as to whether ED is a risk factor. In the study by Rahman et al., bladder injuries were more common in the elective CD than the emergency CD. This could be due to the increased number of elective indications for multiple previous cesarean sections.[6]

Adhesions

The incidence of adhesive disease after a primary CD ranged from 46 to 65%,[7] and are ubiquitously present when there is a history of previous bladder injury.

BOX 1: Risk factors for bladder injury.
- Previous cesarean delivery
- Previous abdominal surgery
- Emergency cesarean delivery
- Adhesions
- Labor

TABLE 1: Timing of bladder injury.

Timing of bladder injury	First time cesarean section	Repeated cesarean section
Opening of the peritoneum	35.7–46.6%	35.7–46.6%
Opening of vesicouterine pouch	23.8–50.0%	32.0–60.0%
The opening of the uterus and the fetus extraction	14.3–28.6%	35.7–46.6%
Closure of the hysterotomy	10%	10%

Labor

Labor was found to be a significant risk factor for bladder injury during cesarean delivery. In a study by Nielsen et al., factors associated with increased complications included: (1) station of the fetal presenting part; (2) patient in active labor; (3) extreme preterm (<32 weeks); (4) premature rupture of membranes (PRM)/preterm premature rupture of the membranes (PPROM); and (5) skill of the operator.[8]

WHEN AND WHERE DOES BLADDER INJURY OCCUR?

Table 1 is showing the timing of bladder injury.[4,6,9]

The time of bladder injury is most commonly during the opening of the peritoneum and during the opening of the UV pouch, as shown in **Table 1**. During a primary CD, bladder injuries have been noted to occur when the peritoneum is opened (46.6%), while the most common step of bladder injury during subsequent CDs occur during formation of the vesicouterine pouch (32–60%).[1,4,6,9]

METHODS TO AVOID BLADDER INJURY

- In subsequent cesarean sections, the Pfannenstiel method of sharp dissection while opening peritoneum as opposed to the blunt dissection as in Joel-Cohen and Misgav-Ladach methods seems to be safer.[6]
- Ensuring a distance of at least 1–2 cm from the dome of the bladder when raising the bladder flap.

TABLE 2: Location of the bladder injury.

Location	First time cesarean delivery	Repeated cesarean delivery
Dome	51.0–76.2%	48.0–53.3%
Body	21.8–24%	46.7–52.0%
Trigone	0–3%	3–8%

- The Misgav-Ladach technique of uterine incision without bladder flap formation is safest mostly for the first cesarean section.[10]

Great care needs to be taken at this important step of a CD, because about 23.8% of injury in a primary CD and up to 60% of injuries in case of subsequent cesarean sections are made during this step.[1,4,6,9]

Table 2 describes the location of the bladder injury.

The most common site of bladder injury is the dome in case of a primary CD. In case of a previous CD, the most common site of injury is the body and the dome, which can be explained due to the fact that the bladder might be pulled up, hence placing the body of the bladder also at risk of injury.[6]

RECOGNITION OF BLADDER INJURIES AND MANAGEMENT (FLOWCHART 1)

In patients with repeat CD, utmost care needs to be taken to prevent bladder injury. In case of injury, it is crucial to recognize and repair intraoperatively after extraction of the baby. Failure to recognize and repair a bladder injury during surgery may later lead

Flowchart 1: Urological assessment of inadvertent cystotomy during cesarean section.

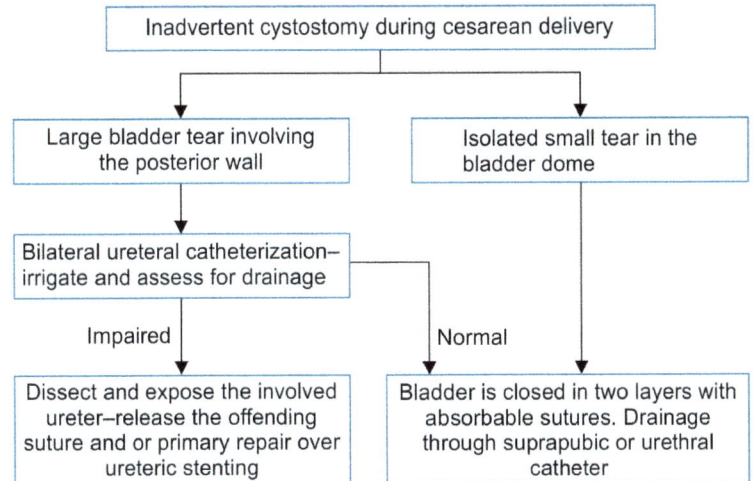

to vesicovaginal, vesicouterine, or ureterovaginal fistula.[11,12]

Some of the signs that suggest bladder injury intraoperatively are:[6]

- Urine extravasation into the peritoneal cavity
- Appearance of the Foley bulb
- Gross hematuria in the Urobag
- Visible detrusor muscle laceration

Confirmation of the suspected bladder injury may be done by filling the bladder through the urethral catheter with saline diluted with methylene blue. To rule out injury to the distal ureter or bladder trigone, an intravenous dye (such as indigo carmine or methylene blue) and/or retrograde ureteral catheterization may be used. If the injury involves trigone and/or ureters and/or urethra, a multidisciplinary approach with the urologist is recommended. When there is suspicion of injury to the urethra or bladder, a cystoscopy should be performed.[13]

Box 2 shows the symptoms of unrecognized bladder injuries (due to urinary ascites) which may manifest in the postoperative period.[13] A cystogram is useful in defining the contour of the bladder and for identifying a cystotomy.[13]

BOX 2: Cystotomy or ureteral defect.

- Profuse drain output
- Profuse wound leakage
- Ileus
- Fever
- Peritonitis
- Hematuria

Repair of Bladder Injuries

- For an injury to the bladder dome, a simple running stitch is used as the first layer to close the mucosa with a 3-0 delayed absorbable suture.[14] Use of permanent suture, especially silk, is contraindicated, as it can serve as a niche for calculi formation **(Fig. 1)**.[15]
- The second layer is closed with a running imbricating stitch using either 2-0 or 3-0 delayed absorbable suture to include the submucosa and muscularis.[14]
- After bladder integrity is confirmed, a third running stitch of the same material can be considered if necessary.[16]
- Indwelling catheter is placed for a period of 7–10 days.

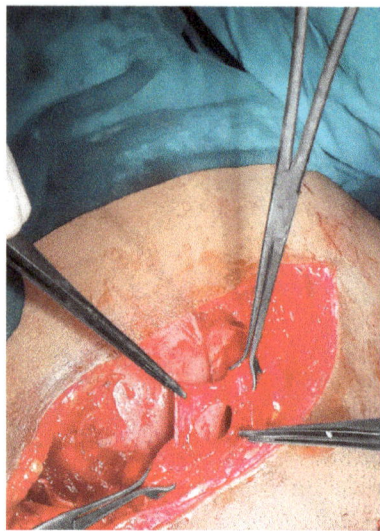

Fig. 1: Bladder injury exposed.

PREVENTION OF BLADDER INJURIES

The pertinent questions that can be asked are:
- Can adhesions be prevented?
- Is bladder flap necessary during CD?

Can Adhesions be Prevented?

Adhesion formation during or after the first CD is an important cause for bladder injury in subsequent CD. Steps that may be adopted to reduce adhesions are:
- Close attention to tissue planes while dissecting
- Avoiding excess blood loss and
- Maintenance of tissue moisture[17,18]

The study by Blumenfeld et al. showed that primary single layer closure of the uterus was associated with increased bladder adhesions during repeat CD.[19] Double layer closure, probably achieves better hemostasis and reduces the exposure of raw surgical surfaces and hence prevents adhesions.

Peritoneal closure during CD has yielded conflicting opinions on whether this step decreases the adhesion rate. A Cochrane review demonstrated that avoiding closure of the peritoneum has been found to have improved short-term benefits such as shorter operative time, reduced incidence of postoperative fever and shorter hospital stay.[20] The study by Alpay et al. showed no difference in adhesion formation when the parietal and visceral peritoneum was closed.[21] The studies by Cheung et al. and Lyell et al. showed decreased risk of adhesions when parietal peritoneum was closed.[22,23]

A number of antiadhesive molecules have been used. Oxidized refined cellulose (Interceed, Ethicon, Johnson & Johnson Company, USA), Sodium hyaluronate and carboxymethylcellulose (Seprafilm Genzyme Biosurgery, Framingham, MA, USA) are the commonly available antiadhesive molecules. The study by Walfisch et al. concluded that the routine use of adhesion barriers during CD is expensive and is not supported by high-quality research.[24]

Is Bladder Flap Necessary during CD?

The initial intention for raising a bladder flap in the preantibiotic era was to prevent spread of intrauterine infection, if any, into the peritoneal cavity. An added advantage is preventing bladder injury during fetus extraction. The study by Hohlagschwandtner et al. concluded that omission of the bladder flap provides short-term advantages such as reduction of operating time and incision-delivery interval, reduced blood loss, and need for analgesics.[25]

In a study by Malvasi et al., women without bladder flap formation had advantages over the women with bladder flap formation in terms of adhesions on the surface of the LUS in repeat CS, and on the uterine scar, and recommended that raising the flap should be avoided during CS in order to prevent inflammatory processes and avoid delayed healing of the uterine scar.

GOOD PRACTICE POINTS

- Previous CD is a risk factor for bladder injury. There is a four-fold increase in bladder injury in a patient with a previous CD.
- Opening the parietal peritoneum, as high as possible in a patient with previous CD may prevent bladder injury.
- When there is suspicion of bladder/urethral/ureteral injury, cystoscopy should be performed.
- Tear in the dome is repaired in two to three layers, using delayed absorbable suture.
- Failure to diagnose a bladder injury during surgery may later lead to vesicovaginal, vesicouterine or ureterovaginal fistula.

REFERENCES

1. Phipps MG, Watabe B, Clemons JL, Weitzen S, Myers DL. Risk factors for bladder injury during cesarean delivery. Obstet Gynecol. 2005;105:156-60.
2. Salman L, Aharony S, Shmueli A, Wiznitzer A, Chen R, Gabbay-Benziv R. Urinary bladder injury during cesarean delivery: maternal outcome from a contemporary large series. Eur J Obstet Gynecol Reprod Biol. 2017;213:26-30.
3. Silver RM, Landon MB, Rouse DJ, Leveno KJ, Spong CY, Thom EA, et al. Maternal morbidity associated with multiple repeat cesarean deliveries. Obstet Gynecol. 2006;107:1226-32.
4. Gungorduk K, Asicioglu O, Celikkol O, Sudolmus S, Ark C. Iatrogenic bladder injuries during caesarean delivery: a case control study. J Obstet Gynaecol. 2010;30:667-70.
5. Rajasekar D, Hall M. Urinary tract injuries during obstetric intervention. Br J Obstet Gynaecol. 1997;104:731-4.
6. Rahman MS, Gasem T, Al Suleiman SA, Al Jama FE, Burshaid S, Rahman J. Bladder injuries during cesarean section in a University Hospital: a 25-year review. Arch Gynecol Obstet. 2009;279(3):349-52
7. Boland GM, Weigel RJ. Formation and prevention of postoperative abdominal adhesions. J Surg Res. 2006;132:3-12.
8. Nielsen TF, Hokegard KH. Cesarean section and intraoperative surgical complications. Acta Obstet Gynecol Scand. 1984;63:103-8.
9. Oliphant SS, Bochenska K, Tolge ME, Catov JM, Zyczynski HM. Maternal lower urinary tract injury at the time of cesarean delivery. Int Urogynecol J. 2014;25(12):1709-14.
10. Korniluk A, Kosiński P, Wielgoś M. Intraoperative damage to the urinary bladder during cesarean section—literature review. Ginekol Pol. 2017; 88(3):161-5.
11. Everett HS, Mattingly RF. Urinary tract injury resulting from pelvic surgery. Am J Obstet Gynecol. 1956;71(3):502-14.
12. Keettel WC. Vesicovaginal and ureterovaginal fistulae. In: Gynecologic and Obstetric Urology. Philadelphia: Saunders; 1978. pp. 267-74.
13. Sharp HT, Adelman MR. Prevention, recognition, and management of urologic injuries during gynecologic surgery. Obstet Gynecol. 2016;127(6):1085-96.
14. Davis JD. Management of injuries to the urinary and gastrointestinal tract during cesarean section. Obstet Gynecol Clin North Am. 1999;26(3):469-80.
15. Morrow FK, Kogan SJ, Freed SZ, Laufman H. In vivo comparison of polygycolic acid, chromic catgut and silk in tissue of the genitourinary tract. An experimental study of tissue retrieval and calcuologenesis. J Urol. 1974;112:655.
16. Tarney CM. Bladder injury during cesarean delivery. Curr Womens Health Rev. 2013; 9(2):70-6.
17. The Practice Committee of the American Society for Reproductive Medicine in collaboration with the Society of Reproductive Surgeons. Pathogenesis, consequences, and control of peritoneal adhesions in gynecologic surgery. Fertil Steril. 2008;90(Suppl):S144-9.
18. Likakos T, Thomakos N, Fine PM, Dervenis C, Young RL. Peritoneal adhesions: etiology, pathophysiology, and clinical significance: recent advances in prevention and management. Dig Surg. 2001;18: 260-73.
19. Blumenfeld YJ, Caughey AB, El-Sayed YY, Daniels K, Lyell DJ. Single versus double layer hysterotomy closure at primary caesarean delivery and bladder adhesions. BJOG. 2010;117:690-4.

20. Bamigboye AA, Hofmeyr GJ. Closure versus non-closure of the peritoneum at caesarean section. Cochrane Database Syst Rev. 2003;(4): CD000163.
21. Alpay Z, Saed GM, Diamond MP. Postoperative adhesions: from formation to prevention. Semin Reprod Med. 2008;26:313-21.
22. Cheung JP, Tsang HH, Cheung JJ, Yu HH, Leung GK, Law WL. Adjuvant therapy for the reduction of postoperative intra-abdominal adhesion formation. Asian J Surg. 2009;32:180-6.
23. Lyell DJ, Caughey AB, Hu E, Daniels K. Peritoneal closure at primary cesarean delivery and adhesions. Obstet Gynecol. 2005;106:275-80.
24. Walfisch A, Beloosesky R, Shrim A, Hallak M. Adhesion prevention after cesarean delivery: evidence, and lack of it. Am J Obstet Gynecol. 2014;211(5):446-52.
25. Hohlagschwandtner M, Ruecklinger E, Husslein P, Joura EA. Is the formation of a bladder flap at cesarean necessary? A randomized trial. Obstet Gynecol. 2001;98:1089-92.
26. Malvasi A, Tinelli A, Guido M, Cavallotti C, Dell'Edera D, Zizza A, et al. Effect of avoiding bladder flap formation in caesarean section on repeat caesarean delivery. Eur J Obstet Gynecol Reprod Biol. 2011;159(2):300-4.

Postpartum Urinary Issues and Management

Ameya C Purandare, Ashwin Shetty

PELVIC FLOOR AND CHILDBIRTH

The pelvic floor consists of the levator ani, which is a complex of the puborectalis, pubococcygeus, and iliococcygeus muscle along with the urethral and anal sphincter, innervated by S2, S3, S4 sacral nerve fibers and the pudendal nerve. The endopelvic connective tissues lie superior to the pelvic floor muscles and connect to the pelvic side walls and sacrum.[1]

Pregnancy and delivery result in stretching, tearing and compression of these muscles and connective tissue causing subsequent nerve injury and denervation. Risk factors include large baby, prolonged second stage and instrumental vaginal delivery. A significant proportion of such injuries resolve by the first postpartum year, however, about 5% such cases will have persistent denervation injury.

Loss of levator support also predisposes to pelvic organ prolapse. Risk factors include operative delivery, prolonged second stage, and high birth weight. Vaginal delivery predisposes to the risk of developing pelvic organ prolapse and stress urinary incontinence with increased risk from forceps delivery. Ventouse delivery is associated with a lesser risk. In some cases, electrophysiological evidence of denervation injury can be seen 5-6 years after delivery

POSTPARTUM URINARY RETENTION

Bladder care is an important aspect of postpartum management. Postpartum voiding dysfunction when unrecognized can result in long-term damage to the detrusor muscle.

Definitions

Urinary retention is defined as an inability to pass urine despite persistent effort.

International Continence Society (ICS) defines acute urinary retention as a painful, palpable or percussable bladder with inability to pass urine. These symptoms might not be present after epidural analgesia. Postpartum urinary retention is an inability to pass urine within 6 hours of delivery. It is a sudden onset voiding disability with significant postvoid residual urine.[2,3]

Chronic urinary retention is not painful and is associated with the postvoid residual urine of more than 150 mL, signs of chronic retention can be frequent urination and the sensation of incomplete voiding.[3]

About 10-15% of women will have postnatal voiding dysfunction. Up to 5% will go on to develop longer lasting dysfunction, which can lead to bladder distention and overflow incontinence.

The Royal College of Obstetricians and Gynaecologists (RCOG) Green-top Guidelines recommend that the women who have had spinal or epidural and instrumental delivery should have an indwelling catheter for at least 12 hours postdelivery to avoid bladder distention.

Risk Factors for Retention

These include the following:
- Nulliparous women
- Prolonged labor (especially a prolonged second stage)

- Assisted/instrumental delivery
- Perineal injury
- Cesarean section
- Regional analgesia

Causes can be due to pudendal nerve injury secondary to stretching of the pelvic floor and transient edema in the urogenital area.[4,5]

Symptoms

Symptoms of retention include the following:
- Difficulty in voiding postpartum
- Sensation of incomplete voiding
- Post-micturition dribble
- Frequent small voids
- Straining while voiding
- Nocturia more than twice

Diagnosis

The patient can be asymptomatic and so the diagnosis is determined by post-void residual urine. Catheterization is the most accurate determinant, however, bladder scanning is a noninvasive method that can be used. Bladder scan may sometimes be inaccurate due to the presence of the postpartum uterus and debris along with the residual urine.

Management

Intrapartum

Prevention of urinary retention by encouraging voiding every 3 hours while in labor is advised. If the patient is unable to void or there is incomplete voiding, intermittent catheterization should be encouraged. In patients with epidural analgesia with a dense block, an indwelling catheter should remain in place for 6 hours or till sensation returns. Catheter should be removed temporarily at time of delivery to avoid urethral injury and reinserted afterwards.

Postpartum

Voiding is to be encouraged every 2–3 hours postpartum. If the patient is unable to pass urine for more than 6 hours than an indwelling Foley catheter is to be inserted and should remain in place for 24–48 hours. A urine sample is to be sent for to rule out infection. In the event of persistently high post-void residual urine, intermittent self-catheterization should be taught or the patient can be discharged to home with the indwelling catheter.

Clean Intermittent Catheterization

If the need for catheterization continues following the immediate postoperative period, clean intermittent catheterization (CIC) is preferred for women who have the mental capability, hand coordination, and body habitus to perform the procedure.

Clean (nonsterile) technique for intermittent catheterization has lower complication rates compared with indwelling urethral or suprapubic catheterization.

Systemic antimicrobial agents are not used in either short- or long-term catheterization settings as prophylactic antibiotic use.

Patients are instructed to record both their voided volumes and post-void residual volumes (PVRs). The combined volume should not exceed the functional bladder capacity, or 400–600 mL, whichever is smaller. This often requires four to five catheterizations daily and varies based on fluid intake patterns and volume. If there is a concern that CIC cannot be performed four to six times a day, then an indwelling catheter should be placed.

POSTPARTUM URINARY INFECTION

Cystitis is defined as symptomatic infection of the bladder. The typical symptoms of acute cystitis in the pregnant woman are the same as in nonpregnant women and include the sudden onset of dysuria and urinary urgency and frequency. Systemic symptoms, such as fevers and chills, are absent in simple cystitis. The presence of fever and chills, flank pain, and costovertebral angle tenderness should raise suspicion for pyelonephritis.

Urine analysis and culture with the midstream specimen of urine is recommended for postnatal women with dysuria.

Symptoms of dysuria, frequency and urgency with colony count of $\geq 10^3$ CFU/mL is an indicator of UTI.

Management of acute cystitis is in the form of empirical antibiotics which are then subsequently modified on the basis the urine culture results and repeat urine culture are to be repeated to confirm cure. Antibiotic treatment options include beta-lactams, nitrofurantoin, fosfomycin and amoxicillin-clavulanate.

Acute pyelonephritis develops with infection of the upper urinary tract and kidneys. Symptoms include high-grade fever (>38°C or 100.4°F), nausea, vomiting and costovertebral angle tenderness associated with dysuria, frequency, and urgency.

About 20% of women with severe pyelonephritis will develop complications such as septic shock syndrome and/or acute respiratory distress syndrome.

Patients admitted in such situations should have a blood culture. Management includes hospital admission for parental antibiotics which are initially empiric and frequent and then converted on the basis of culture results. Third-generation cephalosporins are commonly used for empirical treatment. In patients with a history of infections with extended-spectrum beta-lactamase (ESBL)-producing Enterobacteriaceae (or other risk factors), a carbapenem is an appropriate choice for empiric therapy.

Once afebrile for 48 hours patients can be switched to oral treatment, which is usually for 10-14 days.

POSTPARTUM URINARY INCONTINENCE

Prevalence of stress urinary incontinence (SUI) is in up to 40% of pregnant women.[6] It usually presents antenatally and is more common in multiparous women.

Most complaints resolve by 1 year after delivery. However, with the onset of symptoms developing after delivery, 24% will continue to have symptoms at the end of 1 year.

Viktrup and Lose showed that the length of the second stage correlates with the development of SUI. This risk is increased for vaginal delivery, however, it is important to note that a cesarean delivery does not completely remove risk, indicating that the etiology is multifactorial.[6] A randomized trial of vaginal versus cesarean delivery showed that those who underwent cesarean delivery reported less incidence of urinary incontinence at 3 months postpartum (relative risk 0.62, 95% CI 0.41-0.93), although the difference did not persist 2 years postpartum.[7] Women with cesarean section after labor had a similar incidents of SUI compared to those who had a vaginal birth implying that the labor process may be the cause of pelvic floor damage.[8]

Causes of stress incontinence in pregnancy are thought to be due to the increase in maternal weight, pressure on the bladder by the gravid uterus and increased urinary output. Women with SUI at 3 months postnatal had a 92% risk of having SUI at 5 years.[8] Urge incontinence develops in 30% of postpartum patients. Forceps delivery and episiotomy increase risk and while cesarean section is protective.[8] Large birth weight increases the risk of both stress and urge incontinence.

Management

The International Consultation on Incontinence (ICI) committee (Moore et al., 2013) recommends that pelvic floor muscle training (PFMT) should be offered as first-line therapy to postpartum women with urinary incontinence persisting three months after delivery.

Although PFMT and exercise was originally meant for the treatment of SUI, it is now used as a central element in the treatment of urgency, urge incontinence and overactive bladder (OAB). Patients are taught PFM control and exercise in the same way as for SUI. If symptoms do not respond to conservative measures then a trial of anticholinergic medication for OAB is advised. Stress urinary incontinence will need Burch colposuspension or midurethral sling surgery.

URINARY TRACT TRAUMA DURING DELIVERY

Operative Injuries

Delivery increases the risk of bladder trauma. At cesarean section the bladder can be lacerated at the time of peritoneal entry, development of the bladder flap, uterine incision and adhesiolysis. Incidence of bladder trauma at cesarean section is 0.28%, this risk increases with history of previous cesarean section, prolonged second stage of labor and cesarean hysterectomy.[9] Previous cesarean section increases the risk of urinary injury, with a fourth cesarean section having 1.2% risk of bladder injury compared with just 0.13% for a first cesarean section.[9]

Most often injury to the bladder is at the dome and is easily recognized. Long-term morbidity is minimized when timely repair is done. If in doubt confirmation is by the methylene blue test. Bladder injury when recognized is to be repaired in two layers. If the injury involves the trigone a ureteric stenting may be required. The incidence of ureteric injuries is between 0.02% and 0.1%.[9]

Ureteric injury can present postoperatively with findings of flank tenderness and unilateral hydronephrosis. Recognition and immediate repair is important to avoid complications such as urogenital fistula and urosepsis.[9]

Mid pelvic forceps and rarely ventouse delivery have also been implicated in urinary tract injuries.

Obstetric Fistula

Major degree of trauma during childbirth can result in bladder or ureteric injury. Obstructed labor can cause necrosis of the anterior vagina and bladder resulting in vesicovaginal fistula. This typically presents with continuous incontinence 7–14 days after delivery.[10]

Suspected cases are to be investigated with intravenous urogram, cystoureteroscopy, CT/MRI scan.

Rectovaginal fistula can also rarely develop. A variety of vaginal and abdominal fistula repair surgeries has been described.

These injuries are rare with good obstetric care but are usually a source of lifelong morbidity especially in developing countries. Timely recognition of labor dystocia and access to cesarean section is preventive. The WHO estimates that two million women around the world have untreated fistula, this figure may be an underestimate.[10] These women are then ostracized socially due to the incontinence.

REFERENCES

1. Percy JP, Neill ME, Swash M, Parks AG. Electrophysiological study of motor nerve supply of pelvic floor. Lancet. 1981;1(8210):16-7.
2. Foldspang A, Hvidman L, Mommsen S, Nielsen JB. Risk of postpartum urinary incontinence associated with pregnancy and mode of delivery. Acta Obstet Gynecol Scand. 2004;83(10):923-7.

3. Mulder FE, Hakvoort RA, Schoffelmeer MA, Limpens J, Van der Post JA, Roovers JP. Postpartum urinary retention: a systematic review of adverse effects and management. Int Urogynecol J. 2014;25(12):1605-12.
4. Yip SK, Brieger G, Hin LY, Chung T. Urinary retention in the post-partum period. The relationship between obstetric factors and the post-partum post-void residual bladder volume. Acta Obstet Gynecol Scand. 1997;76(7):667-72.
5. Cunningham FG, Lucas MJ. Urinary tract infections complicating pregnancy. Baillieres Clin Obstet Gynaecol. 1994;8(2):353-73.
6. Granese R, Adile B. Urinary incontinence in pregnancy and in puerperium: 3 months follow-up after delivery. Minerva Ginecol. 2008;60:15-21.
7. Groutz A, Rimon E, Peled S, Gold R, Pauzner D, Lessing JB, et al. Cesarean section: does it really prevent the development of postpartum stress urinary incontinence? A prospective study of 363 women 1 year after their first delivery. Neurourol Urodynam. 2004;23:2-6.
8. Casey BM, Schaffer JI, Bloom SL, Heartwell SF, McIntire DD, Leveno KJ. Obstetric antecedents for postpartum pelvic floor dysfunction. Am J Obstet Gynecol. 2005;192:1655-62.
9. Yossepowitch O, Baniel J, Livine PM. Urological injuries during caesarean section: intraoperative diagnosis and management. J Urol. 2004; 172:196-9.
10. Ahmad S, Nishtar A, Hafeez GA. Management of vesicovaginal fistulas in women. Int J Gynecol Obstet. 2005;68:71-5.

Identification and Management of Genitourinary Fistulae

CHAPTER 21

Madhusudhan Naidu

INTRODUCTION

Fistula is a connection or passage that abnormally connects two organs or vessels. Abnormal connection can develop anywhere between bladder, rectum, vagina, intestine and/or skin, etc.

Urinary fistula is an abnormal connection between bladder, urethra or ureter with vagina or uterus or bowel. Apart from medical sequelae, women experience a significant impact on their quality of life due to physical, mental, social and sexual trauma as a result of a urinary fistula.[1]

Urinary fistulae constitute vesicovaginal, ureterovaginal, urethrovaginal and uterovesical fistula **(Fig. 1)**. Majority of urinary fistulae are vesicovaginal and urethrovaginal. However, the most common type is vesicovaginal fistula (VVF).

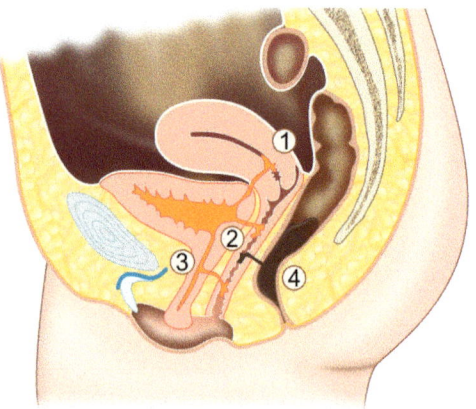

Fig. 1: Urogenital fistula. (1) Vesicouterine fistula; (2) Vesicovaginal fistula; (3) Urethrovaginal fistula; (4) Rectovaginal fistula.

In the developing world (sub-Saharan Africa and Asia), the major cause of urinary fistula [obstetric fistula (OF)] is poor obstetric care and the reported incidence is 3/1,000 women of reproductive age.[2]

In the developed world, the most common cause of urinary fistula is surgical complications (iatrogenic fistula) following hysterectomy or pelvic surgery.

The reported incidence of VVF is between 0.1 and 4%.[3] 1:788 for all types of hysterectomy, 1:540 for abdominal hysterectomy for benign disease, 1:455 for laparoscopic hysterectomy,[4] 1:896 following vaginal hysterectomy for benign disease (excluding prolapse), 1:3,861 following vaginal hysterectomy for prolapse, 1:2,279 for subtotal hysterectomy, 1:486 for endometriosis, 1:1,922 for fibroids and 1:100 for cervical malignancy including radical hysterectomy.[5]

Overall, the rate of urogenital fistula appears to be approximately nine times higher following radical hysterectomy in women with malignant disease as compared to that following simple hysterectomy (abdominal or vaginal) in women with benign conditions.[5]

In addition to surgery, the other known causes of urogenital fistula are surgery for stress urinary incontinence, trauma, CO_2 laser, cone biopsy, foreign bodies, radiation, chronic bladder inflammation, and biopsy.

RISK OF URETERIC INJURIES

Incidence of ureteric injury is 0.6% at laparoscopic hysterectomy versus 0.6% for open hysterectomy, 0.09% for vaginal hysterectomy for prolapse versus 0.2% for vaginal hysterectomy for other benign conditions, 2.2% for laparoscopic procedure for endometriosis versus 1% for open approach to endometriosis.

For malignant surgery, risk of ureteric injury via laparoscopic approach is 0.2% versus 1.3% for open procedure. Higher risk was observed in the radical hysterectomy group for uterine cancer, 2.4–10.6%.[6]

Most common site of injury to the ureter at hysterectomy occurs in the lower one-third and the possible reasons for injury include ligation, kinking by suture, transection/avulsion, partial transection, crush injury, and devascularization.[7] Probably because of these mechanisms, diagnosis of iatrogenic ureteral injury may be delayed or identified after the primary surgery, in 65–80% of cases.

Radiation fistula is higher in postoperative external radiation (1.9%) compared to transvaginal brachytherapy (0.8%).[8]

Uterovesical fistula is observed following cesarean section for placenta accreta or previa when the uterus and bladder are not well separated. About 58% of fistula was observed following second cesarean section.[9]

URETHROVAGINAL FISTULA

This is a rare condition which is mostly iatrogenic secondary to:
- Suburethral sling surgery
- Urethral diverticulum and its repair
- Catheterization
- Radiation
- Trauma
- Foreign body
- Feminizing genital reconstructions surgery

DIAGNOSIS

Symptoms

Involuntary painless leakage of urine, stool or possibly both is a characteristic symptom of fistula. The leakage can be intermittent or may be constant. After TAH, 90% of patients present in second week. After laparoscopic hysterectomy, 36% presented within 1 week and 50% in the second week.[10]

Ureteric injury may occur along the retroperitoneal ureter usually below the pelvic brim. Injury may not be recognized intraoperatively unless there is a complete ureteral transection during surgery, therefore postoperative pain is a key symptom to suggest a possible ureteric injury.

Additional symptoms experienced by patients who developed VVF are excessive postoperative abdominal pain, distension or paralytic ileus, or both. Hematuria, symptoms of irritability of the bladder, prolonged postoperative fever, and increased white blood cell count were also noted more often in the fistula group due to extravasation of urine.[11] Therefore patients who develop any of these symptoms should raise suspicion and initiate investigations to rule out genitourinary tract injury.

CLINICAL ASSESSMENT

Diagnosis of VVF requires clinical assessment in combination with appropriate imaging or laboratory studies. Direct visual inspection of leaking urine or dye or colored fluid extravasation or staining of tampon or pad when the bladder is filled in a retrograde manner with diluted methylene blue or indigo carmine may facilitate the diagnosis of a VVF. However, additional evaluation is required to determine the extent, location, and/or course of the fistula.

Creatinine levels in the collected fluid are checked to confirm suspected extravasation of urine and thereby increasing the suspicion of urinary tract injury.[12]

A *three swab test* (**Fig. 2**) can be done with the most colored swab suggesting the

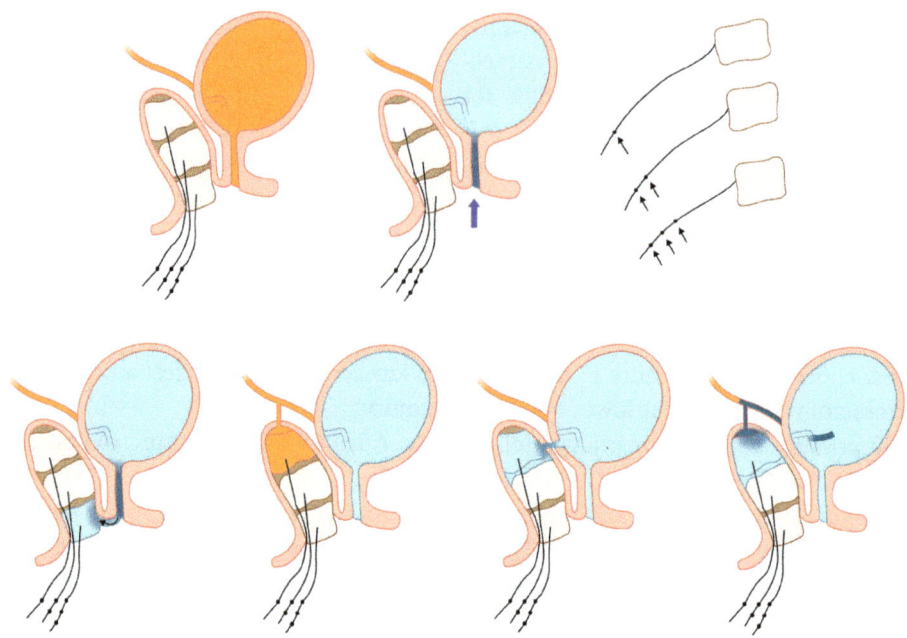

Fig. 2: Three swab test.

presumed location and origin of fistula (proximal, mid or distal vagina).[13] The patient is asked to take oral phenazopyridine three times a day and the bladder is simultaneously filled with methylene blue to differentiate between VVF and ureterovaginal fistula.[14]

Three swabs are placed in the vagina, one above the other, followed by retrograde filling of the bladder with diluted and sterilized methylene blue. Patients are asked to walk around or perform Valsalva maneuver. The swabs are examined for any staining after 15 minutes. Discoloration of lowest swab would suggest a low urethral fistula or back flow from the introitus. Discoloration of the topmost swab indicates a VVF. If the top swab is wet without blue staining, then it indicates a ureterovaginal fistula.

INVESTIGATIONS

Additional tests include performing an examination under anesthesia and performing urethroscopy and cystoscopy to establish the

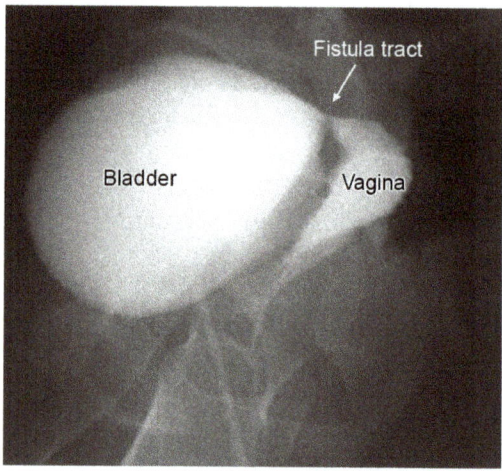

Fig. 3: Voiding cystography demonstrating contrast in the vagina.

diagnosis of fistula along with number and location of fistula in relation to the trigone of the bladder.

Radiologic imaging found to be useful are cystography, urography (ante or retrograde), intravenous urography **(Fig. 3)** and CT urography **(Figs. 4A and B)**.

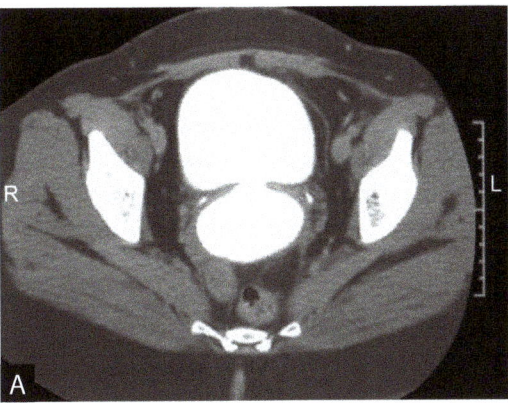
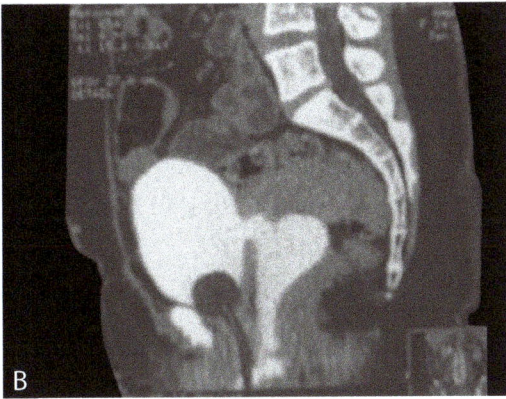

Figs. 4A and B: CT intravenous urography demonstrating contrast in the vagina.

Depending upon availability, MRI with T2 weighting provides optimal diagnostic information regarding fistula associated with pelvic malignancy, however contrast-enhanced CT with late excretory phase is an acceptable alternative.[15]

Performing cystoscopy during the episodes of menouria will help diagnose uterovesical fistula, in addition, simultaneous hysteroscopy or hysterography can be helpful in establishing the location and the size of the fistula.

FISTULA CLASSIFICATION SYSTEMS

Many classifications systems have been reported and mainly developed to classify of obstetric fistula (OF). However, the most common types used are World Health Organization (WHO), Waaldijk and Goh systems. All these systems are based on outcomes of repair which are in turn dependent on the size of the fistula, extent of involvement of urethral closure system, scarring, and length of vagina.

For iatrogenic fistula, the classification is highly variable. OF classifications can be used for iatrogenic fistula, however, use of simple WHO classification is recommended **(Table 1)**.

TABLE 1: WHO classification.[16]

Simple fistula with good prognosis	Complex fistula with uncertain prognosis
• Single fistula < 4 cm • Closing mechanism not involved • No circumferential defect • Minimal tissue loss • Ureters not involved • First attempt to repair	• Fistula > 4 cm • Multiple fistulae • RVF, mixed fistulae, cervical fistula • Closing mechanism involved • Scarring • Circumferential defect • Extensive tissue loss • Involves ureters • Failed previous repair • Radiation fistula

(RVF: rectovaginal fistula)

Waaldijk's Classification System[17]

- *Type 1*: >4 cm away from the urethral meatus
- *Type 2*: 0.5–4 cm from the urethral meatus
  - *2A*: 1–4 cm
  - *2B*: 0.5–1 cm with involvement of urethral closure mechanism
- *Type 3*: All other types of fistula, based on the size of the fistula, they are categorized as:
  - *Small*: <2 cm
  - *Medium*: 2–3 cm
  - *Large*: 4–5 cm
  - *Extensive*: >6 cm

Goh's Classification System[18]
- *Type 1*: >3.5 cm from urethral meatus and no involvement of urethra
- *Type 2*: 2.5–3.5 cm with involvement of proximal urethra
- *Type 3*: 1.5–2.5 cm with involvement of mid urethra
- *Type 4*: <1.5 cm with involvement of mid and distal urethra

Size
- *Type a*: <1.5 cm
- *Type b*: 1.5–3 cm
- *Type c*: >3 cm

Scarring
- None or mild fibrosis with vaginal length > 6 cm, normal caliber of vagina
- Moderate or severe fibrosis, reduced vaginal length or reduced caliber
- Special consideration, e.g., post-radiation, ureteric involvement, circumferential fistula, previous repair

TREATMENT

Conservative Treatment

Spontaneous closure of genital tract fistulae is an exception rather than a rule. Provided the natural outflow is not obstructed before epithelization is complete, the abnormal communication to the viscera will close.

Indwelling catheter drainage should be continued in women who see a progressive reduction in urine leak until to a point of no leakage. Patients with ongoing, continuous vaginal leakage despite a functioning indwelling catheter are unlikely to heal and therefore, must proceed with more definitive repair as soon as medically appropriate, sparing prolonged catheter drainage.

Success of indwelling catheter depends on various factors such as size of fistula, period between injury and initiation of therapy, duration of bladder drainage and mechanism of injury.

Smaller fistulae are known to be successfully managed with indwelling catheters. Sooner insertion and leaving the catheter in situ for at least 2 weeks after the leaking has stopped, is found to have a successful outcome. Injuries secondary to malignancy, radiotherapy, and significant electrical burns will not heal with routine catheterization.

According to Bazi et al., fistula size less than 1 cm secondary to iatrogenic injury is more likely to close spontaneously.[19] Spontaneous healing of obstetric fistulae has been reported in up to 28% of cases in women managed with indwelling catheterization[20] and 13% spontaneous closure rate among surgical fistula group.[2] Patients asymptomatic with small distal urethrovaginal fistulae, uterovesical fistulae with menouria, colovesical fistulae associated with diverticular disease and some low rectovaginal fistula do not require treatment **(Flowchart 1)**.

Medical Treatment

Successful closure of fistula has been reported following amenorrhea due to estrogen, estrogen/progesterone combinations, or luteinizing hormone releasing hormone analogs especially in uretero or vesicouterine fistula following cesarean section. This probably would be successful with a small fistula.

Surgical Treatment

The International Federation of Gynaecology and Obstetrics (FIGO) with the International Society of Obstetric Fistula Surgeon (ISOFS) have created a competency based fistula surgical training manual.

Principles of surgery: The most important principle of fistula repair is to provide a tension-free and watertight closure by an experienced

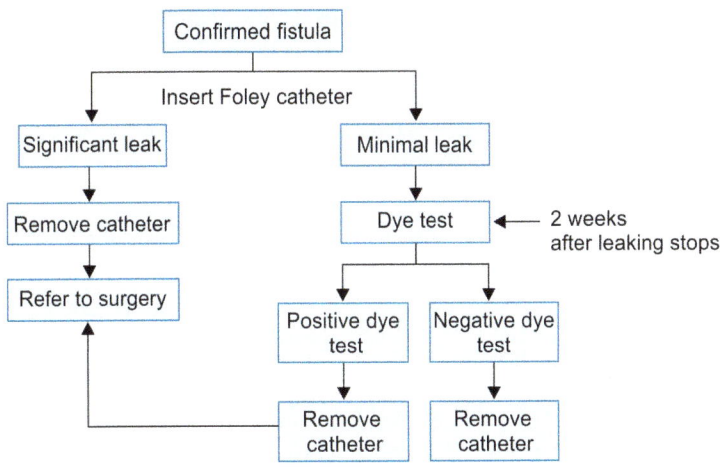

Flowchart 1: Initial management pathway of urinary fistula.

surgeon and the surgical route should be the one that provides the best possible chance of closure at the first attempt. Important steps to be undertaken include adequate mobilization of the bladder from the cervix or vagina. Aim to achieve anatomical apposition to prevent distortion and reduce stricture.

Timing of surgery: The most contentious issue in fistula repair is deciding appropriate timing for surgical repair of fistulae. The advocacy of early intervention groups is to minimize the distress due to continuing urinary leakage. To optimize the outcomes, the delayed intervention groups advocate repair until resolution of inflammation, tissue necrosis, or infection.

According to the data analyzed by De Ridder et al., there is no difference in the outcomes between the early and delayed repair (91% ± 6% vs. 90% ± 27%).[2] However, the majority of surgeons advocate repair after 12 weeks and 12 months post radiation. The exception to this rule is when the fistula is diagnosed within 2 days after surgery, ureteric obstruction in the presence of sepsis, renal failure, or a unilateral kidney, vesicouterine fistulas presenting with severe abdominal pain.

Route of Surgery

The route depends on the characteristics of the fistula and experience of the surgeon. Vaginal, abdominal, abdomino-vaginal, laparoscopic or vesicoscopic approaches have been described.

Most fistulas can be managed vaginally, different techniques have been described and the most commonly used technique is repair in layers or "flap-splitting".[21] Classical saucerization technique described by Sims[22] and subsequently modified as a partial colpocleisis by Latzko[23] has been used in isolation or in combination.

The abdominal route is usually preferred in women with high fistulae inaccessible vaginally, ureteric injury requiring reimplantation or simultaneous VVF and ureterovaginal fistula repair or needing to perform augmentation cystoplasty at the same time. There seems to be no difference in the success rates based on the route of surgery. De Ridder et al. review showed 89% (vaginal) versus 87% (abdominal) success and 93% (transvesical) versus 89% (transperitoneal).[2]

Approach to the fistula transvesically has the advantage of being entirely extraperitoneal.

A transperitoneal repair is relatively uncommonly employed. However, some prefer this technique during laparoscopic approach and this approach also has the advantage to use interposition flaps. The reported success rate of laparoscopic transvesical and extravesical approach were 95.89% and 98.04%.[24]

The laparoscopic approach has an overall cure rate of 92%[2] with advantages of decreased morbidity and a more rapid recovery. Robotic approach has been shown to have a cure rate of 100%[2] with advantages including three-dimensional visualization, increased dexterity, and easier intracorporeal knot tying. Transurethral endoscopic suturing technique described by Mackay showed a cure rate of 80%.[2]

Repeat surgery to repair fistula has been shown to have poor outcomes with success rates falling from 81% for first procedures to 65% for those requiring two or more procedures in obstetric fistula.[25] Similar trend has been observed in surgical fistula.[26]

A randomized controlled trial (RCT) showed no difference in the outcomes based on non-trimming or trimming (75% vs. 67.6%) the edges, suggesting that not trimming would lead to smaller size fistula as a recurrence.[27]

Use of fibrin glue has been reported for the treatment of fistulae. The reported success rate is 77%,[2] however, the indications and selection criteria is not defined and therefore would need to be used on a case by case basis.

Tissue flaps for the repair of fistula is used when managing recurrent fistula related to radiotherapy, ischemic or obstetric fistula, large fistula, and a difficult or weak closure due to poor tissue quality. Tissue flaps that have been used are, labial pad of fat (Martius flap) or a peritoneal flap for transvaginal approach and greater omentum is used for abdominal approach. Other types of flaps that have been reported to be used are gracilis muscle, seromuscular intestinal flaps, rectus abdominis flaps and free grafts of bladder mucosa.[2]

POSTOPERATIVE MANAGEMENT

There is a need for free drainage of urine after the surgery to aid healing of the repaired fistula. The standard practice is to have both urethral as well as suprapubic catheter.[26] The aim of two catheters is to potentially avoid blockage of one of the catheters which can have a detrimental effect on the outcome of fistula repair.

There is no consensus on the duration of bladder drainage following repair, however, according to a survey of obstetric fistula surgeons, standard duration used was 12 days (range 5-21 days); for "large" fistula was 17 days (range 0-30 days); and for "difficult" fistulae, was 21 days (range 14-42 days).[28]

COMPLICATIONS

The complications of fistula repair include:
- Persistence or recurrence of urinary incontinence
- Persistence or occurrence of newer lower urinary tract symptoms, including OAB and stress urinary incontinence
- Wound infection, urinary tract infections (UTI), pyelonephritis and urosepsis
- Ureteric obstruction
- Outlet obstruction
- Bladder contracture
- Vaginal stenosis
- Sexual dysfunction due to dyspareunia
- Granulomas or diverticulum formation
- Complex neuropathic bladder dysfunction and urethral sphincter incompetence
- Psychological trauma
- Infertility

MANAGEMENT

Management of Uterovesical Fistula

The treatment is surgical. Classically a transperitoneal approach will be used, where the plane between bladder and uterus will be developed, the fistula closed and eventually interposition material will be used. The outcome of the surgery is very good. A multidisciplinary approach is advocated to prevent infertility.[29]

Management of Ureteric Fistula

Any identified intraoperative injury should be repaired immediately by an experienced team following the principles of adequate debridement, ensuring blood supply with tension free anastomosis along with establishing drainage using stents.

Initial conservative management with nephrostomy and/or stenting where available and plan surgical repair (early <3 months) or delayed (>6 months).[7] Stenting of ureters following an injury has shown a cure rate of 50% ± 18%.[2] Most commonly, retrograde stenting is performed. However, in cases with difficult retrograde stenting, antegrade stenting with or without nephrostomy or a combination of both techniques can be performed to achieve successful stenting.

If endoluminal techniques fail or result in secondary stricture, the abdominal approach to repair is standard and may require end-to-end anastomosis, reimplantation into the bladder using psoas hitch or Boari flap or replacement with bowel segments with or without reconfiguration.

Routine stenting of ureters prior to hysterectomy is not recommended as there is no difference in the risk of injury with or without stenting.[30] According to an American cost-effectiveness analysis, use of routine ureteric catheterization will be useful when the risk of injury is >3.5%.[31]

Management of Urethrovaginal Fistula

Surgery is offered to women based on the impact on quality of life. Women with distal one-third fistula can avoid surgery as they may be asymptomatic. Vaginal approach, with the same principles of VVF repair, has shown to achieve success up to 90% at first intervention and subsequent improvement following second intervention.[32] Risk of persisting incontinence or de novo stress incontinence is seen in up to 52% of women following the repair.[32]

For a complex fistula, in addition to primary closure, additional techniques of using vaginal flaps, labial pedicle skin flaps, Martius graft (labial bulbocavernosus muscle/fat flap), pedicled rectus abdominis muscle flap and rarely use of rectus fascia sling, omentum (abdominal approach), gracilis muscle or porcine dermis will be needed.

Following the repair, complications that have been reported include fistula recurrence, urethral shortening and retraction, persistent reflux, bladder calculi and bladder cancer.[33]

PREVENTION

Injury to urinary tract is a risk associated with surgery in the pelvis, however, the injury can be mitigated by having a better understanding of anatomy of the renal tract, screening and using strategies to identify or screen women who have risk factors of injury.

CONCLUSION

Urinary tract injury is associated with significant long-term sequelae leading to devastating consequences. Identification and appropriate management with a skilled multidisciplinary team will help to mitigate the consequences. However, prevention of injury by having a high degree of suspicion and undertaking steps to recognize and initiate timely correct management will have better short- and long-term outcomes in women with urinary tract injuries.

REFERENCES

1. Sharma S, Rizvi SJ, Bethur SS, Bansal J, Qadri SJ, Modi P. Laparoscopic repair of urogenital fistulae: a single centre experience. J Minim Access Surg. 2014;10(4):180-4.
2. De Ridder D, Mourad M, Stanford E, Ioposso M, Muleta M, Badlani G, et al. Fistula. In: Abrams LP, Wagg A, Wein A (Eds). Incontinence. Bristol: ICS; 2017. p. 40.
3. Forsgren C, Altman D. Risk of pelvic organ fistula in patients undergoing hysterectomy. Curr Opin Obstet Gynecol. 2010;22(5):404-7.
4. Harkki-Siren P, Sjoberg J, Tiitinen A. Urinary tract injuries after hysterectomy. Obstet Gynecol. 1998;92(1):113-8.
5. Hilton P, Cromwell DA. The risk of vesicovaginal and urethrovaginal fistula after hysterectomy performed in the English National Health Service—a retrospective cohort study examining patterns of care between 2000 and 2008. BJOG. 2012;119(12):1447-54.
6. Kiran A, Hilton P, Cromwell DA. The risk of ureteric injury associated with hysterectomy: a 10-year retrospective cohort study. BJOG. 2016;123(7):1184-91.
7. Brandes S, Coburn M, Armenakas N, McAninch J. Diagnosis and management of ureteric injury: an evidence-based analysis. BJU Int. 2004;94(3):277-89.
8. Kucera H, Skodler W, Weghaupt K. Complications of postoperative radiotherapy in uterine cancer. Geburtshilfe Frauenheilkd. 1984;44(8):498-502.
9. Rao MP, Dwivedi US, Datta B, Vyas N, Nandy PR, Trivedi S, et al. Post caesarean vesicouterine fistulae—Youssef syndrome: our experience and review of published work. ANZ J Surg. 2006;76(4):243-5.
10. Kochakarn W, Pummangura W. A new dimension in vesicovaginal fistula management: an 8-year experience at Ramathibodi hospital. Asian J Surg. 2007;30(4):267-71.
11. Kursh ED, Morse RM, Resnick MI, Persky L. Prevention of the development of a vesicovaginal fistula. Surg Gynecol Obstet. 1988;166(5):409-12.
12. Kruger PS, Whiteside RS. Pseudo-renal failure following the delayed diagnosis of bladder perforation after diagnostic laparoscopy. Anaesth Intens Care. 2003;31(2):211-3.
13. Gannon MJ. The three swab test using knots for urovaginal fistula. Surg Gynecol Obstet. 1990;170(2):171.
14. O'Brien, WM, Lynch JH. Simplification of double-dye test to diagnose various types of vaginal fistulas. Urology. 1990;36(5):456.
15. Narayanan P, Nobbenhuis M, Reynolds KM, Sahdev A, Reznek RH, Rockall AG. Fistulas in malignant gynecologic disease: etiology, imaging, and management. Radiographics. 2009;29(4):1073-83.
16. de Bernis L. Obstetric fistula: guiding principles for clinical management and programme development, a new WHO guideline. Int J Gynaecol Obstet. 2007;99(Suppl 1):S117-21.
17. Waaldijk K. Surgical classification of obstetric fistulas. Int J Gynaecol Obstet. 1995;49(2):161-3.
18. Goh JT. A new classification for female genital tract fistula. Aust NZJ Obstet Gynaecol. 2004;44(6):502-4.
19. Bazi T. Spontaneous closure of vesicovaginal fistulas after bladder drainage alone: review of the evidence. Int Urogynecol J Pelvic Floor Dysfunct. 2007;18(3):329-33.
20. Waaldijk K. Immediate indwelling bladder catheterization at postpartum urine leakage-personal experience of 1200 patients. Trop Doct. 1997;27(4):227-8.
21. Wall LL. Dr. George Hayward (1791-1863): a forgotten pioneer of reconstructive pelvic surgery. Int Urogynecol J Pelvic Floor Dysfunct. 2005;16(5):330-3.
22. Sims JM. On the treatment of vesico-vaginal fistula. 1852. Int Urogynecol J Pelvic Floor Dysfunc. 1998;9(4):236-48.
23. Latzko W. Postoperative vesicovaginal fistulas. Am J Surg. 2004;58(2):17.
24. Miklos JR, Moore RD, Chinthakanan O. Laparoscopic and robotic-assisted vesicovaginal fistula repair: a systematic review of the literature. J Minim Invas Gynecol. 2015;22(5):727-36.
25. Hilton P, Ward A. Epidemiological and surgical aspects of urogenital fistulae: a review of 25 years' experience in Southeast Nigeria. Int Urogynecol J Pelvic Floor Dysfunct. 1998;9(4):189-94.
26. Hilton P. Urogenital fistula in the UK: a personal case series managed over 25 years. BJU Int. 2012;110(1):102-10.
27. Shaker H, Saafan A, Yassin M, Idrissa A, Mourad MS. Obstetric vesicovaginal fistula repair: should we trim the fistula edges? A randomized prospective study. Neurourol Urodyn. 2011;30(3):302-5.
28. Arrowsmith SD, Ruminjo R, Landry EG. Current practices in treatment of female genital fistula: a cross sectional study. BMC Pregnancy Childbirth. 2010;10:73.

29. Wiedemann A, Karroum S, Kociszewski J, Fabian G, Füsgen I. The uterovesical fistula–report of a rare cause of incontinence and review of the literature. Aktuelle Urol. 2014; 45(1):48-9.
30. Chou MT, Wang CJ, Lien RC. Prophylactic ureteral catheterization in gynecologic surgery: a 12-year randomized trial in a community hospital. Int Urogynecol J Pelvic Floor Dysfunct. 2009;20(6):689-93.
31. Schimpf MO, Gottenger EE, Wagner JR. Universal ureteral stent placement at hysterectomy to identify ureteral injury: a decision analysis. BJOG. 2008;115(9):1151-8.
32. Pushkar DY, Dyakov VV, Kosko JW, Kasyan GR. Management of urethrovaginal fistulas. Eur Urol. 2006;50(5):1000-5.
33. Tehan TJ, Nardi JA, Baker R, Complications associated with surgical repair of urethrovaginal fistula. Urology. 1980;15(1):31-5.

CHAPTER 22

Genital Prolapse

Manish Machave

"Our strength grows out of our weakness."
—Ralph Waldo

INTRODUCTION

Pelvic organ prolapse (POP) is a major public health issue that will continue to grow due to the increasing proportion of ageing population as a result of better overall geriatric care. There is a pressing need to better understand its pathogenesis, not only for its treatment but also for its prevention. Proper diagnosis is the first step toward achieving these goals.

This chapter aims to highlight the understanding of the Pelvic Organ Prolapse Quantification (POP-Q) system and its evolution, relevant anatomy, and application for management approach. It also encompasses its limitations and need for improvisation.

PELVIC ORGAN PROLAPSE BURDEN

Pelvic organ prolapse affects 50% of parous women with a 10–20% lifetime risk for surgical repair. In actuality, the true prevalence is difficult to ascertain because of different classification systems, symptomatic versus asymptomatic, etc. However, worldwide prevalence is 3–6% based on symptoms and 41–50% based on clinical findings. In low-income countries, mean prevalence is 19.7% (3.4–56.4%).

Nulliparous prolapse is seen in 2% and vault prolapse in 0.5%.

ETIOLOGY OF PELVIC ORGAN PROLAPSE

The most important etiological factors in POP are atonicity and asthenia that follow menopause. Some women experience minor degrees of POP soon after childbirth but in majority of patients, this can be improved with pelvic floor exercises.

Birth injury in the form of excessive stretching and prolonged bearing down can lead to prolapse, while a perineal tear rarely leads to POP.

RISK FACTORS FOR PELVIC ORGAN PROLAPSE

The risk factors for POP have been described in **Box 1**.

SYMPTOMS OF PELVIC ORGAN PROLAPSE

Symptoms associated with prolapse are often difficult to correlate with the anatomical site or severity of the "bulge" and are often nonspecific.[1]

BOX 1: Risk factors for pelvic organ prolapse (POP).

Nulliparous prolapse:
- Spina bifida occulta and split pelvis
- Congenital weakness of pelvic floor muscles

Risk factors in multipara:
- Pudendal nerve injury during childbirth
- Ventouse extraction before full cervical dilatation
- Crede's method of placental extraction
- Delivery of big baby
- Short interpregnancy intervals
- Raised intra-abdominal pressure due to chronic cough, large tumors, obesity
- Abdominoperineal resection of rectum and radical vulvectomy

Genital Prolapse

The common symptoms of POP have been described in **Box 2**.

TYPES OF PELVIC ORGAN PROLAPSE

Types of POP have been shown in **Box 3** and **Figures 1 to 4**.

BOX 2: Common symptoms of pelvic organ prolapse.
- Sensation of a "lump" or vaginal "heaviness"
- Recurrent irritative bladder symptoms
- Voiding difficulty, incontinence or defecatory difficulty and low back or pelvic pain, decubitus ulcer, infection, discharge
- Sensation of laxity of vagina by patient or sexual partner
- Rectal symptoms are infrequent and constipation is rare

BOX 3: Types of pelvic organ prolapse.
- *Anterior vaginal wall*:
  - Upper two-thirds—cystocele
  - Lower one-third—urethrocele
- *Posterior vaginal wall*:
  - Upper one-third—enterocele
  - Lower two-thirds—rectocele
- *Uterine descent*:
  - First-degree—descent of cervix in the vagina
  - Second-degree—descent of cervix up to introitus
  - Third-degree—descent of cervix outside the introitus
  - Procidentia—entire uterus outside the introitus

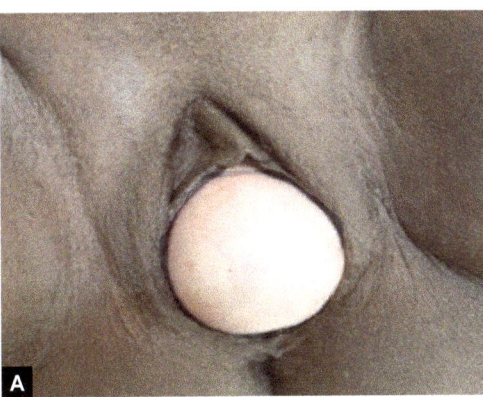
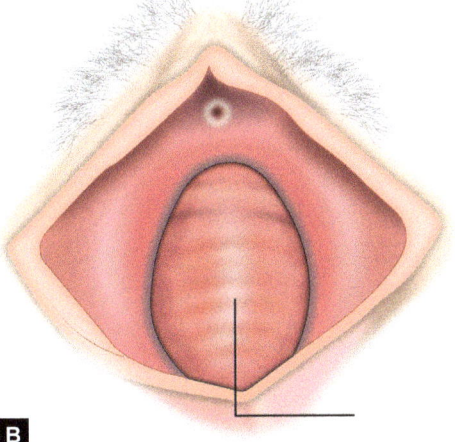

Figs. 1A and B: Anterior vaginal wall prolapse.

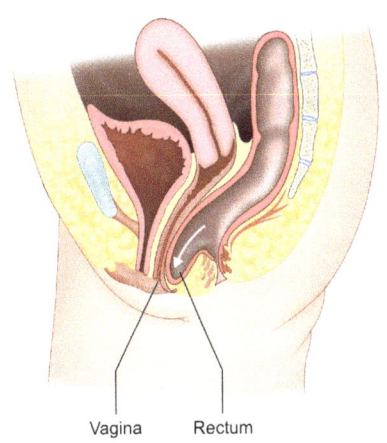
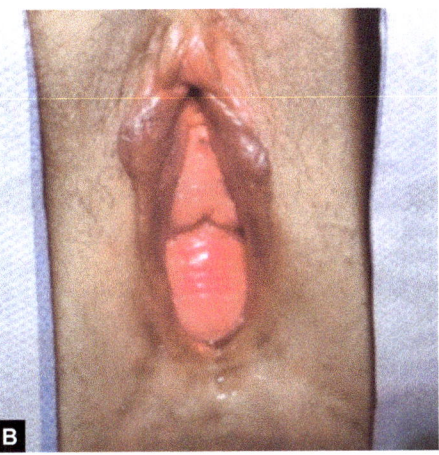

Figs. 2A and B: Posterior vaginal wall prolapse.

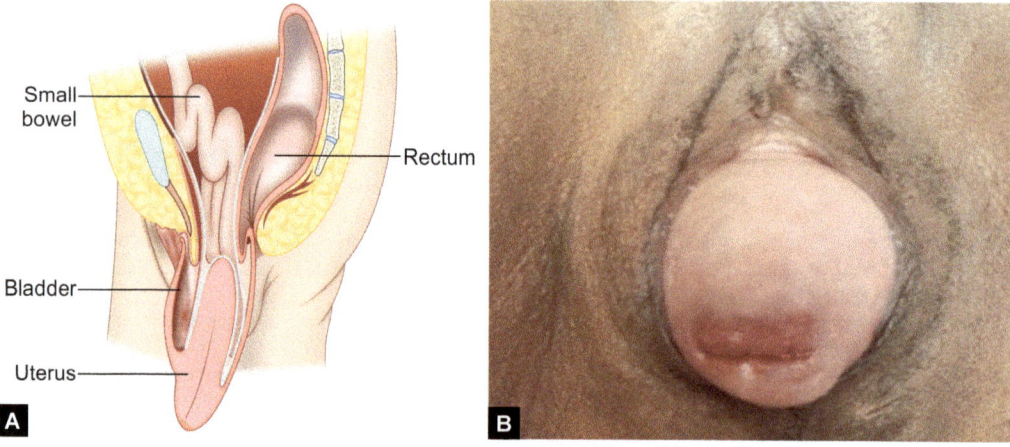

Figs. 3A and B: Apical prolapse.

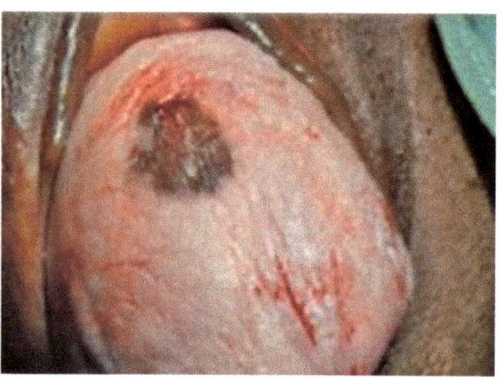

Fig. 4: Vault prolapse.

Figs. 5A and B: Pelvic floor map.

EVOLUTION OF CLASSIFICATION SYSTEMS FOR PELVIC ORGAN PROLAPSE

One of the main problems concerning the prolapse of pelvic organs is the need for a universal, clear, and reliable staging method.

Common method is depending on the degree of anatomical deformity and depending on the site of the defect and the presumed pelvic viscera that are involved. The terms "anterior vaginal wall prolapse," "posterior vaginal wall prolapse," and "apical prolapse" are often preferred because of the uncertainty as to the anatomical structures on the other side of the vaginal bulge.

The Baden–Walker Halfway Scoring System (1972)

Figures 5A and B depicts the map of pelvic floor according to this scoring system. The system has shortcomings in that it tends to oversimplify the staging and adversely affect the management. A small increase in prolapse results in an increase in the assigned stage.

In addition, interobserver agreement is not perfect with the Baden–Walker system.

Classification of Vault Prolapse

- *First-degree:* Vaginal apex is visible when perineum is depressed.

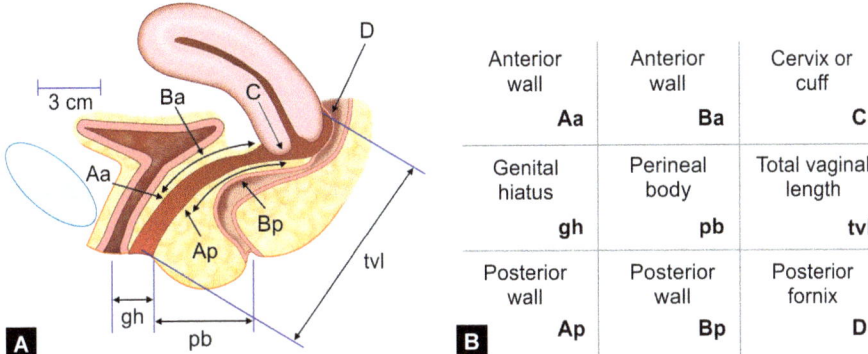

Figs. 6A and B: Pelvic Organ Prolapse Quantification (POP-Q) examination.

- *Second-degree:* Apex extends just through the introitus.
- *Third-degree:* Upper two-thirds of vagina is outside the introitus.
- *Fourth-degree:* Whole vagina is outside the introitus.

Pelvic Organ Prolapse Quantification System (1996)

In an effort to create an encoding tool useful to both the clinician and researcher, the Standardization Subcommittee of the International Continence Society created the POP-Q system in 2002.[2] Detailing of the grid can be complicated and time consuming; but regular incorporation into practice has known to reduce the time for POP-Q examination from 3.7 to 2 minutes per patient **(Figs. 6A and B)**.[3]

INVESTIGATIONS AND DIAGNOSIS

The key in diagnosis of prolapse lies in a systematic and thorough examination.

Examination should be performed with an empty bladder. A full bladder is potentially associated with underestimation of the POP-Q severity.

Any position that best demonstrates the maximum extent of the prolapse and which can be confirmed by the woman, by digital palpation or use of a mirror, should be used (left lateral, standing, lithotomy, or standing).

BOX 4: Examination of pelvic organ prolapse.
- Vulva—perineal laceration
- Genital hiatus—dimensions
- Perineal body and levator muscles for tone and dimensions of hiatus urogenitalis
- Tests to elicit urinary incontinence
- Speculum examination to quantify prolapse
- Cervical cytology
- Adnexal mass/size of uterus and mobility
- Superficial and deep perineal reflexes
- Thorough general and systemic examination for fitness for surgery

Use a Sims' speculum if necessary to retract the anterior and posterior vaginal walls to assess for prolapse. **Box 4** depicts the systematic examination of POP.

Along with relevant preoperative investigations, an ultrasound of the pelvis is done to rule out associated uterine/adnexal pathology and hydroureteronephrosis due to long-standing prolapse. A perineal ultrasound helps in exact assessment of points of detachment.

The minimal investigations for POP have been described in **Box 5**.

DIFFERENTIAL DIAGNOSIS

- Vulval cyst or tumor
- Cyst of anterior vaginal wall
- Urethral diverticula
- Congenital elongation of cervix
- Chronic uterine inversion
- Fibroid or polyp
- Rectal prolapse

PROPHYLAXIS OF PELVIC ORGAN PROLAPSE

- Antenatal physiotherapy/correction of anemia/due attention to weight gain
- Proper management of labor—timely and adequate episiotomy, low forceps delivery, anatomic repair of perineal tears
- Postnatal exercises/early ambulation
- Increasing interpregnancy interval
- Hormone replacement therapy (HRT) to menopausal women

MANAGEMENT OF PELVIC ORGAN PROLAPSE

- Postnatal POP—conservative management for 4–6 months
- Pregnant woman/postnatal women/women not willing for surgery—pessary treatment
- Women who want to retain uterus—apical suspension procedures
    - Isolated cervical elongation: Fothergill's repair (Manchester operation) or Shirodkar's operation
- Women with childbearing over—Ward Mayo's hysterectomy
- Elderly women in whom sexual activity is not required—colpocleisis/Le Fort's operation and modifications

Adjunctive Management of POP

Changes in diet and lifestyle may help relieve some symptoms. If a woman is overweight or obese, weight loss can help improve her overall health and prevent worsening her prolapse symptoms. In patients with chronic cough and chronic constipation, treatment of these aggravating factors will prevent upstaging the prolapse.

Asymptomatic patient with stage I and II prolapse and desirous of conservative treatment should be advised to abstain from aggravating conditions (heavy weight lifting, coughing, constipation, excess weight gain, etc.), employ use of Kegel's exercises and pessary treatment.

Pessary Treatment of POP

Ring pessary, made up of plastic polyvinyl chloride, is available in various sizes. Pessary treatment is now to be offered to patients having other comorbidities and pose a risk or contraindication for surgery and those with short vaginal length and previous vaginal surgery.

Limitations of pessary treatment of POP have been listed in **Box 6**.

PELVIC ORGAN PROLAPSE IN PREGNANCY

Conservative management and use of vaginal pessary are the most common modalities used for POP in pregnancy. Although in rare cases, laparoscopic uterine suspension and concomitant cesarean hysterectomy with abdominal sacrocolpopexy (SCP) have also been used.

When conservative management fails and prolonged bed rest is impossible, another treatment choice may be laparoscopic uterine

---

BOX 5: Preoperative investigations.

- Complete blood count (CBC)
- Urine—routine and microscopy (R/M)-culture and sensitivity (C/S) if infection is present
- Blood urea nitrogen (BUN) and blood sugar level (BSL)
- Chest x-ray, ultrasonography (USG) and electrocardiography (ECG)
- High vaginal swab in cases of vaginitis

BOX 6: Limitations of pessary treatment of pelvic organ prolapse.

- It is never curative, only palliative
- It can cause vaginitis
- There is a chance of slippage
- Not useful if vagina is patulous
- Forgotten pessary is associated with ulcers and sometimes cancer of vagina
- It rarely treats urinary incontinence

suspension during early pregnancy. This procedure should be performed in experienced hands since several failed laparoscopic uterine suspension cases have been reported.[4]

PREOPERATIVE TREATMENT

- Treatment of urinary infection
- Local estrogen cream for senile vaginitis which should be stopped a few days prior to surgery.
  - Identifying the aggravating factors if any and control them.
- Determine preoperatively whether lower urinary tract dysfunction and defecatory dysfunction coexist.

Surgical Decision-making for Symptomatic POP: Evidence-based Approach

Surgery is the mainstay of treatment for symptomatic POP. Epidemiologic studies have shown that women have an 11–19% risk of undergoing operation for POP during their lifetime,[5,6] and up to one-third of them undergo additional operation for disease recurrence.

Goal of treatment for POP is to:
- Alleviate symptoms
- Restore anatomical structure
- Restore/preserve sexual function

There are various vaginal and abdominal surgical approaches for the treatment of POP. Important considerations for deciding the type and route of surgery include the location and severity of prolapse, the nature of the symptoms (e.g., presence of urinary, bowel, or sexual dysfunction), the patient's general health, patient preference, and the surgeon's expertise. Surgical techniques for POP have been shown in **Table 1**.

The choice of treatment depends on symptoms severity, prolapse severity, and fertility desire. When deciding on the proper surgical procedure to be performed, the surgeon must take into consideration the individual patient's risk for surgical complication and prolapse recurrence and her preference.

Synthetic Mesh and Biologic Graft Materials in Vaginal POP Surgery

Suspension Procedures (Figs. 7 to 11)

Use material which is either synthetic material-mesh (polypropylene mesh) or a Graft—xenograft or allograft-harvested rectus fascia.

The US Food and Drug Administration (FDA) (April 2019) ordered manufacturers of synthetic mesh for POP to discontinue sale and distribution in the United States.

TABLE 1: Surgical techniques for pelvic organ prolapse.

Surgical technique	Compartment	Indication
Abdominal sacral colpopexy	Apical prolapse	Most commonly used in women with recurrent cystocele, vault prolapse, or enterocele
Uterosacral ligament suspension	Apical prolapse	Performed at the time of hysterectomy or in patients with posthysterectomy vaginal vault prolapse
Sacrospinous fixation	Apical/anterior vaginal wall prolapse	Performed at the time of hysterectomy or in patients with posthysterectomy vaginal vault prolapse
Anterior vaginal repair (anterior colporrhaphy)	Anterior vaginal wall prolapse	May be used for the treatment of prolapse of the bladder or urethra (bladder, urethra, or both herniate downward into the vagina)
Posterior vaginal repair (posterior colporrhaphy) and perineorrhaphy	Posterior vaginal wall prolapse	May be used for the treatment of rectocele (rectum bulges or herniates forward into the vagina), defects of the perineum, or both

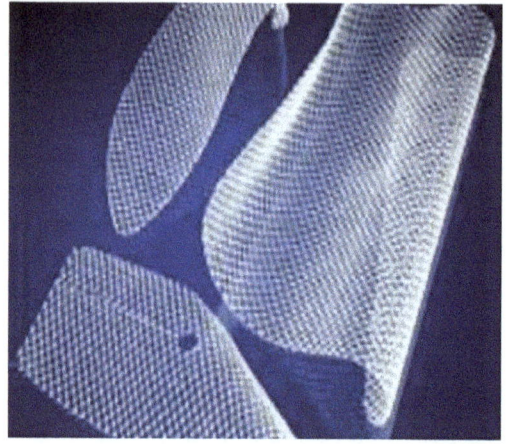

Fig. 7: Mesh.   Fig. 8: Pessary.

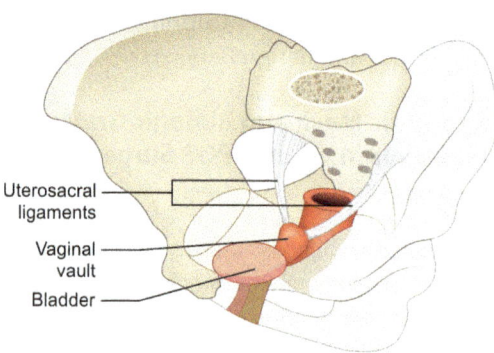 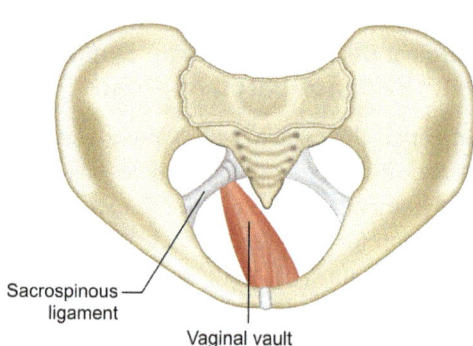

A *The prolapsed vaginal vault is attached to a ligament called the uterosacral ligament.*

B *The prolapsed vaginal vault is attached to the sacrospinous ligament on one side* (shown) *or both sides* (not shown).

Figs. 9A and B: Apical suspension procedures: (A) Uterosacral ligament suspension; (B) Sacrospinous colpopexy.

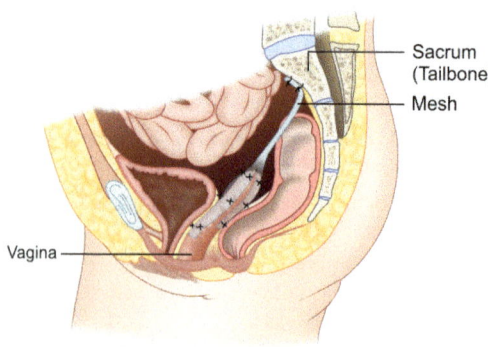 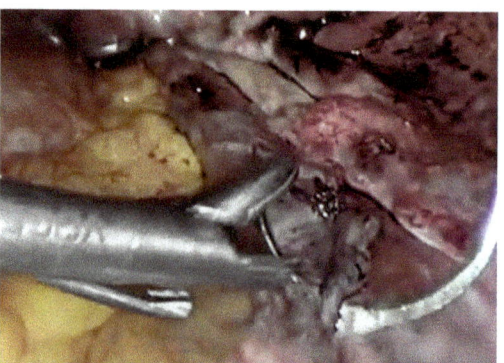

Fig. 10: Sacral colpopexy.   **Fig. 11:** Laparoscopic sacrocolpopexy.

This order applies to transvaginal mesh only and not transabdominal use for POP or stress urinary incontinence (SUI).

Vaginal prolapse repair:
- Both mesh and biologic grafts are associated with greater likelihood of repeat surgery for combined outcomes of prolapse, stress incontinence, or mesh exposure.
- Data on biologic grafts (e.g., cadaver) are limited and of low quality (most no longer available for use).

Posterior wall prolapse:
- Use of synthetic mesh or biologic grafts is associated with increased complications (mesh exposure) and no improvement in outcome.
- Mesh or grafts should not be used routinely in the primary repair of posterior wall prolapse.

Anterior wall prolapse:
- Biologic grafts show minimal/no difference in recurrence risk versus native tissue repair.
- Synthetic mesh improves anatomic outcome, but is associated with:
  - Increased risk of repeat surgery for prolapse, urinary incontinence, and mesh exposure
  - Longer operating times and greater blood loss
  - 11% risk of mesh erosion following anterior vaginal repair
  - 7% of cases that will require surgical correction
  - Dyspareunia rate of approximately 9%.

Use of mesh or biologic grafts should only be undertaken by surgeons who have training specific for these procedures. Training should include patient selection, anatomy, intraoperative and postoperative techniques, and treatment of any adverse outcomes. Routine intraoperative cystoscopy should be performed during POP surgery when there is risk to the bladder or ureter.

PROVIDING MECHANICAL SUPPORT

Anterior Colporrhaphy (Fig. 12A)

This procedure is done to repair cystocele and cystourethrocele. Pubovesicocervical fascia is used to support the weakness in anterior vaginal wall after dissecting bladder away. Kelly's stitch was taken for SUI, which is now obsolete.

Posterior Colpoperineorrhaphy (Fig. 12B)

Procedure done to repair rectocele and enterocele is culdoplasty.

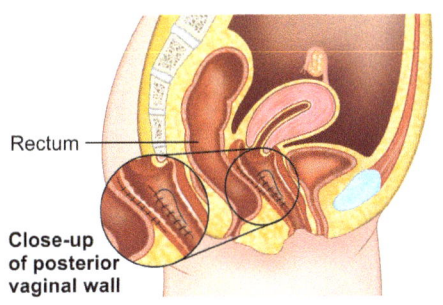
A. The posterior wall of the vagina is strengthened with stitches so that it once again supports the rectum.

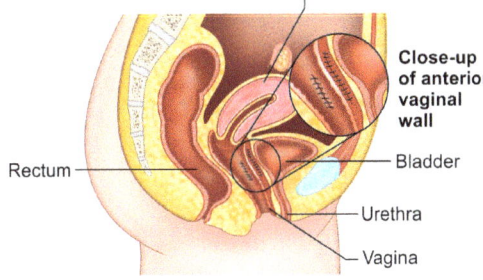
B. The anterior wall of the vagina is strengthened with stitches so that it once again supports the bladder.

Figs. 12A and B: (A) Anterior colporrhaphy; (B) Posterior colporrhaphy.

McCall culdoplasty: A wedge of posterior vaginal wall and peritoneum is removed. Enterocele sac is freed and excised. Two internal sutures (permanent) placed approximately using both uterosacral ligament (USL) and peritoneum. One external suture is taken through the USL and posterior peritoneum and brought out through the posterior vaginal wall. This obliterates cul-de-sac, supports vaginal apex, and lengthens posterior vaginal wall.

Obliterative Procedures (Figs. 13 to 15)

- Le Fort's colpocleisis
- Goodall-Power modification of Le Fort's colpocleisis—for sexually active females

RECONSTRUCTIVE VERSUS OBLITERATIVE SURGERY

If a woman has an isolated anterior or posterior vaginal wall prolapse without apical prolapse, surgical decision-making is easy. Traditional anterior or posterior colporrhaphy can be performed to treat this condition. The choice depends on the medical condition and sexual function of the patient. Reconstructive surgery corrects the prolapse while restoring the normal vaginal anatomy, whereas obliterative surgery does so by closing off the vaginal canal either partly (Le Fort's colpocleisis) or totally (total colpocleisis).[7]

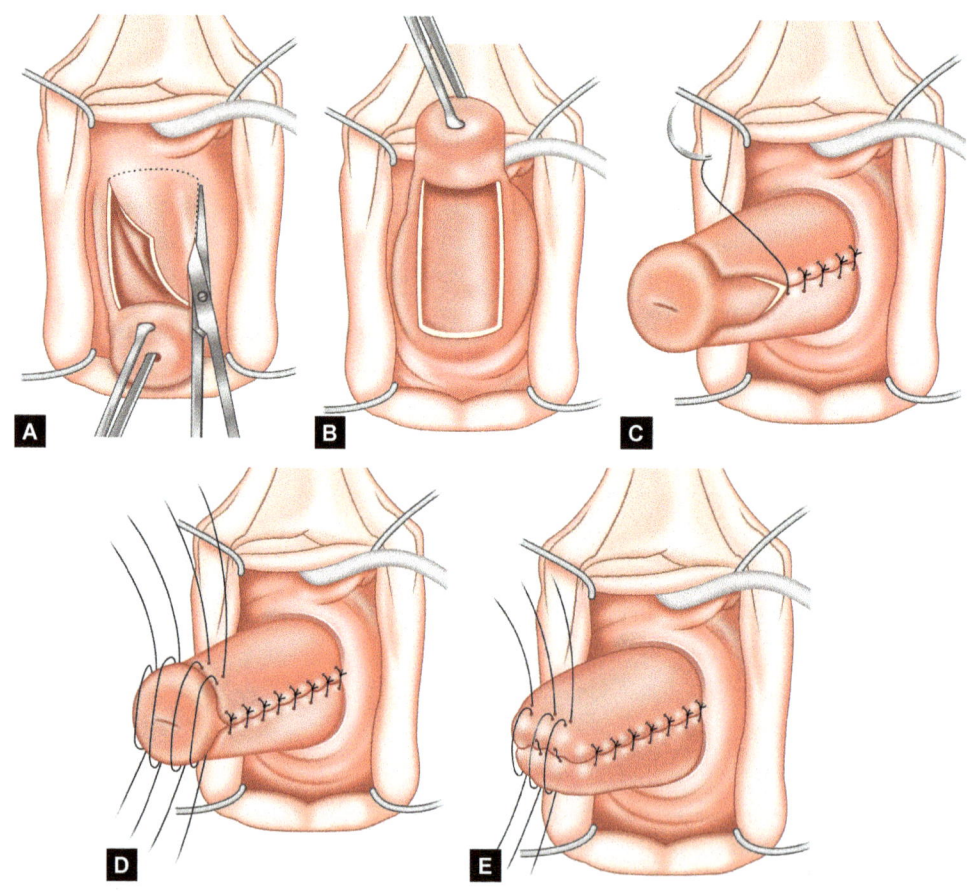

Figs. 13A and E: Colpocleisis.

This order applies to transvaginal mesh only and not transabdominal use for POP or stress urinary incontinence (SUI).

Vaginal prolapse repair:
- Both mesh and biologic grafts are associated with greater likelihood of repeat surgery for combined outcomes of prolapse, stress incontinence, or mesh exposure.
- Data on biologic grafts (e.g., cadaver) are limited and of low quality (most no longer available for use).

Posterior wall prolapse:
- Use of synthetic mesh or biologic grafts is associated with increased complications (mesh exposure) and no improvement in outcome.
- Mesh or grafts should not be used routinely in the primary repair of posterior wall prolapse.

Anterior wall prolapse:
- Biologic grafts show minimal/no difference in recurrence risk versus native tissue repair.
- Synthetic mesh improves anatomic outcome, but is associated with:
  - Increased risk of repeat surgery for prolapse, urinary incontinence, and mesh exposure
  - Longer operating times and greater blood loss
  - 11% risk of mesh erosion following anterior vaginal repair
  - 7% of cases that will require surgical correction
  - Dyspareunia rate of approximately 9%.

Use of mesh or biologic grafts should only be undertaken by surgeons who have training specific for these procedures. Training should include patient selection, anatomy, intraoperative and postoperative techniques, and treatment of any adverse outcomes. Routine intraoperative cystoscopy should be performed during POP surgery when there is risk to the bladder or ureter.

PROVIDING MECHANICAL SUPPORT

Anterior Colporrhaphy (Fig. 12A)

This procedure is done to repair cystocele and cystourethrocele. Pubovesicocervical fascia is used to support the weakness in anterior vaginal wall after dissecting bladder away. Kelly's stitch was taken for SUI, which is now obsolete.

Posterior Colpoperineorrhaphy (Fig. 12B)

Procedure done to repair rectocele and enterocele is culdoplasty.

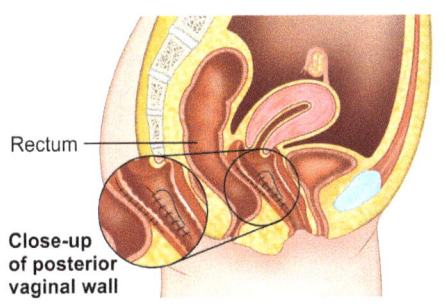

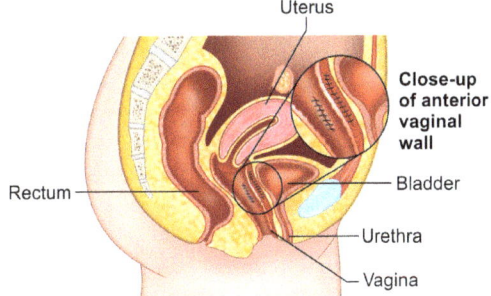

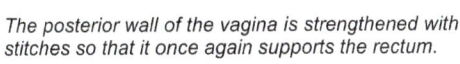

Figs. 12A and B: (A) Anterior colporrhaphy; (B) Posterior colporrhaphy.

McCall culdoplasty: A wedge of posterior vaginal wall and peritoneum is removed. Enterocele sac is freed and excised. Two internal sutures (permanent) placed approximately using both uterosacral ligament (USL) and peritoneum. One external suture is taken through the USL and posterior peritoneum and brought out through the posterior vaginal wall. This obliterates cul-de-sac, supports vaginal apex, and lengthens posterior vaginal wall.

Obliterative Procedures (Figs. 13 to 15)

- Le Fort's colpocleisis
- Goodall–Power modification of Le Fort's colpocleisis—for sexually active females

RECONSTRUCTIVE VERSUS OBLITERATIVE SURGERY

If a woman has an isolated anterior or posterior vaginal wall prolapse without apical prolapse, surgical decision-making is easy. Traditional anterior or posterior colporrhaphy can be performed to treat this condition. The choice depends on the medical condition and sexual function of the patient. Reconstructive surgery corrects the prolapse while restoring the normal vaginal anatomy, whereas obliterative surgery does so by closing off the vaginal canal either partly (Le Fort's colpocleisis) or totally (total colpocleisis).[7]

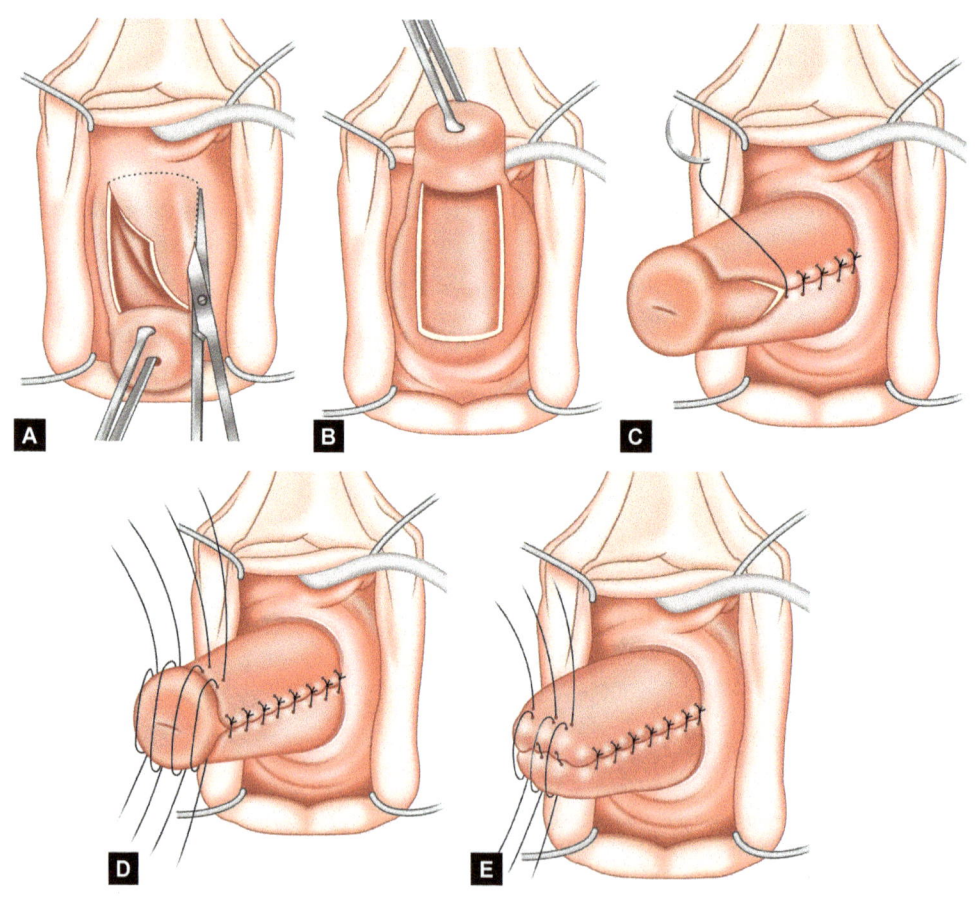

Figs. 13A and E: Colpocleisis.

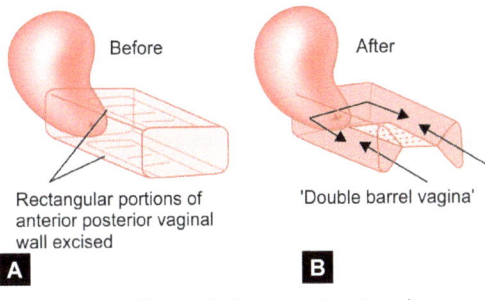

Figs. 14A and B: Colpocleisis principle.

Therefore, reconstructive surgery is appropriate for a woman who is sexually active or may be sexually active in the future. Fragile, older women cannot tolerate an extensive reconstructive procedure, which may involve an attempt to correct more than one sites.[8-10] Hence, less invasive, obliterative surgery may be an appropriate option for these women. Additionally, obliterative surgery has an extremely low risk of prolapse recurrence.

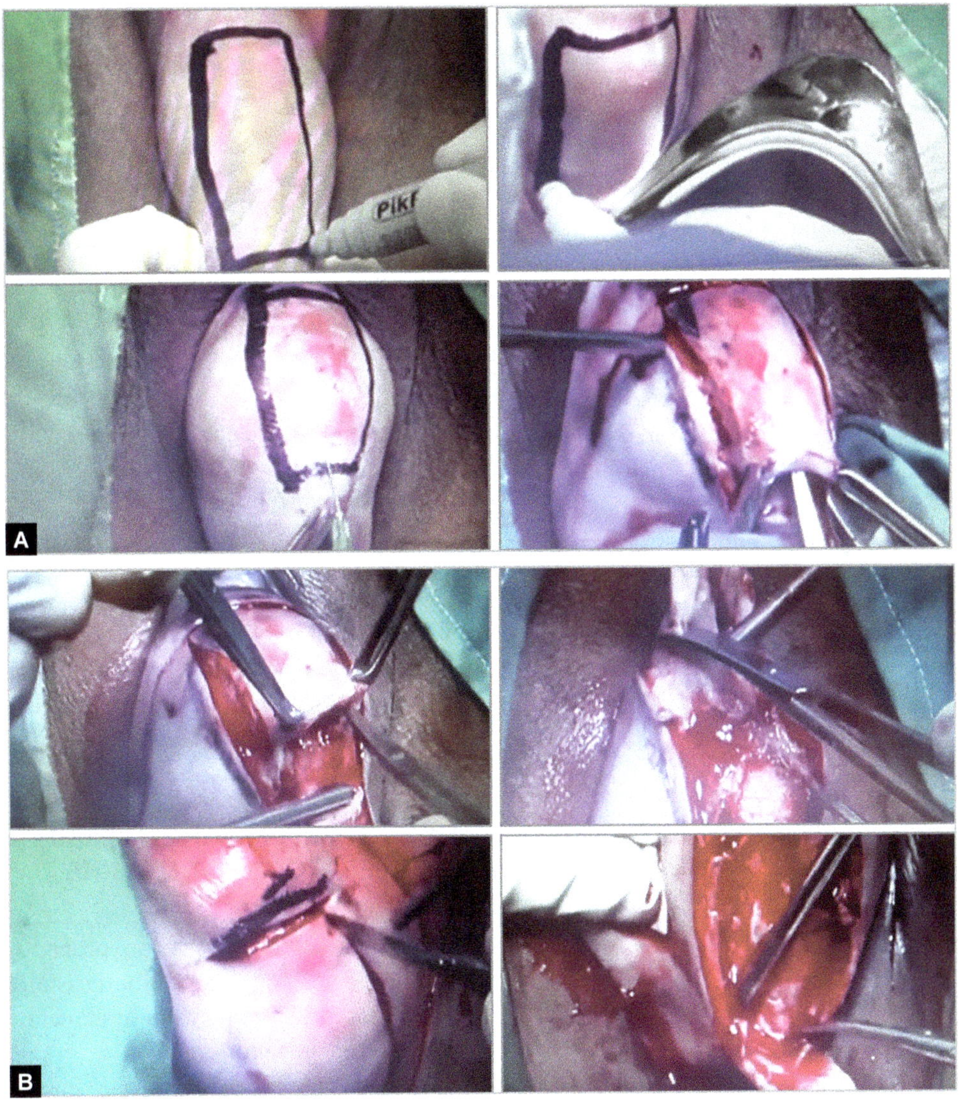

Figs. 15A and B: Obliterative procedures.

Decision-making in Reconstructive Surgery

There is growing recognition that adequate support for the vaginal apex is essential for a durable surgical repair. Because of the significant contribution of the vaginal apex to anterior and posterior vaginal support, surgical correction of the anterior and posterior walls may fail unless the apex is adequately supported.

Although there are no consensus statements or guidelines about the degree of apical support severe enough to warrant surgical correction, the descent of the vaginal apex at least halfway into the vaginal canal (i.e., POP-Q point C > −0.5 × total vaginal length) needs to be corrected because it is closely linked with prolapse symptoms.[11]

SURGICAL ROUTE FOR APICAL SUSPENSION: ABDOMINAL VERSUS VAGINAL

Apical suspension procedures can be performed either transvaginally or abdominally.

Abdominal procedures, including sacrocolpopexy (SCP) and uterosacral ligament (USL) suspension, can be performed via laparotomy or laparoscopy (with or without robotic assistance).

Transvaginal procedures include native tissue repair (USL suspension, sacrospinousligament fixation, or iliococcygeus suspension) and mesh repair. The choice of an apical suspension procedure should be individualized to the specific patient because each procedure carries its own risk and benefit.

For SCP, minimally invasive approach (laparoscopy with or without robotic assistance) begins to gain popularity.

A systematic review[12] found that minimally invasive SCP and open SCP had a similar efficacy in terms of apical support and recurrence rate.

BOX 7: Laparoscopic sacrocolpopexy.
- Y-shaped mesh is used.
- One proximal and two distal arms
- Bowel and bladder dissected off the vault
- Distal arms sutured to anterior and posterior vaginal wall
- Proximal arm sutured or fixed with tackers to sacral promontory
- Reperitonization is done

Given the current data, SCP may be more appropriate for women with risk factors for prolapse recurrence, including young age, obesity, and advanced prolapse (POP-Q stage 3 or 4), and the preferred approach to SCP is laparoscopy.

Laparoscopic Approach

This has been found to have a lot of benefits over vaginal or open approaches that improved visualization of anatomy, reduced hospital stay, less postoperative pain, and reduced cost. Only limitation is steep learning curve, increased operative time, and injuries to vital organs.

Laparoscopic approach to SCP has been given in **Box 7**.

Abdominal Sacral Colpopexy

Subumbilical midline vertical incision taken. 3 × 15 cm tape or mesh sutured to the vaginal vault after dissecting off the bladder and rectum, with nonabsorbable sutures and then secured to the sacrum.

UTERINE PRESERVATION VERSUS HYSTERECTOMY FOR UTERINE PROLAPSE

When the apical suspension procedure is planned for uterine prolapse, the decision must be made whether to perform hysterectomy as a part of the procedure.

There is a considerable desire for uterine preservation among patients.

The most common procedures for correcting uterine prolapse with uterine preservation include sacrospinous hysteropexy (transvaginal), transvaginal mesh hysteropexy, USL uterine suspension (transvaginal or abdominal), and sacrohysteropexy with mesh (abdominal).

Given the current data, concomitant hysterectomy is recommended over uterine preservation at the time of apical suspension. Hysteropexy may be a reasonable alternative for women who have mild uterine prolapse and desire to preserve their uterus if they have no contraindications for uterine preservation.[13]

Contraindications to preservation of the uterus are enlarged fibroids, adenomyosis, endometrial hyperplasia, current or recent cervical dysplasia, abnormal uterine bleeding or postmenopausal bleeding, BRCA1 and 2 mutations, hereditary nonpolyposis colorectal cancer (Lynch syndrome), taking tamoxifen therapy, unable to comply with routine gynecologic surveillance, and cervical elongation (relative contraindication).

CONCOMITANT REPAIR OF ANTERIOR OR POSTERIOR PROLAPSE

As with apical prolapse, there is no consistent recommendation on which degree of anterior or posterior prolapse is to be corrected during reconstructive surgery. Nonetheless, when stage 2 or greater anterior or posterior vaginal prolapse (i.e., point Ba or Bp ≥ −1) is detected during the preoperative POP-Q examination, several surgeons think that it needs to be addressed at the time of reconstruction.[14]

An effective apical suspension can correct other sites of vaginal prolapse, but this is not always the case. Therefore, the decision must be made whether to perform an additional procedure to correct anterior or posterior prolapse. Simulated apical support during the preoperative POP-Q examination can mimic the results following apical suspension and may help in this decision-making.

Surgical decision-making for POP requires a complex process. It is important that a surgeon provides adequate information on the risks and benefits of options available for correcting prolapse and guides a patient's decision-making. Recommendations based on the current scientific evidence are summarized in **Box 8**.[15]

COMPLICATIONS OF PELVIC ORGAN PROLAPSE SURGERY

Complications after native tissue POP surgery include bleeding, infection (typically urinary tract), and voiding dysfunction (which usually is transient). Less common complications include rectovaginal or vesicovaginal fistula, ureteral injury, foreshortened vagina, or a restriction of the vaginal caliber.

In the operations and pelvic muscle training in the management of apical support loss trial, dyspareunia was noted in 16% of women 24 months after native tissue POP surgery. Changes in vaginal anatomy may lead to pelvic pain and pain with intercourse. Fistula and ureteral injury require prompt referral to specialists with expertise in managing these conditions. A short vagina or vaginal constriction after POP surgery often can be managed with vaginal estrogen and progressive dilators.

There are unique complications associated with synthetic mesh when they are used in POP surgery. These include mesh contracture and erosion into the vagina, urethra, bladder, and rectum. The rate of mesh erosion is approximately 12% after vaginal mesh prolapse surgery. When mesh is used for anterior vaginal wall prolapse repair, there is an 11% risk of mesh erosion, with 7% of these cases requiring surgical correction. The rate of dyspareunia is approximately 9% after vaginal

BOX 8: Recommendations based on the current scientific evidence.

ACOG PRACTICE BULLETIN
Clinical Management Guidelines for Obstetrician–Gynecologists

Number 185, November 2017　　　　　　　　　　　　(Replaces Practice Bulletin Number 176, April 2017)

Committee on Practice Bulletins–Gynecology and American Urogynecologic Society. This Practice Bulletin was developed by the Committee on Practice Bulletins—Gynecology and the American Urogynecologic Society in collaboration with Paul Tulikangas, MD

The following recommendations and conclusions are based on good and consistent scientific evidence (Level A):
1. Uterosacral and sacrospinous ligament suspension for apical POP with native tissue are equally effective surgical treatments of POP, with comparable anatomic, functional, and adverse outcomes
2. The use of synthetic mesh or biologic grafts in transvaginal repair of posterior vaginal wall prolapse does not improve outcomes
3. Compared with native tissue anterior repair, polypropylene mesh augmentation of anterior vaginal wall prolapse repair improves anatomic and some subjective outcomes but is associated with increased morbidity

The following recommendations and conclusions are based on limited or inconsistent scientific evidence (Level B):
1. Many women with POP on physical examination do not report symptoms of POP. Treatment is indicated only if prolapse is causing bothersome bulge and pressure symptoms, sexual dysfunction, lower urinary tract dysfunction, or defecatory dysfunction
2. Women considering treatment of POP should be offered a vaginal pessary as an alternative to surgery
3. Vaginal apex suspension should be performed at the time of hysterectomy for uterine prolapse to reduce the risk of recurrent POP
4. Abdominal sacrocolpopexy with synthetic mesh has a lower risk of recurrent POP but is associated with more complications than vaginal apex repair with native tissue
5. Obliterative procedures––which narrow, shorten, or completely close the vagina—are effective for the treatment of POP and should be considered a first-line surgical treatment for women with significant medical comorbidities who do not desire future vaginal intercourse or vaginal preservation
6. The use of synthetic mesh or biologic grafts in POP surgery is associated with unique complications not seen in POP repair with native tissue
7. Hysteropexy is a viable alternative to hysterectomy in women with uterine prolapse, although there is less available evidence on safety and efficacy compared with hysterectomy

The following recommendations are based primarily on consensus and expert opinion (Level C):
1. A POP-Q examination is recommended before treatment for the objective evaluation and documentation of the extent of prolapse
2. A pessary should be considered for a woman with symptomatic POP who wishes to become pregnant in the future
3. Pelvic organ prolapse vaginal mesh repair should be limited to high-risk individuals in whom the benefit of mesh placement may justify the risk, such as individuals with recurrent prolapse (particularly of the anterior or apical compartments) or with medical comorbidities that preclude more invasive and lengthier open and endoscopic procedures
4. Before placement of synthetic mesh grafts in the anterior vaginal wall, patients should provide their informed consent after reviewing the benefits and risks of the procedure and discussing alternative repairs. Surgeons who perform POP surgery with biologic grafts or synthetic mesh grafts should have training specifically for these procedures and should be able to counsel patients regarding the risk-benefit ratio for the use of mesh compared with native tissue repair
5. Routine intraoperative cystoscopy during POP surgery is recommended when the surgical procedure performed is associated with a significant risk of injury to the bladder or ureter. These procedures include suspension of the vaginal apex to the uterosacral ligaments, sacrocolpopexy, and anterior colporrhaphy and the placement of mesh in the anterior and apical compartments
6. All women with significant apical prolapse, anterior prolapse, or both should have a preoperative evaluation for occult SUI, with cough stress testing or urodynamic testing with the prolapse reduced
7. Patients with POP but without SUI who are undergoing either abdominal or vaginal prolapse repair should be counseled that postoperative SUI is more likely without a concomitant continence procedure but that the risk of adverse effects is increased with an additional procedure

mesh prolapse surgery. Multiple procedures often are required to manage mesh-related complications.

RECURRENCE OF PELVIC ORGAN PROLAPSE AFTER SURGERY

Recurrence of POP is possible after any POP surgery. Recurrence rates between 6 and 30% have been reported. Women should be counseled about the risk of recurrence before undergoing POP surgery. Women who present with recurrent POP should undergo counseling similar to that for women who present with primary POP. It is helpful to review the preoperative examination results and prior surgical reports. Many patients may choose not to undergo a repeat surgery. They may choose instead to monitor the prolapse or to use a pessary. If a patient chooses to undergo surgery for recurrent vaginal apex prolapse, abdominal SCP, vaginal colpopexy with possible mesh or graft augmentation, or colpocleisis may be considered if the patient has failed a vaginal native tissue apical suspension. If the surgeon is not comfortable performing these procedures, referral of the patient to a surgeon who subspecializes in pelvic reconstructive surgery and can offer these procedures is recommended.

PREVENTION OF VAULT PROLAPSE (RCOG 2011)

Primary prevention is feasible through modification of obstetric management. The main modifiable risk factor for pelvic floor trauma and later POP is forceps, whereas vacuum is not associated with increased risk.

Secondary prevention is feasible through pelvic floor physiotherapy, which requires provision of adequate diagnostic and therapeutic postnatal services. Such services do not currently exist. Until they are established, women with psychological or somatic morbidity due to POP will benefit from a greater awareness early diagnosis, and customized treatment approach.

1. McCall culdoplasty with vaginal hysterectomy—Grade A evidence.
2. Suturing the cardinal—uterosacral ligament complex to the vaginal cuff during hysterectomy—Grade B evidence.
3. If the vault descends to the introitus during closure at vaginal hysterectomy, simultaneous sacrospinous fixation is recommended—Grade B evidence.

REFERENCES

1. Swift SE, Tate SB. Correlation of symptoms with degree of pelvic organ support in a general population of women: What is pelvic organ prolapse? Am J Obstet Gynecol. 2003;189: 372-9.
2. Abrams P, Cardozo L. The standardisation of terminology of lower urinary tract function: Report from the Standardisation Subcommittee of International Continence Society. Am J Obstret Gynecol. 2002;187:116-26.
3. Persu C, Chapple CR, Cauni V, Gutue S, Geavlete P. Pelvic Organ Prolapse Quantification System (POP-Q)—a new era in pelvic prolapse staging. J Med Life. 2011;4(1):75-81.
4. Matsumoto T, Nishi M, Yokota M, Ito M. Laparoscopic treatment of uterine prolapse during pregnancy. Obstet Gynecol. 1999;93:849.
5. Smith FJ, Holman CD, Moorin RE, Tsokos N. Lifetime risk of undergoing surgery for pelvic organ prolapse. Obstet Gynecol. 2010;116: 1096-100.
6. Løwenstein E, Ottesen B, Gimbel H. Incidence and lifetime risk of pelvic organ prolapse surgery in Denmark from 1977 to 2009. Int Urogynecol J Pelvic Floor Dysfunct. 2015;26:49-55.
7. Jelovsek JE, Maher C, Barber MD. Pelvic organ prolapse. Lancet. 2007;369:1027-38.
8. Stepp KJ, Barber MD, Yoo EH, Whiteside JL, Paraiso MF, Walters MD. Incidence of perioperative complications of urogynecologic surgery in elderly women. Am J Obstet Gynecol. 2005;192:1630-6.

9. Sung VW, Weitzen S, Sokol ER, Rardin CR, Myers DL. Effect of patient age on increasing morbidity and mortality following urogynecologic surgery. Am J Obstet Gynecol. 2006;194:1411-7.
10. Bretschneider CE, Robinson B, Geller EJ, Wu JM. The effect of age on postoperative morbidity in women undergoing urogynecologic surgery. Female Pelvic Med Reconstr Surg. 2015;21:236-40.
11. Lowder JL, Oliphant SS, Shepherd JP, Ghetti C, Sutkin G. Genital hiatus size is associated with and predictive of apical vaginal support loss. Am J Obstet Gynecol. 2016;214:718.e1-718.e8.
12. De Gouveia De Sa M, Claydon LS, Whitlow B, Dolcet Artahona MA. Laparoscopic versus open sacrocolpopexy for treatment of prolapse of the apical segment of the vagina: a systematic review and meta-analysis. Int Urogynecol J Pelvic Floor Dysfunct. 2016;27:3-17.
13. Gutman RE. Does the uterus need to be removed to correct uterovaginal prolapse? Curr Opin Obstet Gynecol. 2016;28:435-40
14. Jeon MJ. Surgical decision making for symptomatic pelvic organ prolapse: evidence based approach. Obstet Gynecol Sci. 2019;62(5):307-12.
15. Jelovsek JE. Pelvic organ prolapse in women: Choosing a primary surgical procedure. Waltham: UpToDate; 2018.

CHAPTER 23

Vaginal Apical Suspension Procedures

T Srikala Prasad

INTRODUCTION

Pelvic organ prolapse (POP) is one of the most common conditions which necessitate women to seek professional assistance. Roughly 50% of parous women suffer from this condition which, although not fatal, significantly affects their quality of life. The life time risk of surgery for either POP or stress urinary incontinence is 20% by the age of 80 years.[1] The fact that 30% of them will require repeat surgery for recurrence is a matter of concern.[2] Apical defects need to be identified so that concomitant procedures for apical support can be performed at the time of initial surgery, thereby minimizing recurrence.

APICAL SUSPENSION PROCEDURES

Ensuring adequate apical support forms an important step in successful prolapse surgery. Apical suspension procedures can be done via the vagina, abdominal, laparoscopic, or robotic methods.

Vaginal apical suspension procedures	Transabdominal/ Laparoscopic/ Robotic procedures
McCall culdoplasty	Sacrocolpopexy
High uterosacral ligament suspension	Uterosacral ligament colposuspension
Sacrospinous ligament suspension	
Iliococcygeus suspension	
Transvaginal mesh placement to augment apical suspension	

The apical support, Delancey level 1, comprises the uterosacral and the cardinal ligaments. Not addressing deficient apical support at the time of surgery for POP markedly increases the chances of recurrence. Sacrocolpopexy is the gold standard procedure for apical suspension. However, the vaginal approach may be favored by gynecologists as the operating time is shorter, has less blood loss, can be done under regional anesthesia, has less postoperative morbidity, reduced hospital stay, less painful recovery and does not require the equipment associated with a laparoscopy or robot. It is also possible to repair other compartment defects concomitantly.[3] The abdominal approach is preferred in patients having orthopedic deformities precluding lithotomy positioning, coexisting intra-abdominal pathology and patients with reduced vaginal length.[3]

Methods which can be used at the time of hysterectomy to prevent vault prolapse:[4]
- McCall culdoplasty at the time of vaginal hysterectomy is effective in preventing subsequent post hysterectomy vault prolapse (PHVP).
- Suturing the cardinal and uterosacral ligaments to the vaginal cuff at the time of hysterectomy is effective in preventing PHVP at the time of both abdominal and vaginal hysterectomies.
- Sacrospinous ligament suspension at the time of vaginal hysterectomy should be considered when the vault descends to the introitus during closure.[4]

Traditionally sacrocolpopexy is considered the gold standard for apical suspension. With the use of mesh, high success rate and low recurrence was found.[5] However, it is associated with prolonged operating time, increased blood loss, longer hospital stay, higher complication rates and the potential need for repeat operation to address mesh complications which are far more difficult to manage than a recurrence.[5]

SACROSPINOUS LIGAMENT SUSPENSION

This technique was first described by Richter but popularized by Nichols and Randall. This technique may be preferred by some surgeons because it can be performed vaginally and is an extraperitoneal approach. The main indications are procidentia, PHVP, post hysterectomy enterocele and sacrospinous hysteropexy in women who wish to retain the uterus. This procedure can be done unilaterally or bilaterally and via an anterior or posterior approach.[6] When the procedure is done unilaterally, the right side is preferred because of the anatomic advantage of the sigmoid colon being on the left and that the majority of the surgeons are right-handed. The relative contraindications to this procedure are a short vagina (due to the inability to reach the sacrospinous ligament), failed previous repairs and surgeon inexperience.[6]

Anatomy

The sacro-spinous ligament extends from the ischial spine bilaterally and courses medially under the coccygeus muscle before it inserts into the lower portion of the sacrum and coccyx. The sacrospinous ligament lies within the substance of the coccygeus muscle and is referred to as coccygeus-sacrospinous ligament complex (CSSL) **(Fig. 1)**. This can be identified by palpating the ischial spine and tracing the free, triangular thickening posterior to the sacrum.[7]

Technique

This procedure can be done under regional or general anesthesia. Routine preprocedural antibiotics are given as well as consideration of venous thromboembolism prophylaxis. The patient is positioned in lithotomy and surgically prepped and draped. **Figures 2 to 6** show steps of vaginal sacrospinous ligament fixation.

Sacrospinous suspension can be approached anteriorly or posteriorly. For the posterior approach, the posterior vaginal wall

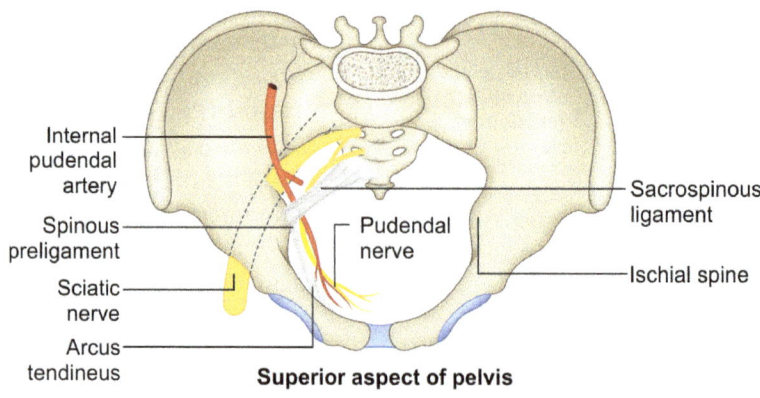

Fig. 1: Anatomy of sacrospinous ligament.[8]

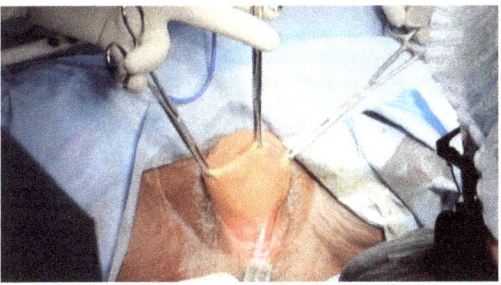

Fig. 2: Hydrodissection.

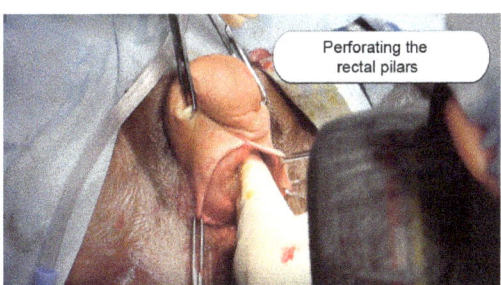

Fig. 4: Blunt dissection through rectal pillars.

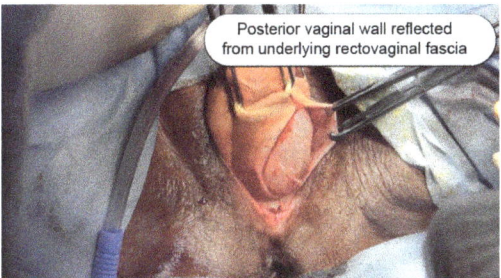

Fig. 3: Posterior vaginal wall deflection.

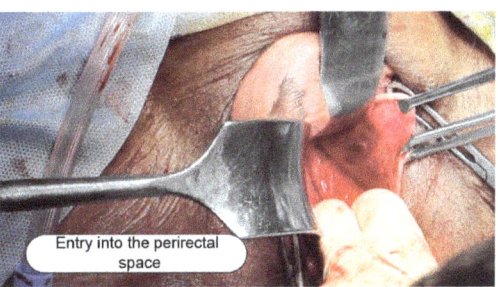

Fig. 5: Entry into perirectal space.

is grasped and local anesthetic is infiltrated for hydrodissection **(Fig. 2)**. A vertical midline incision is made and the rectovaginal fascia separated from the vaginal wall by either blunt or sharp dissection **(Figs. 3 and 4)**.

The loose areolar tissue that extends from the rectum to the arcus tendineus fasciae pelvis (ATFP) and overlies the levator muscle is called the rectal pillar **(Fig. 4)**.

This rectal pillar separates the rectovaginal space from the perirectal space. Entry into the perirectal space is achieved by bluntly perforating the rectal pillars and gently mobilizing the rectum medially until the ischial spine and the sacrospinous ligament is palpated **(Fig. 5)**. Breisky-navratil retractors can be used to retract the rectum medially and help in visualizing the ligament to the point of stitch.[7]

A No. 1 prolene suture is placed approximately one to two finger breadths medial to the spine and passed through the ligament and coccygeus muscle complex **(Fig. 6)**. Care

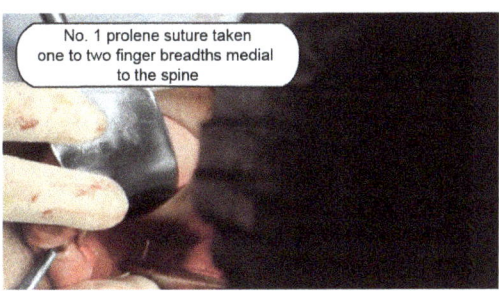

Fig. 6: Suture placement through sacrospinous ligament.

is taken in avoiding injury to the pudendal nerve and vessels which are just below the ischial spine.

Suture placement devices are now available to help with this suturing process. Placement can be confirmed by pulling both ends of the threads. The ligament is a tough structure and pulling on the prolene threads will cause movements of the patient's body. If the suture is placed incorrectly on loose fascia or muscle tissue, it will come away with this maneuver **(Fig. 7)**.

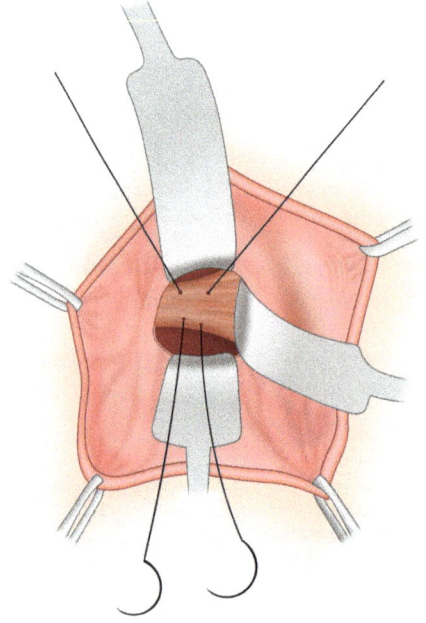

Fig. 7: Sacrospinous ligament suspension.

The sutures are then attached to the apex of the vaginal vault, with care taken not to pass the suture through the vagina as it is a non-absorbable suture. If this is accidentally done, it may cause discomfort to the patient. If there is a rectocele, it can now be repaired. The vaginal walls should be approximated about one third to half way down the vagina before the prolene suture is tied. This suggestion is made because on tying the sacrospinous suture, the vault will be suspended or elevated making it difficult to close the cranial portion of the vagina, if not done prior.

It is important to note that unilateral sacrospinous suspension alters the vaginal axis posteriorly and laterally. This may result in anterior compartment prolapse.

ANTERIOR SACROSPINOUS SUSPENSION TECHNIQUE

For the anterior approach, which is used in patients with anterior compartment defects, the same initial steps are taken, but the midline vaginal incision is made anteriorly. With this approach, the rectopubic space is entered and the ipsilateral paravesical and paravaginal areas are dissected from the level of bladder neck to the ischial spine along the arcus tendineus fasciae pelvis. A large space is now available to place the suture through the sacrospinous ligament in the same way as previously described.[9]

Michigan Four-wall Technique

A diamond shape is marked at the most dependent portion of the prolapsed vaginal cuff and dissection performed. The enterocele, if present, is dealt with in the usual way. The SSL is approached by posterolateral dissection and stitch taken as described earlier. The anterior vaginal wall, with the underlying pubocervical fascia, and the posterior vaginal wall, with the underlying rectovaginal fascia, is exposed with this technique. The sacrospinous ligament sutures can be anchored through both of these cuff edges.[9]

Complications

Most of the complications, similar to pudendal, sciatic and sacral neuropathies, are mild and self-limiting. However, if there is any evidence of direct injury to the pudendal or sciatic nerve, the patient must return to theater to remove the stitch.

Bleeding is usually not a major concern however, if there is significant bleeding the dissected space must be systematically examined and hemostasis secured. Bleeding usually occurs as a result of injury to the small vessels along the medial side of the rectum, possibly as a result of over enthusiastic retraction. The presacral vessels may also be injured in the same way. If it is not possible to locate the bleeder, prolonged pressure packing, tying the sacrospinous suture just placed or hemostatic agents may be useful.

In the rare event of hemodynamic instability, blood transfusion and radiological guided embolization may be needed. Voiding dysfunction, rectal injury, infection, and dyspareunia are other complications.[9]

BILATERAL ILIOCOCCYGEUS FASCIA SUSPENSION (FIG. 8)

This procedure was first described by Inmon in 1963[10] and popularized by Shull et al.[11]

The risk of damage to the pudendal neurovascular bundle and the possibility of anterior compartment prolapse occurring after sacrospinous ligament suspension led to the method of iliococcygeus fascia suspension or prespinous fixation.

Surgical Procedure

A vertical midline incision is made in the posterior vaginal wall after hydro dissection and the posterior vagina is separated from the underlying rectovaginal fascia. Dissection is continued laterally all the way to the pelvic side wall. The perirectal space is then entered. The rectal pillars are perforated and the ischial spine is reached. This is done by following the steps described in the sacrospinous suspension procedure. The fascia of the iliococcygeus muscle is identified lateral to the rectum and distal to the ischial spine. The rectum is safe guarded by the surgeon's non-dominant hand. The delayed absorbable suture is placed in the exposed iliococcygeus muscle and fascia 1–2 cm caudal and posterior to the ischial spine, near the insertion of the ATFP. This suture is now passed through the condensation of connective tissue at the apex of the vagina anteriorly through the pubocervical fascia and posteriorly through the rectovaginal fascia. This procedure is then repeated on the opposite side. The posterior colporrhaphy is completed and the vaginal wall approximated. Concomitant repair of other compartment defects can also be done. If a non-absorbable suture material like prolene is used, a pulley stitch technique is

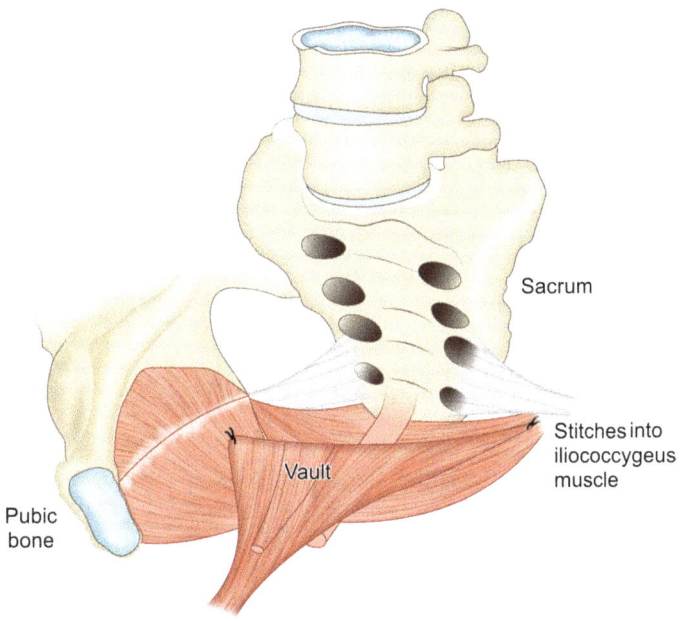

Fig. 8: Bilateral iliococcygeus fascia suspension.

applied with the knot being tied internally. The vaginal walls should be approximated at least halfway before the sutures are tightened, otherwise the suspended apex may be difficult to approximate.

A retrospective study by Maher et al. did not find any significant difference in efficacy or complications between iliococcygeus and sacrospinous suspension.[12] A recent retrospective study by Milani et al. which compared iliococcygeus and abdominal sacrocolpopexy did not find any significant differences in subjective or objective outcomes and both procedures were effective in restoring normal anatomy in patients with vaginal vault prolapse.[13]

Advantages and Disadvantages

The iliococcygeus fascia does not have important structures like the pudendal nerve and vessels, or the ureter immediately adjacent to it. Hence, this procedure is associated with a lower rate of pelvic pain from nerve entrapment, bleeding and ureteric injury. Furthermore, the surgery is technically easier to perform because of the lateral position of the iliococcygeus fascia in relation to the other anchoring pelvic structures such as the sacrospinous ligament, uterosacral ligament and the sacrum. The final surgical result more closely mimics the normal anatomy of the upper vagina. This surgery can be done in women with restricted vaginal mobility or a short vagina that cannot be attached to sacrospinous ligament/uterosacral ligament without tension. It also maintains the normal vaginal axis because this procedure is performed bilaterally.

A potential disadvantage of this approach is vaginal shortening attributable to the position of the ischial spines inferior to the normal position of the vaginal apex.[10] Potential complications include rectal and/or bladder lacerations, bleeding, vaginal cuff abscesses and transient femoral neuropathy.[12]

McCALL CULDOPLASTY (FIG. 9)

This procedure was first described by Dr Milton McCall in 1957 as a technique to address the cul-de-sac during a vaginal hysterectomy.[14]

The McCall culdoplasty is the most common procedure used to suspend the vaginal apex at the time of vaginal hysterectomy and prevent PHVP with minimal morbidity. The aim of the procedure is to obliterate the cul-de-sac by pulling the uterosacral ligaments across the midline and attaching the posterior vaginal cuff and the cul-de-sac peritoneum. By closing off the cul-de-sac a subsequent prolapse can be prevented.

The surgeon needs to assess whether a patient requires a formal vaginal vault suspension or obliteration of the cul-de-sac by McCall culdoplasty to achieve adequate support and vaginal length. For example, patients who present with procidentia or stage IV POP, or women with a vaginal vault that descends to the level of the introitus will require a formal apical suspension procedure. The McCall culdoplasty is usually

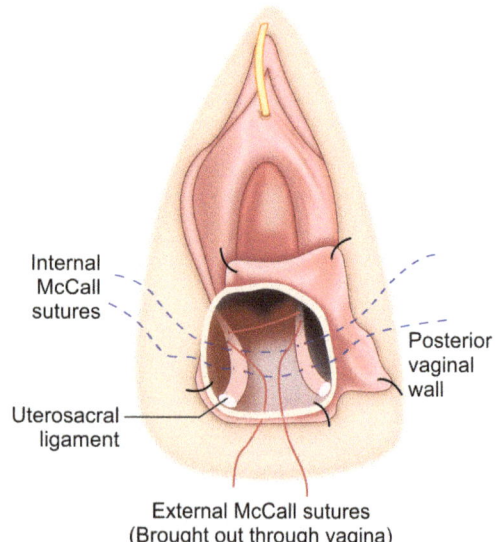

Fig. 9: McCall culdoplasty.

sufficient for patients with stage I-III POP and those undergoing hysterectomy for other conditions.[15]

There is an increasing trend toward laparoscopic hysterectomy without an increase in the number of concomitant procedures to support the vaginal vault. McCall culdoplasty can also be done during laparoscopic procedures and has been found to be a safe, simple and efficient technique in preventing apical prolapse without severe morbidity, or significant blood loss.[16]

Technique of the McCall Culdoplasty

The McCall culdoplasty is performed after the removal of the uterus and the cervix from the apex of the vagina. The traditional McCall culdoplasty involves both internal and external McCall sutures.

The *internal McCall sutures*—the suture (monofilament 0 suture) is passed through the left uterosacral ligament, roughly 2 cm above its cut edge, and tacking sutures are taken across the posterior peritoneum until the right uterosacral ligament is reached. A suture is placed through the cut end of the ligament but not tied. Additional sutures, a second or even a third row, are placed above this and the ends also left untied.

The *external McCall sutures* are placed with a delayed absorbable suture beginning with the posterior vaginal wall, left uterosacral ligament, and peritoneum with bites continued across the peritoneum over the sigmoid colon to the right uterosacral ligament. The suture is then brought out through the vagina where it is tagged. Depending on the redundancy of the posterior vaginal wall, an additional second or third external McCall sutures is performed and tagged. Some portion of the vagina and peritoneum can be removed in case of marked redundancy.[15] The internal McCall sutures are now tied thereby creating a firm, shelf-like midline structure.[14]

If required, anterior or posterior colporrhaphy is performed at this point. The vaginal walls are then approximated with interrupted 2-0 delayed absorbable sutures. The vaginal vault should be closed prior to tying the external McCall sutures. As a result, the posterior vaginal wall is anchored to the uterosacral ligaments, the cul-de-sac is well obliterated and the vaginal cuff is well supported. Check cystoscopy is done to ensure ureteric patency.

The modified McCall culdoplasty is much simple in that it involves placing a suture through one uterosacral ligament incorporating the cul-de-sac peritoneum and vaginal cuff before continuing the suture through the opposite uterosacral ligament.

Pictures of Modified McCall Culdoplasty (Figs. 10 to 13)

The vaginal apex is suspended with the incorporation of the uterosacral ligaments and the risk of enterocele formation is minimized because the cul-de-sac peritoneum is also incorporated.[17,18]

The procedure begins with taking a bite on the posterior vaginal wall and then on the left Mackenrodt's ligament, uterosacral ligament complex and then the apex of the peritoneum is taken and bite taken on the edge of the peritoneum and the posterior vaginal wall and tied.

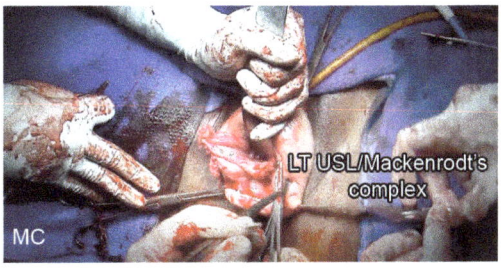

Fig. 10: Left uteroscacral/Mackenrodt's complex.

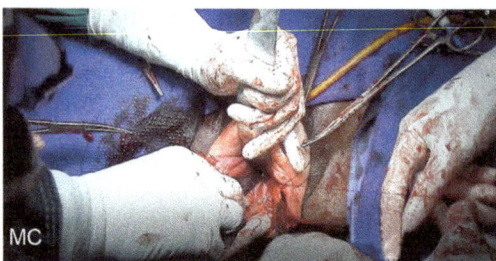

Fig. 11: Peritoneal apex.

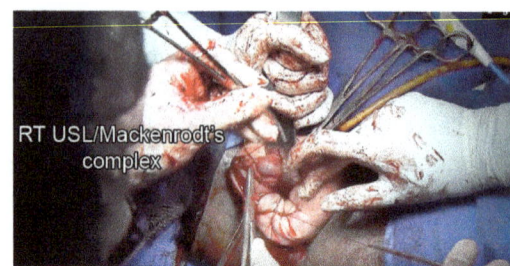

Fig. 13: Suture exiting through right uterosacral/Mackenrodt's complex.

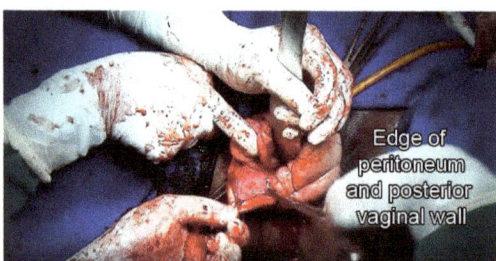

Fig. 12: Suture through peritoneum and posterior vaginal wall.

This is now continued by taking a bite on the peritoneum as high as possible and taking a bite on the edge of the peritoneum and vaginal wall and tied. This procedure is continued till the right uterosacral/Mackenrodt's ligament complex is anchored to the posterior vaginal wall.

Any such modifications of the McCalls procedure where in the supporting structures (uterosacral-cardinals) are attached to the vault will achieve the purpose of apical suspension.[18,19] Kathy Niblock et al. have compared vaginal McCall culdoplasty to laparoscopic uterosacral plication to prophylactically address vaginal vault prolapse and found the McCall culdoplasty to be a superior surgery in preventing PHVP with no difference in complications.[16]

Various authors have compared the modified McCall culdoplasty to Shull suspension (uterosacral ligament suspension) in POP primary repair and found both procedures to be safe and equally effective.[20,21]

Vaginal Mesh to Augment Apical Suspension

Because of the inherent connective tissue defects that lead to POP and the failures seen with traditional repair, pelvic surgeons have looked for ways to augment repairs resulting in longer lasting outcomes. Transvaginal mesh (TVM) to treat POP was very popular in the yesteryear because it was considered to be "less invasive" with good durability. Standardized technique, standardization of the mesh and the fact that it was possible to repair multiple compartment defects through a vaginal approach was attractive. These mesh surgeries also had complications which included vaginal mesh erosion or extrusion, pelvic pain, dyspareunia and rarely injury and/or perforation to the bladder and bowel.[22]

The 2017 Cochrane review demonstrated that the use of TVM in POP repairs decreases subjective awareness of a vaginal bulge at 1-3 years postoperatively as well as the need for repeat surgery for prolapse, and recurrent prolapse (stage II or greater) in any compartment when compared to native tissue repairs. However, these patients had a significantly increased operating time, increased bleeding, SUI and higher rates of repeat surgery to tackle mesh complications.[23] Complications such as mesh erosions (12%)[24] and dyspareunia were reported and these led to an increased number of litigations worldwide. The United States Food and Drug

Administration (US FDA) reclassified the surgical mesh into type III on January 5th 2016 and mandated that premarket approval is required. Hence, all manufacturers stopped marketing of TVM kits intended for transvaginal repair of posterior compartment prolapse by July 2018. On April 16, 2019, the FDA ordered manufacturers of TVM kits used for transvaginal repair of anterior compartment prolapse to stop selling and distributing their products immediately. Therefore, at the present time, there are no FDA approved TVM kits for transvaginal repair of prolapse.

"The recent 2017 International collaboration of Incontinence Evidence-based Pathway did not recommend transvaginal mesh for any primary prolapse intervention".[25] Today, transvaginal mesh for prolapse is not approved for use in Australia, New Zealand, USA and currently paused in England, Scotland and Ireland while it remains available in Europe.[26] In 2015, the European Commission indicated that synthetic meshes may be used in complex cases of POP, recurrent POP or in difficult cases where a conventional procedure is expected to fail. In keeping with good medical practice, such complicated cases should be managed in high volume units by experts after adequate selection and counseling of patients so as to minimize any possible adverse sequelae.[15] There is a need for long-term data and follow-up before we draw conclusions about safely using mesh for apical support. The surgeon must discuss in detail with their patients all possible complications including mesh extrusion, erosion into the genitourinary tract and the rectum, infections, dyspareunia and pelvic pain, along with other viable options.

CONCLUSION

There are multiple factors to be considered in surgical planning. The decision regarding the route of surgery and the method depends on the age of the patient, weight, associated comorbidities, sexual activity, and surgical history.

The need for concomitant or prophylactic apical suspension in the form of sacrospinous ligament suspension, high uterosacral ligament suspension or iliococcygeus suspension needs to be considered. The McCall culdoplasty, or its modification, would be sufficient for lesser degrees of prolapse and at the time of laparoscopic hysterectomy.[17]

ACKNOWLEDGMENT

Sincere thanks to Dr S Anitha for the illustrations.

REFERENCES

1. Wu JM, Matthews CA, Conover MM, Pate V, Jonsson Funk M. Lifetime risk of stress urinary incontinence and pelvic organ prolapse surgery. Obstet Gynecol. 2014;123(6):1201-6.
2. Bradley CS, Nygard IE. Vaginal wall descensus and pelvic floor symptoms in older women. Obstet Gynecol. 2005;106:759-66.
3. May A, Salomon Z, Drutz HP. Vaginal Approach to Fixation of vaginal Apex. In: Cardozo L, Staskin D (Eds). Textbook of Female Urology and Urogynaecology, 4th edition. New York: CRC Press; 2019.
4. RCOG. Post Hysterectomy Vaginal Vault Prolapse (Green top Guideline No. 46, RCOG/BSUG Joint Guideline). London: RCOG; 2015.
5. Cardozo L, Staskin D. Open abdominal approach to supporting the vaginal apex. Randomized controlled trial comparing abdominal sacrocolpopexy to sacrospinous vaginal vault. In: Textbook of Female Urology and Urogynaecology, 4th edition. New York: CRC Press; 2019.
6. Alas AN, Anger JT. Management of apical pelvic organ prolapsed. Current Urol Rep. 2015;16:33.
7. Karram MM. Vaginal operations for prolapsed. In: Atlas of Pelvic anatomy and Gynecologic surgery, 2nd edition. Gurugram: Elsevier India; 2015.
8. Katke RD, Kiran U. Sacrospinous fixation: an efficient technique for prevention and treatment of vault prolapsed. IJRHS. 2016;4(3):60-4.

9. Botros SM, Goldberg RP, Sand PK. Sacrospinous ligament suspension for vaginal vault prolapsed. In: Raz S, Rodriguez CV. Female Urology. Gurugram: Elsevier India; 2018.
10. Krissi H, Stanton S. Bilateral iliococcygeus fixation technique for enterocele and vaginal vault prolapse repair. Pelviperineology. 2010;29:11-4.
11. Shull BL, Capen MD, Riggs MW, Kuehl TJ. Bilateral attachment of the vaginal cuff to iliococcygeus fascia: an effective method of cuff suspension. Am J Obstet Gynecol 1993;168:1669-74.
12. Maher CF, Murray CJ, Carey MP, Dwyer PL, Ugoni AM. Iliococcygeus or sacrospinous fixation for vaginal vault prolapse. Obstet Gynecol. 2001;98:40-4.
13. Milani RI, Cesana MC, Spelzini F, Sicuri M, Manodoro S, Fruscio R. Iliococcygeus fixation or abdominal sacral colpopexy for the treatment of vaginal vault prolapse: a retrospective cohort study. Int Urogynecol J. 2014;25(2);279-84.
14. Smilen SW. How to manage the cuff at vaginal hysterectomy. OBG Manag. 2007;19(2):45-53.
15. Afifi R, Sayed AT. Post-hysterectomy vaginal vault prolapsed: review. Obstet Gynecol. 2005;7:89-97.
16. Gencdal S, Demirel E, Soyman Z, Kelekci S. Prophylactic McCall Culdoplasty by a vaginal approach during mini-laparoscopic hysterectomy. Biomed Res Int. 2019;8047924.
17. University of North Carolina. Prophylactic modified McCall's Culdoplasty during total laparoscopic hysterectomy. Bethesda: NIH US National Library of Medicine; 2017.
18. Cruishank S. Operations for support of the vaginal wall. Glob Libr Wome Med. 2009.
19. Cruishank, S, Kovac SR. Randomised comparison of 3 surgical methods used at the time of vaginal hysterectomy to prevent posterior enterocele. Am J Obstet Gynecol. 1999;180:859-65.
20. Spelzini F, Frigerio M, Manodoro S, Interdonato ML, Cesana MC, Verri D, et al Modified McCall Culdoplasty versus Shull suspension in pelvic prolapse primary repair: a retrospective study. Int Urogynecol J. 2017;28(1):65-71.
21. Schiavi MC, Savone D, Di Mascio D, Di Tucci C, Perniola G, Zullo MA, et al. Long term experience of vaginal vault prolapse prevention at hysterectomy time by modified McCall culdoplasty or Shull suspension: clinical, sexual & quality of life assessment after surgical intervention. Eur J Obstet Gynecol Reprod Biol. 2018;223:113-8.
22. Abed H, Rahn DD, Lowenstein L, Balk EM, Clemons JL, Rogers RG, et al. Incidence in management of graft erosion, wound granulation and dyspareunia following vaginal prolapse repair with graft materials: a systematic review. Int Urogynecol J. 2011;22(7):789-98.
23. Moen M, Gebhart J, Tamussino K. Systematic reviews of apical prolapse surgery: are we being misled down a dangerous path? Int Urogynecol J. 2015;26(7):937-9.
24. Izett M, Kupelian A, Vashist A. Safety and efficacy of non-absorbable mesh in contemporary gynecological surgery. Gynecol Surg. 2018;15:20.
25. Maher C, Feiner B, Baessler K, Christmann-Schmid C, Haya N, Marjoribanks J. Transvaginal mesh or grafts compared with native tissue repair for vaginal prolapsed. Cochrane Database Syst Rev. 2016;2(2):CD012079.
26. Maher C. There is still a place for vaginal mesh in urogynaecology: FOR: There is still a place for vaginal mesh in urogynaecology. BJOG. 2019;126(8):1074.

CHAPTER 24

High Uterosacral Ligament Suspension for Apical Prolapse

N Rajamaheswari

INTRODUCTION

Pelvic organ prolapse (POP) is a common gynecological problem observed in 40–60% of parous women during clinical examination.[1,2]

Apical support is provided by uterosacral cardinal ligament complex and it forms the keystone of pelvic organ support. Apical defect results in uterine and vault descent and surgical correction of the apex is of paramount importance in prolapse repair **(Fig. 1)**.

In advanced prolapse, providing adequate apical support is essential to ensure durable success.[3,4]

Anterior vaginal prolapse is most common in women. If anterior vaginal prolapse extends beyond hymen, associated loss of apical support is customary.[5,6]

Because apex offers significant support to anterior vaginal wall, unless apex is adequately supported, even the best repairs of anterior/posterior walls may fail.[3,4,7-9]

Even though several vaginal, abdominal, and laparoscopic surgical procedures are available to repair apical defect, 80–90% of procedures are performed by the vaginal approach.[10-13]

Among the available vaginal native tissue apical suspension procedures, high uterosacral ligament suspension (HUSLS) and sacrospinous ligament suspension are in regular use.

HIGH UTEROSACRAL LIGAMENT SUSPENSION

Miller[14] in 1927 first described USLS and later Shull[15] popularized it in the late 1990s.

Shull suspended vaginal apex to the proximal remnants of the intermediate part of uterosacral ligaments [(USL) above the level of ischial spine] using an intraperitoneal approach. This procedure restores the vagina to the hollow of the sacrum and restores normal vaginal axis. There is no retroflexion and distortion of the vaginal axis with HUSLS as seen in the sacrospinous ligament suspension.

Vaginal transperitoneal HUSLS is used as a therapeutic surgical procedure to correct the apical defect of advanced stages of uterine and vault prolapse **(Figs. 2 and 3)**.

As most of the patients have mixed defects, anterior and posterior repairs are combined with HUSLS.

Though abdominal, laparoscopic, and extraperitoneal vaginal HUSLS have been reported, transperitoneal vaginal HUSLS is commonly practiced.

Fig. 1: Delancey's levels of support.

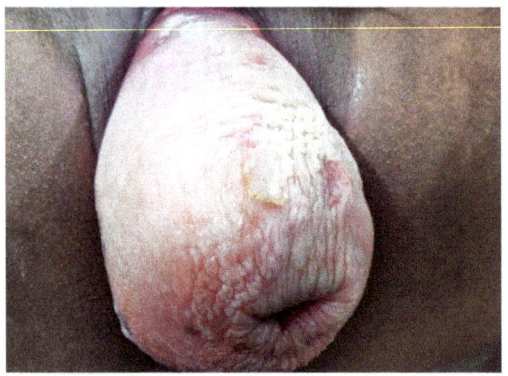

Fig. 2: Stage IV pelvic organ prolapse (POP).

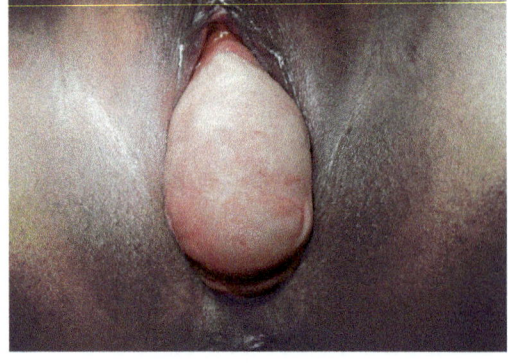

Fig. 3: Stage III vault prolapse.

If future child bearing is desired, vaginal HUSLS can be considered to correct apical prolapse while preserving the uterus.

The Uterosacral Ligament

It is a major suspensory structure of the female pelvic floor, providing support to the cervix and upper vagina. It plays a pivotal role in surgical procedures for pelvic organ prolapse intended at restoring apical support. Buller et al.[16] performed suture pullout studies on cadavers and concluded that the intermediate segment of USL was the optimal site to anchor the apex. The ischial spine was found to be a good marker of the intermediate segment, which has good strength and fewer vital, subjacent vessels and nerves. He advocated placing the suture 1 cm posterior to its most palpable anterior margin of the USL (when the ligament is in tension).

Technique: Vaginal Transperitoneal HUSLS

In women with stage III/IV uterovaginal prolapse, vaginal hysterectomy is done prior to HUSLS. In women with vault prolapse, vaginal wall incised and dissected from the underlying bladder and enterocele sac. The sac is then opened to gain intraperitoneal access to the USL.

Visualization of Uterosacral Ligament

Packing of bowels, retraction at 12 and 9/3 o'clock position (depending on right/left USL) using long Deaver's retractor and a Sim's speculum at 6 o'clock position facilitates access to the uterosacral ligament.

Transperitoneal palpation of the ischial spine can be a guide to reach uterosacral ligament.

In addition, gentle traction on the tag holding the remaining uterosacral ligament or upward traction of the Allis clamp placed (approximately at 4 and 7 o'clock position) enables the identification of the uterosacral ligament.

Placement of Sutures on USL

Using 2-0 polyglactin, the first suspension suture is placed just above and medial to the ischial spine on the tissue lying over the groove next to bowel with visual check on the course of the ureter. Similarly, second and third 2-0 delayed absorbable sutures are placed one above the other aided by gentle traction on the previous suture. The sutures are placed from lateral to medial to minimize ureteral inclusion. The procedure is repeated on the contralateral side **(Fig. 4)**.

High Uterosacral Ligament Suspension for Apical Prolapse

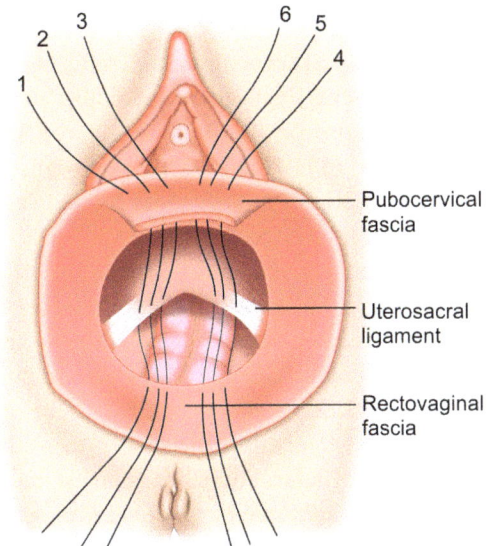

Fig. 4: Placement of sutures on uterosacral ligament (USL). The numbers indicate no. of suture exit points through pubocervical fascia.

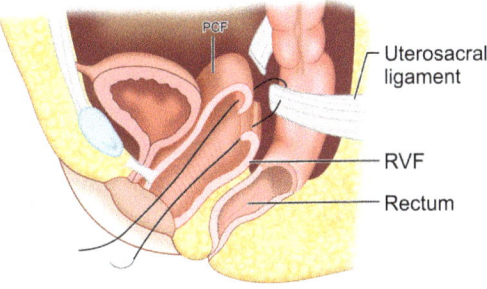

Fig. 5: Sutures on the uterosacral ligament passed through the vaginal apex to suspend the apex to the ligament. (PCF: pubocervical fascia; RVF: rectovaginal fascia)

Anterior fascial repair: Midline approximation of pubocervical fascia is done halfway through using 2-0 polyglactin suture material.

Exteriorizing sutures (anchoring) on USL: The anterior limb of the first suspension suture is passed through the pubocervical fascia and through the anterior vaginal wall at the future apex of the vault. The posterior limb of the same suture is passed through the posterior vaginal wall close to the apex **(Fig. 5)**.

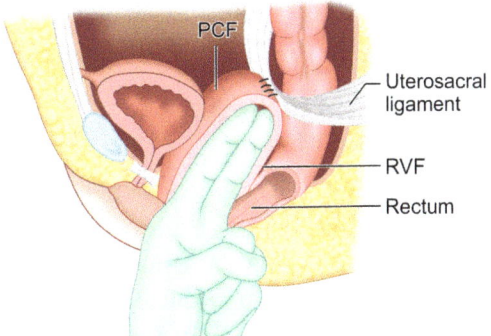

Fig. 6: Vaginal apex anchored to the uterosacral ligament along with the pubocervical and rectovaginal fascia. (PCF: pubocervical fascia; RVF: rectovaginal fascia)

No attempt is made to dissect the rectovaginal fascia from the posterior vaginal wall. The second and third sutures are passed through the pubocervical fascia and rectovaginal fascia but not through the vaginal wall. After trimming redundant anterior vaginal wall, closure of the anterior vaginal wall is accomplished halfway before tying the suspension sutures.

Anchoring vaginal apex along with pubocervical and rectovaginal fascia to the USL: The anterior and posterior limbs of all three pairs of the sutures were tied together on both sides **(Fig. 6)**.

By tying these sutures, the vault with pubocervical and rectovaginal fascia gets anchored to the USL, which elevates the apex above the ischial spine.

Evaluation of Ureteric Patency

In order to confirm ureteric patency, cystoscopy is done to look for urinary efflux. Oral preoperative administration of phenazopyridine 200–400 mg 6 hours prior to surgery enables recognition of orange colored urinary efflux with postoperative cystoscopy. Intravenous indigo carmine may clearly reveal the blue efflux from the ureteric orifices. Alternatively, filling the bladder with

100–150 mL of 50% dextrose solution may clearly reveal the low viscous urinary efflux.

Management of Ureteric Obstruction/Kinking

Absence of efflux or sluggish efflux indicates ureteric inclusion and warrants removal of the distal uterosacral sutures. Usually, it relieves the obstruction caused by kinking of the ureter and a repeat cystoscopy confirms it. Even after removal of distal USL sutures, if efflux is absent or unsatisfactory, ureteroscopic stenting should be done.

Posterior colpoperineorrhaphy is done after closure of the remaining anterior vaginal wall and the vault. Postoperatively, vaginal pack is left for 12 hours and Foley catheter is left indwelling for 24–48 hours.

Surgical Outcome of HUSLS

The current evidence on USLS is limited to uncontrolled retrospective case-series and it reveals an objective success rate of 85% and a reoperation rate for prolapse of 5.8% **(Table 1)**.

Pooled rates of a meta-analysis by Margulies et al. found anatomical success (POP-Q Stage 0–1) of 81.2% for the anterior segment, 98.3% of the apical segment, and 87.4% of the posterior segment.[33]

A retrospective review of over 900 patients receiving USLS[30] found an overall adverse event rate of 31.2% with 20.3% being attributed to perioperative urinary tract infection.

Rates of pulmonary and cardiac events were 2.3%, whereas the rate of ileus and small bowel obstruction were less than 0.5%.

Margulies et al. identified 10 studies on perioperative complications of USLS which included a total of 820 women.[33] Blood transfusions were reported in 1.3% and bowel injury in 0.2%.

Level 1 Evidence for HUSLS

1. **Abdominal sacrocolpopexy (ASC) versus uterosacral ligament suspension:**
   A small prospective RCT[32] compared ASC ($N = 54$) to HUSLS ($N = 56$) and reported an objective 100 % success for ASC and 82.5% for HUSLS.
   The recurrence and reoperation rate for prolapse were significantly lower in the ASC arm. Both intraoperative and postoperative complications were higher in the HUSLS arm.
   Level 1 evidence from this small prospective RCT is not in favor of HUSLS as a first line of treatment in women with vault prolapse.

2. **Sacrospinous Ligament Suspension (SSLS) versus Uterosacral Ligament Suspension:**
   The NICHD Pelvic Floor Disorders Network reported the results of the OPTIMAL trial in 2014[31]
   This RCT compared the safety and efficacy of the SSLS to USLS in women with uterine or post hysterectomy apical prolapse.
   A total of 374 patients were randomized (188 ULS and 186 SSLF) and at the end of 2 years:
   - There was no statistical difference between the two groups for the composite outcome (ULS 64.5% vs. SSLF 63.1%)
   - No differences between groups with reference to bothersome vaginal bulge symptoms (18%), anterior or posterior prolapse beyond the hymen (17.5%) and retreatment with pessary or surgery (5.1%)
   - Neurological pain requiring medical, behavioral or surgical intervention was higher in the SSLS group (12.4% vs. 6.9%).

   Neuropathic pain with HUSLS reported from entrapment or direct injury to sacral nerve roots S2 and S3 which is vulnerable with deep suture placement at USL sites closer to sacrum.[34,35]

TABLE 1: Outcome of transvaginal high uterosacral ligament suspension procedures.

First author	Year	No. of Pts.	Mean follow-up months (range)	Definition of anatomic success	Anatomic success-all segments	Anatomic recurrence by segment	Reoperation for prolapse
Jenkins[17]	1997	50	(6–48)	Not defined	48/50 (96%)	Anterior 4%	NR
Comiter[18]	1999	100	17 (6.5–35)	Grade 0–1	96/100 (96%)	Apex 4%	4/100 (4%)
Barber[19]	2000	46	15.5 (3.5–40)	Stage 0/1 or Stage 2 without symptoms	41/46 (90%)	Apex 5% Anterior 5% Posterior 5%	3/46 (6.5%)
Shull[15]	2000	289	Not stated	Grade 0–1	275/289 (95%)	Apex 1% Anterior 3.5% Posterior 1.4%	NR
Karram[20]	2001	168	21.6 (6–36)	Grade 0–1	148/168 (88%)	Apex 1% Anterior or Posterior 11%	11/168 (5.5%)
Amundsen[21]	2003	33	28 (6–43)	Stage 0 or 1	27/33 (82%)	Apex 6% Posterior 12%	NR
Silva[22]	2006	72	61.2 (42–90)	Symptomatic Stage 2 or greater	61/72 (85%)	Apex 3% Anterior 7% Posterior 14%	2/72 (3%)
Antovska[23]	2006	32	25 (9–42)	Stage 0 or 1	NR	Apex 0%	NR
Wheeler[24]	2006	35	24 (0–46)	Stage 0 apical prolapse	28/35 80%	Apex 20%	0/0 (0%)
De Boer[25]	2009	48	12	Stage 0–1	23/48 (48%)	Apex 4.2% Anterior 47.9% Posterior 14.6%	NR
Doumouchtsis[26]	2011	42	60	Grade 0 of vaginal vault	36/84 (84.6%)	Apex 15.4%	5/42 (11.9%)
Wong[27]	2011	57	12	Apical stage 0–1	4/57 (93%)	NR	1/57 (1.8%)
Cunjian[28]	2012	31	14 +/-6	Stage 0–1	31/31 (100%)	NR	NR
Edenfield[29]	2013	219	14 (8.5–26.5)	Beyond the hymen or retreatment	54/219 (24.7%)	Apical 8.7% Anterior 17.4% Posterior 6.8%	33.219 (15%)
Unger[30]	2015	983	6.9	Beyond hymen	875/983 (89%)	NR	3.4%
Barber[31] (OPTIMAL trial) RCT USLS vs. SSLS	2014	188	24	*Absence of:* 1. Apical descent 1/3 into vaginal canal 2. Anterior or posterior prolapse beyond hymen 3. Bothersome vaginal bulge symptoms and 4. Retreatment	100/155 (64.5%)	Apical 2% Anterior 12.9% Posterior 1.9%	51/61 (3.1%)
Rondini[32] RCT ASC vs. USLS	2015	56	12	Apex stage 0 or 1	46/56 (82%)	Apex 18% Anterior 34% Posterior 6.3%	10/56 (17%)

Source: Christopher M, et al. Pelvic organ prolapse surgery, Incontinence, 6th edition; 2017. 6th International Consultation on Incontinence, ICS & ICUD.

Level 1 evidence from this small RCT concludes that uterosacral ligament suspension and sacrospinous ligament suspension have similar efficacy for apical suspension (GoR B).

HUSLS and Ureteral Injuries

Although 80–100% of success rate with low morbidity and mortality reported by various retrospective series[15,17,21,36] favor HUSLS, pelvic surgeons are concerned about 1–11% of ureteral kinking/injury rate reported.[15,19]

A review of 700 consecutive vaginal prolapse surgeries found 5.9% of intraoperative ureteral kinking/injury to be directly attributable to USLS.

However, 87% were identified during cystoscopy before the completion of the index surgery and corrected by removing suspension sutures intraoperatively with no long-term consequence to the patient.[36]

Only 3 of 355 USLS (0.9%) performed in this series required additional procedures to relieve or correct ureteral obstruction or injury.

A retrospective review of over 900 patients receiving ULS found the intraoperative bladder injury rate at 1%. There were no intraoperative ureteral injuries. However, 4.5% of cases were complicated by ureteral kinking, all of which were resolved with intraoperative suture removal, with or without replacement of the vault suspension stitches.[30]

Margulies et al. identified 10 studies involving a total of 820 women that reported on perioperative complications of USLS.[33] The ureteric reimplantation rate in this series was only 0.6% and cystotomy in 0.1%. Shull et al.[15] reported the lowest of 1% ureteric injury rate (n = 289). Barber et al.[19] reported the highest rate of 11% ureteric injury. Amundsen et al.[21] reported ureteric kinking in 3%. In 2001, Karram et al.[20] reported a 2.4% risk of ureteric injury/kinking.

By restricting his bite to deep, dorsal, posterior part of the ligament, Aronson succeeded in reducing ureteric injury rate nearly fivefold.[37]

By comparing sacrospinous ligament suspension to uterosacral ligament suspension, OPTIMAL trial[31] reported intraoperative ureteric obstruction in five patients (3.2%) in the USLS group (n = 188) and none in the SSLF (n = 186).

Avoiding Ureteric Complications

Shull's vaginal HUSLS, is an effective native tissue repair procedure used for apical suspension.[15] Restoration of vaginal axis and feasibility of combining repair of level 2 anterior and posterior defects makes HUSLS procedure appealing. Despite its advantages, vaginal HUSLS received restricted acceptance as a primary procedure due to the potential inclusion of ureters and difficulties in defining the uterosacral ligament.

During the surgery, pelvic surgeons are expected to execute two essential steps to achieve successful anchorage without any ureteral complications.
1. Identification of the uterosacral ligament
2. Identification of the ureter

Identification of USL

It is not easy to identify the ligament, particularly in vault prolapse cases. To facilitate recognition of USL, the following measures are used.
- Packing and retracting the bowels
- Gentle traction on the tag holding uterosacral ligament or upward traction of the Allis clamp placed approximately at 4 and 7 o'clock position.
- Transperitoneal palpation of the ischial spine and identifying Uterosacral ligament which lies posterior and medial to the ischial spine.

Identification of Ureter

Performing vaginal HUSLS without encountering any ureteral injury will make the technique universally acceptable and fetch it its due recognition.

Shull and others[15,20,37] localized the uterosacral ligament prior to placement of suspension sutures by packing and retracting bowel combining it with gentle traction on the remaining uterosacral ligament. Even after adopting these measures, often the ligament cannot be defined, especially when we move cephalad. When the ligament is not distinctly seen, suspension sutures are placed under assumption, which enhances the vulnerability of the ureter.

Though it would be ideal to visualize the course of the ureter and then to place sutures on the USL, visual recognition of the ureter lying lateral to the USL may not be possible in all cases.

Attempt to stent the ureters pre or per operatively may not be successful with advanced stage III/IV POP.

Combining laparoscopic assistance while placing the suspension sutures is an option but it may undermine the benefits of vaginal approach.

The course of the ureter and USL diverges as we proceed from the cervical segment towards the sacrum.

It is worth remembering that ureter descends postero laterally along the anterior border of greater sciatic notch **(Fig. 7)**.

Ureter lies in the pelvic side wall from 2 to 5 cm ventral and lateral to the ischial spine.

Opposite the ischial spine, the ureter turns anteromedially above the levator ani to reach the base of the bladder.

Besides applying anatomical knowledge, the pelvic surgeon must be skilled at visual identification of the pelvic ureter and should implement it routinely while placing the suspension sutures on USL during HUSLS.

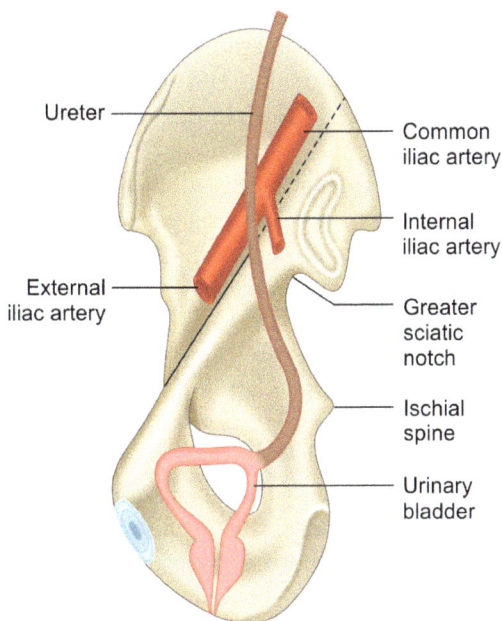

Fig. 7: Anatomy of ureter in the pelvis.

If identifying USL is difficult, it is worth retracting the sigmoid colon medially and with a constant visual guard over the course of the ureter, sutures are placed on the tissue lying over the groove lateral to the colon between these two vital structures, i.e., colon and ureter.

This step is beneficial in eliminating the inclusion of ureter particularly when USL is unidentifiable.

During transperitoneal abdominal surgery, the ureter being retroperitoneal, is inconspicuous and not easily seen in the operative field unless effort is taken.

Similarly, it is difficult to visualize ureters during vaginal surgery and most of us are not familiar with identifying ureters. It is more difficult to visualize a normal ureter than a dilated ureter.

Though hydroureter of long standing stage III/IV POP may facilitate the recognition, associated ureteral distortion may increase its vulnerability.

It is imperative that the surgeon is forewarned about the anatomical proximity and intimacy of the ureter to USL especially while performing HUSLS than in other vaginal surgeries.

During vaginal intraperitoneal HUSLS, it is possible for a pelvic surgeon to eliminate ureteral injury if constant visual guidance over the course of ureter is used while placing sutures on the USL. This step does not involve additional dissection and hence worth adopting routinely.

Extraperitoneal HUSLS

Dwyer & Fatton have described extra peritoneal USLS[38,39] in a series of 123 consecutive cases (93 received anterior and or posterior synthetic mesh). They have reported anatomical success of 85.5 % and apical success of 95.4 %. The reoperation rate for recurrent prolapse was 7%.

Abdominal and Laparoscopic USLS

Abdominal USLS has been used prophylactically after hysterectomy and therapeutically for apical prolapse. It can be done by laparotomy or laparoscopy.[38,39] Women with POP desiring childbearing can consider uterus conservation with high USLS. Results from a follow-up of a short-term small series indicate similar success to laparoscopic uterosacral hysteropexy.[40,41]

Lowenstein et al. reported a retrospective review of 107 women who underwent prolapse surgery that included abdominal USLS.[42]

In the 75 patients who completed 1 year follow up, 12% reported recurrent/persistent prolapse symptoms and 7% had anatomical failure. Complications were few, however, erosion of apical suture occurred in 9% (Gortex, expanded PTFT).

Vaginal versus Laparoscopic USLS

There were two retrospective comparisons between vaginal and laparoscopic USLS procedure. Both found no significant differences in perioperative morbidity or anatomical or subjective outcomes.[43,44]

CONCLUSION

Vaginal high USLS is a promising native tissue apical suspension technique performed to correct the apical defect induced prolapse. Anterior and posterior repairs should be combined.

It is a mesh and a gadget independent procedure, but warrants postoperative cystoscopy.

It offers long term objective and subjective success with an acceptable rate of complications. Pelvic surgeons are encouraged to identify the ureter while placing the suspension sutures on USL to avoid ureteral complications.

HUSLS involves a learning curve, but is well within the reach of most of the pelvic surgeons.

REFERENCES

1. Handa VL, Garrett E, Hendrix S, Gold E, Robbins J. Progression and remission of pelvic organ prolapse: a longitudinal study of menopausal women. Am J Obstet Gynecol. 2004;190(1):27-32.
2. Hendrix SL, Clark A, Nygaard I, Aragaki A, Barnabei V, McTiernan A. Pelvic organ prolapse in the Women's Health Initiative: gravity and gravidity. Am J Obstet Gynecol. 2002; 186(6):1160-6.
3. Shull BL. Pelvic organ prolapse: anterior, superior, and posterior vaginal segment defects. Am J Obstet Gynecol. 1999;181(1):6-11.
4. Eilber KS, Alperin MM, Khan AM, Wu NP, Pashos CL, Clemens JQ, et al. Outcomes of Vaginal Prolapse Surgery Among Female Medicare Beneficiaries: the Role of Apical Support. Obstet Gynecol. 2013;122(5):2-9.
5. Swift SE. The distribution of pelvic organ support in a population of female subjects seen for routine gynecologic health care. Am J Obstet Gynecol. 2000;183(2):277-85.
6. Delancey JO. Fascial and muscular abnormalities in women with urethral hypermobility and anterior vaginal wall prolapse. Am J Obstet Gynecol. 2002;187(1):93-8.

7. Rooney K, Kenton K, Mueller ER, FitzGerald MP, Brubaker L. Advanced anterior vaginal wall prolapse is highly correlated with apical prolapse. Am J Obstet Gynecol. 2006;195(6):1837-40.
8. Hsu Y, Chen L, Summers A, Ashton-Miller JA, Delancey JO. Anterior vaginal wall length and degree of anterior compartment prolapse seen on dynamic MRI. Int Urogynecol J Pelvic Floor Dysfunct. 2008;19(1):137-42.
9. Toozs-Hobson P, Boos K, Cardozo L. Management of vaginal vault prolapse. Br J Obstet Gynaecol. 1998;105(1):13-7.
10. Olsen AL, Smith VJ, Bergstrom JO, Colling JC, Clark AL. Epidemiology of surgically managed pelvic organ prolapse and urinary incontinence. Obstet Gynecol. 1997;89(4):501-6.
11. Boyles SH, Weber AM, Meyn L. Procedures for pelvic organ prolapse in the United States, 1979-1997. Am J Obstet Gynecol. 2003;188(1):108-15.
12. Brown JS, Waetjen LE, Subak LL, Thom DH, Van den Eeden S, Vittinghoff E. Pelvic organ prolapse surgery in the United States, 1997. Am J Obstet Gynecol. 2002;186(4):712-6.
13. Brubaker L. Burch Colposuspension at the time of sacrocolpopexy in stress continent women reduces bothersome stress urinary symptoms: The CARE randomized trial. J Pelvic Surg. 2005;11(Suppl 1):S5.
14. Miller N. A new method of correcting complete inversion of the vagina. Surg Gynecol Obstet. 1927;44:550-4.
15. Shull BL, Bachofen C, Coates KW, Kuehl TJ. A transvaginal approach to repair of apical and other associated sites of pelvic organ prolapse with uterosacral ligaments. Am J Obstet Gynecol. 2000;183:1365-73.
16. Buller JL, Thomson JR, Cundiff GW, Krueger Sullivan L, Schön Ybarra MA, Bent AE. Uterosacral ligament: description of Anatomic relationships to optimise surgical safety. Obstet Gynecol. 2001;97:873-9.
17. Jenkins VR 2nd. Uterosacral ligament fixation for vaginal vault suspension in uterine and vaginal vault prolapse. Am J Obstet Gynecol. 1997;177(6):1337-44.
18. Comiter CV, Vasavada SP, Raz S. Transvaginal culdosuspension: technique and results. Urology. 1999;54(5):819-22.
19. Barber MD, Visco AG, Weidner AC, Amundsen CL, Bump RC. Bilateral uterosacral ligament vaginal vault suspension with site-specific endopelvic fascia defect repair for treatment of pelvic organ prolapse. Am J Obstet Gynecol. 2000;183(6):1402-11.
20. Karram M, Goldwasser S, Kleeman S, Steele A, Vassallo B, Walsh P. High uterosacral vaginal vault suspension with fascial reconstruction for vaginal repair of enterocele and vagina vault prolapse. Am J Obstet Gynecol. 2001;185(6):1339-43.
21. Amundsen CL, Flynn BJ, Webster GD. Anatomical correction of vaginal vault prolapse by uterosacral ligament fixation in women who also require a pubovaginal sling. J Ural. 2003;169(5):1770-4.
22. Silva WA, Pauls RN, Segal JL, Rooney CM, Kleeman SD, Karram MM. Uterosacral ligament vault suspension: five-year outcomes. Obstet Gynecol. 2006;108(2):255-63.
23. Antovska SV, Dimitrov DG. Vaginosacral colpopexy (VSC)—a new modification of the Mc Call operation using vaginosacral ligaments as autologous sliding grafts in posthysterectomy vault prolapse. Bratisl Lek Listy. 2006;107(3):62-72.
24. Wheeler TL 2nd, Richter HE, Duke AG, Burgio KL, Redden DT, Varner RE. Outcomes with porcine graft placement in the anterior vaginal compartment in patients who undergo high vaginal uterosacral suspension and cystocele repair. Am J Obstet Gynecol. 2006;194(5):1486-91.
25. De Boer TA, Milani AL, Kluivers KB, Withagen MI, Vierhout ME. The effectiveness of surgical correction of uterine prolapse: cervical amputation with uterosacral ligament plication (modified Manchester) versus vaginal hysterectomy with high uterosacral ligament plication. Int Urogynecol J Pelvic Floor Dysfunct. 2009;20(11):1313-9.
26. Doumouchtsis SK, Khunda A, Jeffery ST, Franco AV, Fynes MM. Long-term outcomes of modified high uterosacral ligament vault suspension (HUSLS) at vaginal hysterectomy. Int Urogynecol J. 2011;22(5):577-84.
27. Wong MT, Abet E, Rigaud J, Frampas E, Lehur PA, Meurette G. Minimally invasive ventral mesh rectopexy for complex rectocoele: impact on anorectal and sexual function. Colorectal Dis. 2011;13(10):e320-6.
28. Cunjian Y, Li L, Xiaowen W, Shengrong L, Hao X, Xiangqiong L. A retrospective analysis of the effectiveness of a modified abdominal high uterosacral colpopexy in the treatment of uterine prolapse. Cell Biochem Biophys. 2012;64(2):95-9.
29. Edenfield AL, Amundsen CL, Weidner AC, Wu JM, George AM, Siddiqui NY. Vaginal prolapse recurrence after uterosacral ligament suspension in normal weight compared with overweight and obese women. Obstet Gynecol. 2013;121(3):554-9.

30. Unger CA, Walters MD, Ridgeway B, Jelovsek JE, Barber MD, Paraiso MF. Incidence of adverse events after uterosacral colpopexy for uterovaginal and posthysterectomy vault prolapse. Am J Obstet Gynecol. 2015;212(5):603.e1-7.
31. Barber MD, Brubaker L, Burgio KL, Richter HE, Nygaard I, Weidner AC, et al. Factorial comparison of two transvaginal surgical approaches and of perioperative behavioral therapy for women with apical vaginal prolapse: the OPTIMAL Randomized Trial. JAMA. 2014;311(10):1023-34.
32. Rondini C, Braun H, Alvarez J, Urzua MJ, Villegas R, Wenzel C, et al. High uterosacral vault suspension vs sacrocolpopexy for treating apical defects: a randomized controlled trial with twelve months follow-up. Int Urogynecol J. 2015;26(8):1131-8.
33. Margulies RU, Rogers MA, Morgan DM. Outcomes of transvaginal uterosacral ligament suspension: systematic review and meta-analysis. Am J Obstet Gynecol. 2010;202(2):124-34.
34. Siddique SA, Gutman RE, Schon Ybarra MA, Rojas F, Handa VL. Relationship of the uterosacral ligament to the sacral pexus and to the pudendal nerve. Int Urogynecol J Pelvic Floor Dysfunct. 2006;17:642-5.
35. Flynn M, Amundsen C, Weidner A. Sensory nerve injury after uterosacral ligament suspension. Am J Obstet Gynecol. 2006;195(6):1869-72.
36. Gustilo-Ashby AM, Jelovsek JE, Barber MD, Yoo EH, Paraiso MF, Walters MD. The incidence of ureteral obstruction and the value of intraoperative cystoscopy during vaginal surgery for pelvic organ prolapse. Am J Obstet Gynecol. 2006;194(5):1478-85.
37. Aronson MP, Aronson PK, Howard AE, Morse AN, Baker SP, Young SB. Low risk of ureteral obstruction with "deep" (dorsal/posterior) uterosacral ligament suture placement for transvaginal apical suspension. Am J Obstet Gynecol. 2005;192(5):1530-6.
38. Dwyer PL, Fatton B. Bilateral extraperitoneal uterosacral suspension: a new approach to correct posthysterectomy vaginal vault prolapse. Int Urogynecol J Pelvic Floor Dysfunct. 2008;19(2):283-92.
39. Fatton B, Dwyer PL, Achtari C, Tan PK. Bilateral extraperitoneal uterosacral vaginal vault suspension: a 2-year follow-up longitudinal case series of 123 patients. Int Urogynecol J Pelvic Floor Dysfunct. 2009;20(4):427-34.
40. Maher CF, Carey MP, Murray CJ, Laparoscopic suture hysteropexy for uterine prolapse. Obstet Gynecol. 2001;97:1010-4.
41. Diwan A, Rardin CR, Strohsnitter WC, Weld A, Rosenblatt P, Kohli N. Laparoscopic uterosacral ligament uterine suspension compared with vaginal hysterectomy with vaginal vault suspension for uterovaginal prolapse. Int Urogynecol J Pelvic Floor Dysfunction. 2006;17:79-83.
42. Lowenstein L, Fitz A, Kenton K, FitzGerald MP, Mueller ER, Brubaker L. Transabdominal uterosacral suspension: outcomes and complications. Am J Obstet Gynecol. 2009;200(6):656.e1-5.
43. Rardin CR, Erekson EA, Sung VW, Ward RM, Myers DL. Uterosacral colpopexy at the time of vaginal hysterectomy: comparison of laparoscopic and vaginal approaches. J Reprod Med. 2009;54(5):273-80.
44. Turner LC, Lavelle ES, Shepherd JP. Comparison of complications and prolapse recurrence between laparoscopic and vaginal uterosacral ligament suspension for the treatment of vaginal prolapse. Int Urogynecol J. 2016;27(5):797-803.

25. Abdominal Apical Suspension Procedures for Pelvic Organ Prolapse

Bimal M John, Raji S

INTRODUCTION

Advances in health care have made women lead longer and healthier life. However, the issue of pelvic organ prolapse has increased due to increasing age, the management of which is demanding due to coexistent defects in different compartment. Consequently, it is pertinent to have an in-depth understanding of the anatomy and relationship of the surrounding structures of the vagina.

Normal anatomical position of the vagina is 5 cm inferior to the 2nd sacral vertebra and 5 cm medial to ipsilateral ischial spine.

DeLancey classified supports of the vagina into three levels **(Table 1)**.

ABDOMINAL/LAPAROSCOPIC/ROBOTIC PROCEDURE

1. Sacrocolpopexy
2. Abdominal uterosacral ligament suspension
3. Pectopexy

The object of prolapse surgeries is to restore normal anatomy, minimizing symptoms, improving quality of life, and reducing recurrences. Prior to deciding on procedure, the patient's expectation and priority should be discussed.

ABDOMINAL SACROCOLPOPEXY (FIG. 1)

Abdominal sacrocolpopexy, introduced by Lane in 1962, is a widely accepted procedure to suspend the vaginal vault to the sacrum using natural/synthetic grafts.[1-3]

Long-term success rate ranges nearly up to 90%. It can be used as primary surgery for prolapse or even as surgery to treat relapse, in addition it can be used in patients with increased risk of recurrence [patients with chronic obstructive pulmonary disease (COPD), obesity, constipation, etc.].

Sacrocolpopexy provides a substantial support by attaching the vaginal apex and

TABLE 1: DeLancey's three levels of vaginal support.

DeLancey's levels	Defects	Structures comprising
Level 1	Suspension/apical defect	• Uterosacral ligaments • Paracolpium • Parametrium
Level 2	Attachment defect	• Arcus tendineus fascia pelvis • Arcus tendineus rectovaginalis
Level 3	Fusion defect	• Levator ani • Perineal body

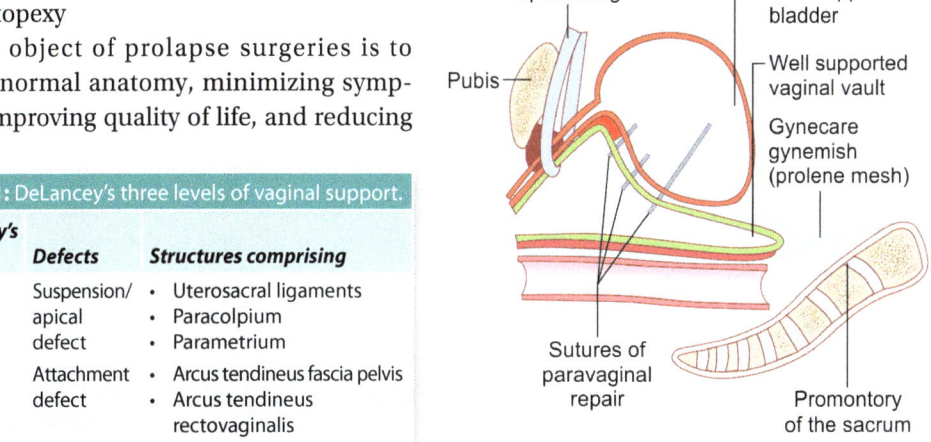

Fig. 1: Level of apical restoration with sacrocolpopexy versus paravaginal repair versus sparc sling.

the anterior and posterior vaginal walls to the anterior longitudinal ligament of the ischial spine at the level of the sacrum using a mesh.

Despite autologous, cadaveric, or synthetic graft materials may be used, permanent (synthetic) mesh has the best success rate and should be used if not contraindicated.[4]

Patient Evaluation

Women are advised preoperative urodynamic studies. In those with symptoms of urinary incontinence, it is to determine need for corrective procedures and in those without urinary symptoms to assess if after reducing the prolapse, the repair may unmask incontinence.[5,6]

Comprehensive assessment should be performed preoperatively to identify the concurrent defects in other compartment for repair.

Patient Preparation

- A detailed informed consent encompassing procedure, complication, and recurrence risk to be obtained.
- Use of vaginal estrogen cream 6–8 weeks preprocedure may be recommended. It is opined that estrogen treatment enhances vascularity to promote healing and improve tissue strength, despite no data to suggest it is beneficial.
- Bowel preparation given on eve of operative day.
- Antibiotics and thromboprophylaxis should be given.[7]

Technique

Anesthesia and Positioning

Following general anesthesia, the patient is positioned supine in Allen stirrups. It is imperative to ensure no pressure on the calf/thigh, maintaining the thigh parallel to the ground to reduce the risk of nerve injury. The buttocks are placed at the edge of the table to aid in full range of vaginal stent manipulation. Parts surgically prepared, and an indwelling catheter inserted.

Incision

An incision used to be placed so as to allow access to both vaginal apex and promontory. A vertical or transverse abdominal incision may be used. A Pfannenstiel incision provides sufficient access to the sacrum and deep pelvis.

Bowel Packing

After placing a self-retaining retractor (Balfour or Bookwalter type), the bowel is packed with laparotomy sponges up and out of the pelvis.

Bowel packing is aimed at shifting the sigmoid colon farther to the patient's left thereby allowing access to the sacrum.

Identification of Anatomic Structures

The aortic bifurcation and iliac vessels are identified and middle sacral vessels palpated ventral to the sacral promontory in the midline.

Tracing of the ureters at this level aids in reducing their injury. The right being at a greater risk of injury during suture placement at the sacrum.

Peritoneal Incision

A peritoneal tunnel is created by elevating the peritoneum overlying the promontory and incising it sharply. This incision is then extended caudally into the Douglas' cul-de-sac.

This tunnel will house the mesh and its closure at the end of the surgery allows the mesh to lie beneath the peritoneum which reducing the risk of adhesion of bowel to mesh.

Selection of Sacral Suture Site

Suture placement at S1/sacral promontory risks laceration of the middle sacral vessels/

left common iliac vein.[8] Whereas placement at S3 or S4 vertebral bodies increases age risk of injury to presacral venous plexus.

Many surgeons presently prefer to place sutures at the level of S1/sacral promontory.[9] Reason being that at S1 level the middle sacral vessels are readily visible, easily isolated thus injury can be avoided. Also, the anterior longitudinal ligament at this level thicker and stronger therefore affixing the sutures at this portion will minimize the risk of suture avulsion.

However, few cases of discitis and sacral osteomyelitis have been reported related to suture placement at this site.[10] Thus, care should be taken to suture only the anterior longitudinal ligament thereby avoiding deep suture placement into the disc.

Bleeding Complications

The most common vessels lacerated during sacrocolpopexy are the presacral venous plexus and the middle sacral vessels.[11]

Although suturing and clipping may be useful, suturing of small veins worsens bleed. Additionally, vessels retract into the bone making isolation and ligation difficult.

Sterile thumbtacks may be used directed through the lacerated vessels and pushing into the sacrum compressing the vessels.[12]

Local hemostatic agents may also be considered.[13,14]

Placement of Sacral Sutures

A Kittner sponge is used to separate and remove fat gently dissect fat and areolar tissue from the sacrum.

The shiny white anterior longitudinal ligament identified overlying the bone in the midline.

Sutures may be placed at S1 through S4. Three sutures approximately 0.5 cm apart of 2-0 gauge permanent material is used. The needle driven either horizontally or vertically through the ligament.

Dissection of Anterior Vaginal Wall

A vaginal stent is placed to elevate the vaginal apex, and the peritoneum covering it is incised transversely. Peritoneum and bladder are separated from the anterior vaginal wall.

Dissection of the Posterior Vaginal Wall

The vaginal apex is grasped with Allis clamps, peritoneum covering the posterior vaginal wall is then opened.

The rectovaginal space is identified and entered.

Posterior Mesh Placement

Synthetic, nonabsorbable, macroporous, monofilament polypropylene mesh is preferred. The large pore size allows host tissue ingrowth and monofilament decreases bacterial adherence.

Mesh is prepared as two separate straps, each 2-3 cm wide. Alternatively, "Y" mesh is used.

Anterior Mesh Placement

The length of the mesh used on the anterior vaginal wall is shorter than on the posterior vaginal wall. Two rectangular pieces of mesh are then cut to the width of the dissected anterior and posterior vaginal wall surfaces. They are left long to allow fixation to the sacrum later in the procedure. Mesh is attached using 2-0 nonabsorbable suture. Six sutures are used at the edges of the mesh to secure it to the posterior vaginal wall's fibromuscular layers.

Suturing the vaginal apex should be avoided as it is the least vascular region, thus most susceptible for suture and mesh erosion.

Vaginal epithelial penetration should be avoided during suturing, however, if the fibromuscular layer is thin, the epithelium may be incorporated. These vaginal sutures will generally be epithelialized postoperatively.

Passage of Mesh into Peritoneal Tunnel

After securing the anterior and posterior meshes, both are passed through the peritoneal tunnel to the sacral sutures.

Vaginal Peritoneal Closure

The peritoneum over the vaginal apex with 2-0 delayed-absorbable running sutures.

Mesh Sizing and Placement

After removing the vaginal stent, digital examination of the vagina is done. The length of mesh is estimated holding the megs to the sacrum with the hand over the abdomen while palpating prolapse improvement vaginally. Care executed to avoid tension on the mesh and cut to the appropriate length.

Peritoneal Closure

The mesh is buried retroperitoneally by closing the peritoneum over it at the level of sacral promontory.

Cystoscopy

Cystoscopy is performed to ensure ureteral integrity.

Abdominal Closure

The abdomen is closed in a standard fashion.

Postoperative Care

If concomitant incontinence procedure is not performed, catheter can be routinely removed at first. Care to avoid constipation is advised at discharge.

Complications

- Hemorrhage from presacral venous plexus and presacral arteries can be life-threatening.
- Ureteric injuries, bladder injury (<3%), bowel injury, and sacral osteomyelitis.[10]
- Postoperative complications include ileus, small bowel obstruction, and wound complications.
- Long-term complication includes mesh erosion (3-4%).

Mesh Erosion

Occurrence can be years after procedure.
- Symptoms develop 14 months following surgery and classically are vaginal bleeding and discharge.[15]
- The diagnosis is easy, as mesh or sutures can be seen directly on speculum examination.

Management

- Initially treated with 6-week course of intravaginal estrogen cream.
- Removal of eroded mesh can be done by abdominal/vaginal route.

For those in whom epithelium fails to cover the mesh, surgical removal is performed vaginally.

The mucosal edges surrounding the erosion site are dissected away from the mesh, undermined, and reapproximated.

Failure to heal is a sign of graft infection, and the graft material should be completely removed either vaginally or abdominally (MaCox, 2004).

Suture erosion may be managed by removal in the office.

Satisfyingly, postoperative scarring may continue to hold the vagina; apex and thus removal of the mesh does not compromise the prolapse repair.

Advantages

High success rate and low recurrence rate. Sacrocolpopexy maintains genital tract anatomy, so dyspareunia is less.[16]

Disadvantages

Greater blood loss accounting to bleeding from presacral venous plexus and presacral arteries and postoperative development of stress urinary incontinence. Chance of ureteric injury is also a disadvantage.

Recent long-term data provided by the Pelvic Floor Disorders committee, New York which followed 215 women for 7 years after the procedure. Out of which, 149 underwent physical examination for prolapse assessment. It was found that 31 of 149 women (21%) had anatomic prolapsed recurrence, of which 16 (52%) were symptomatic, and 11 (7%) had apical recurrence.

Minimally Invasive Sacrocolpopexy

Sacrocolpopexy may also be performed with a minimally invasive technique using laparoscopy or robotic surgery. The basic steps are the same and differ mainly by the method of abdominal entry.

Port placement: A 10-mm incision is made in the base of the umbilicus, and a 10-mm trocar I placed to gain abdominal access and after safe abdominal entry, a diagnostic laparoscopy is performed. Three accessory ports are then usually placed under direct laparoscopic visualization. We typically place a 5-mm port in the upper abdomen and two 10-mm ports in the right and left lower abdomen. Remaining steps are same as abdomen sacrocolpopexy.

Minimally invasive procedures are associated with shorter hospitalization, though with longer operating time and greater cost.[17]

ABDOMINAL UTEROSACRAL LIGAMENT SUSPENSION

Anatomy: Uterosacral ligaments extend from the posterior aspect of supravaginal cervix to sacrum and lie on either side of rectosigmoid forming the lateral boundaries of cul-de-sac. It is done in patients with well-defined uterosacral ligaments, often preferred in those undergoing hysterectomy as there is higher chance of mesh erosion in abdominal sacrocolpopexy if done along with hysterectomy. Procedure involves suturing the uterosacral ligaments to the anterior and posterior vaginal walls at the vaginal apex such that enteroceles are effectively closed. Consequently, Halban or Moschcowitz culdoplasty enterocele repairs are not required (**Fig. 2**).

Preoperative

Patients with symptoms of urinary incontinence should undergo simple or complex urodynamic testing.

Intraoperative

Anesthesia and Patient Position

Performed under general or regional anesthesia. Position same as in abdominal sacrospinous colpopexy. Foley catheter is placed in situ.

Incision

Midline vertical or Pfannenstiel incision put, abdomen opened, a self-retaining retractor is placed, bowel is packed from the operative field.

Uterosacral ligament suspension is done usually at the completion of abdominal hysterectomy.[18]

Identification of Uterosacral Ligaments

The ureters are identified bilaterally because of an increased risk of ureteral injury during suturing of the uterosacral ligaments.

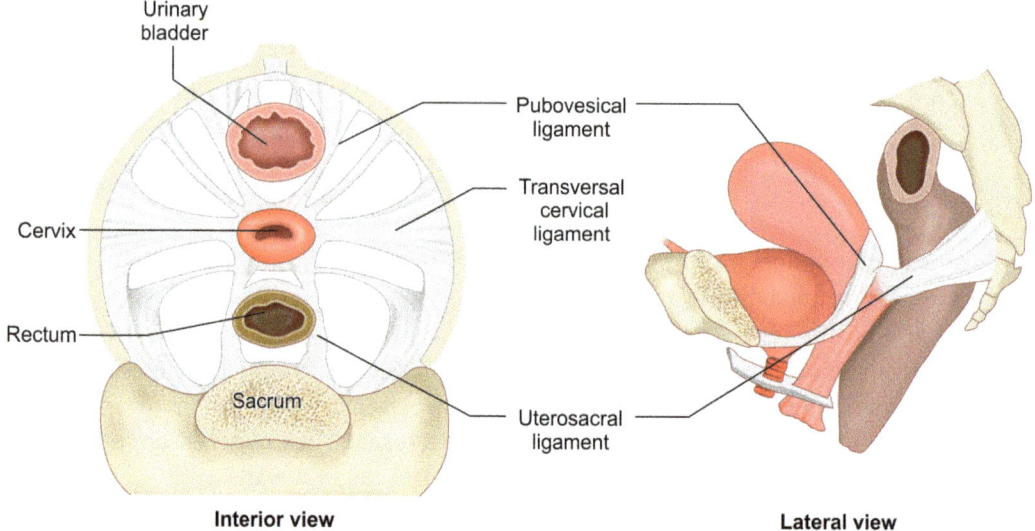

Fig. 2: Anatomy of uterosacral ligament.

Uterosacral ligaments are identified prior to hysterectomy by applying contralateral upward traction to the uterine fundus. The uterosacral ligaments are placed on stretch and can be identified.

These ligaments originate from the lower and posterior uterine surface and extend to the sacrum. They also lie medial and posterior to the ischial spines.

Three double-armed sutures of 2-0 permanent suture are placed 1 cm apart in each uterosacral ligament and held. This is the step of greatest risk to the ureters.

Nonetheless, it should be reiterated that if sutures are placed medial and posterior to the ischial spines, the ureters will not be in jeopardy.

Hysterectomy

If hysterectomy is planned, it is now completed, cuff is left open. A purse-string suture of 2-0 delayed-absorbable suture is placed 1.5 cm from the edge of the cuff in the vaginal epithelium to close the vaginal apex. This step will prevent erosion of permanent vaginal uterosacral ligament suspension (USLS) sutures through the vaginal epithelium.

Suture Placement

Six sutures are placed equidistant along the horizontal length of the vaginal cuff. These sutures are placed through the fibromuscular layer above the prior purse-string.

Knots secured starting with most medial to lateral sutures. Care is taken to firmly secure all knots and to ensure that vaginal wall is directly approximated to the uterosacral ligaments **(Figs. 3A and B)**.

Cystoscopy

Cystoscopy is done to document ureteral patency. After which vaginal examination may be performed to assess the need for additional prolapse repair of the anterior and posterior vaginal walls.

Concurrent Procedures

If posterior repair or anti-incontinence surgery is required, these will follow abdominal incision closure.

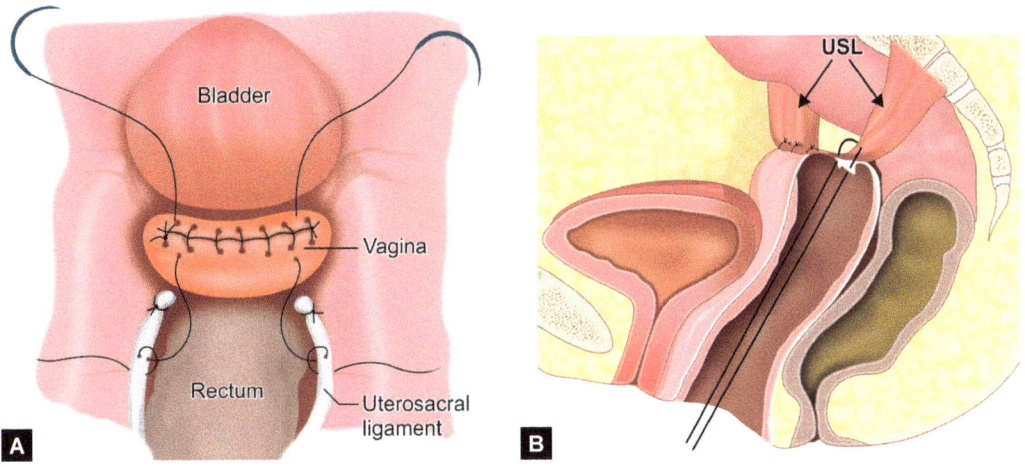

Figs. 3A and B: Uterosacral ligament (USL) fixation.

Complications

- Recurrence of approximately 10–15%.
- Uterosacral ligament suspension has a possibility to shorten and fix the upper vagina. The possibility of postprocedural dyspareunia must be discussed with the patient.
- Sacral plexus nerve injury with consequential neuropathy has been reported.

PECTOPEXY

A more recent approach to apical prolapse described first in 2007. This method mobilizes the iliopectineal ligament on both sides for the mesh fixation, so there is no restriction created by the mesh.

The mesh follows natural structures (round and broad ligaments) without crossing delicate spots, such as the ureter or bowel.[19] The hypogastric trunk is at a comfortable distance and out of danger. The iliopectineal ligament is considerably stronger than the sacrospinous ligament and the arcus tendineus fascia pelvis.

To maintain a physiological axis of the vagina, the cranial anchor point should be at the S2 level. As opposed to sacrocolpopexy, pectopexy has lesser chance of relapse and better long-term outcome because of the lower likelihood of disorders caused by narrowing of the pelvis.[20]

Anatomy

The pectineal ligament (inguinal ligament of Cooper) is an extension of the lacunar ligament which runs on the pectineal line of the pubic bone and is a thickening in the pubic bone periosteum **(Figs. 4A and B)**.

Technique

After administering general anesthesia, patient positioned as in abdominal sacrocolpopexy. Laparoscopic entry into the abdomen as in standard gynecological laparoscopic approach. The peritoneal layer along the right round ligament toward the pelvic side wall identified and opened. Incision is made in the medially and caudally using a harmonic scalpel and the right external iliac vein visualized.

About 4–5 cm of right iliopectineal ligament adjacent to insertion of iliopsoas muscle identified. Same repeated on the left side. The peritoneal layers on either side opened toward the vaginal apex, vaginal apex was prepared for mesh preparation. If the uterus is preserved, anterior peritoneum of the uterus is opened and lower uterine segment of uterus

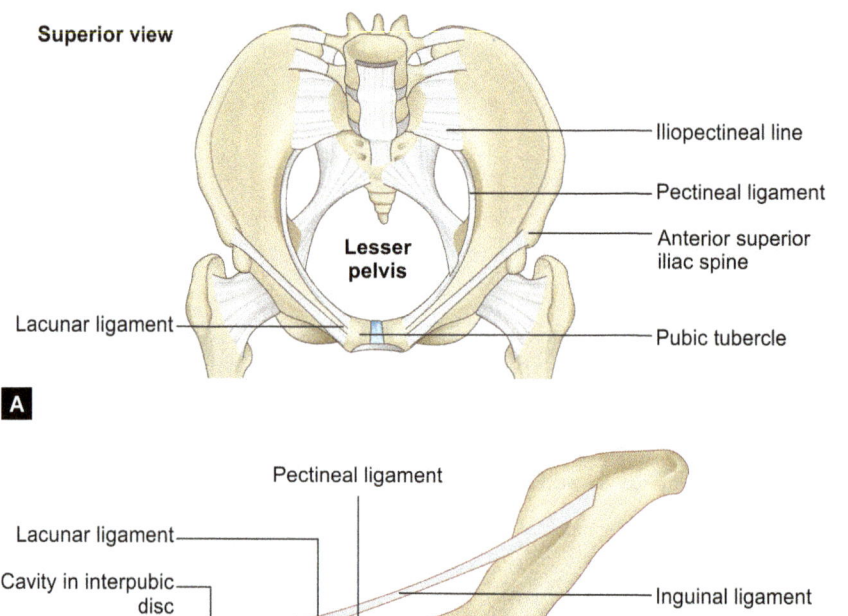

Figs. 4A and B: Anatomy of pectineal ligament.

is prepared for mesh fixation. A monofilament mesh is inserted, same sutured to both iliopectineal ligaments using nonabsorbable sutures. Mesh is fixed tension-free to vaginal apex or uterus. Finally, peritoneum above the mesh is sutured with absorbable sutures **(Fig. 5)**.

Advantages

- Procedure does not reduce pelvic space.
- Lesser chance of defecation disorders.
- Incidence of defecation disorders and urinary incontinence was found to be lesser in comparison to sacropexy.
- Risk of recurrence lesser than sarcopexy.

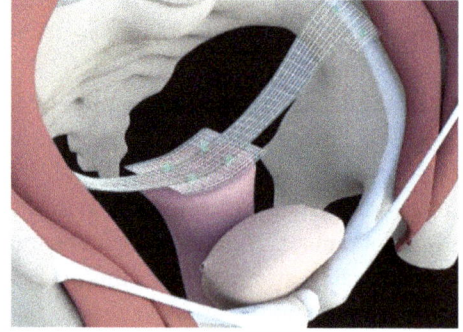

Fig. 5: Iliopectineal ligament fixation.

REFERENCES

1. Lane FE. Repair of posthysterectomy vaginal-vault prolapse. Obstet Gynecol. 1962;20:72-7.

2. Maher CF, Qatawneh AM, Dwyer PL, Carey MP, Cornish A, Schluter PJ. Abdominal sacral colpopexy or vaginal sacrospinous colpopexy for vaginal vault prolapse: a prospective, randomized study. Am J Obstet Gynecol. 2004; 190:20-6.
3. Mattox TF, Stanford EJ, Varner E. Infected abdominal sacrocolpopexies: diagnosis and treatment. Int Urogynecol J Pelvic Floor Dysfunct. 2004;15(5):319-23.
4. Culligan PJ, Blackwell L, Goldsmith LJ, Graham CA, Rogers A, Heit MH. A randomized controlled trial comparing fascia lata and synthetic mesh for sacral colpopexy. Obstet Gynecol. 2005;106:29-37.
5. Chaikin DC, Groutz A, Blaivas JG. Predicting the need for anti-incontinence surgery in continent women undergoing repair of severe urogenital prolapse. J Urol. 2000;163:531-4.
6. Brubaker L, Cundiff GW, Fine P, Nygaard I, Richter HE, Visco AG, et al. Abdominal sacrocolpopexy with Burch colposuspension to reduce urinary stress incontinence. N Engl J Med. 2006;354:1557-66.
7. American College of Obstetricians and Gynecologists. ACOG practice bulletin No. 104: antibiotic prophylaxis for gynecologic procedures. Practice Bulletin No. Obstet Gynecol. 2009;113(5):1180-9.
8. Wieslander CK, Rahn DD, McIntire DD, Marinis SI, Wai CY, Schaffer JI, et al. Vascular anatomy of the presacral space in unembalmed female cadavers. Am J Obstet Gynecol. 2006;195:1736-41.
9. Nygaard IE, McCreery R, Brubaker L, Connolly A, Cundiff G, Weber AM, et al. Abdominal sacrocolpopexy: a comprehensive review. Obstet Gynecol. 2004;104:805-23.
10. Weidner AC, Cundiff GW, Harris RL, Addison WA. Sacral osteomyelitis: an unusual complication of abdominal sacral colpopexy. Obstet Gynecol. 1997;90:689-91.
11. Galloway NT, Davies N, Stephenson TP. The complications of colposuspension. Br J Urol. 1987;60:122-4.
12. Oz MC, Cosgrove DM 3rd, Badduke BR, Hill JD, Flannery MR, Palumbo R, et al. Controlled clinical trial of a novel hemostatic agent in cardiac surgery. The Fusion Matrix Study Group. Ann Thorac Surg. 2000;69(5): 1376-82.
13. Kheirabadi BS, Field-Ridley A, Pearson R, MacPhee M, Drohan W, Tuthill D. Comparative study of the efficacy of the common topical hemostatic agents with fibrin sealant in a rabbit aortic anastomosis model. J Surg Res. 2002;106:99-107.
14. Weaver FA, Hood DB, Zatina M, Messina L, Badduke B. Gelatin-thrombin-based hemostatic sealant for intraoperative bleeding in vascular surgery. Ann Vasc Surg. 2002;16:286-93.
15. Kohli N, Walsh PM, Roat TW, Karram MM. Mesh erosion after abdominal sacrocolpopexy. Obstet Gynecol. 1998;92:999-1004.
16. Given FT Jr, Muhlendorf IK, Browning GM. Vaginal length and sexual function after colpopexy for complete uterovaginal eversion. Am J Obstet Gynecol. 1993;169:284-8.
17. Judd JP, Siddiqui NY, Barnett JC, Visco AG, Havrilesky LJ, Wu JM. Cost-minimization analysis of robotic-assisted, laparoscopic, and abdominal sacrocolpopexy. J Minim Invasive Gynecol. 2010;17(4):493-9.
18. Zullo F, Palomba S, Russo T, Sbano FM, Falbo A, Morelli M, et al. Laparoscopic colposuspension using sutures or prolene meshes: a 3-year follow-up. Eur J Obstet Gynecol Reprod Biol. 2004;117:201-3.
19. Ross JW. Apical vault repair, the cornerstone or pelvic vault reconstruction. Int Urogynecol J Pelvic Floor Dysfunct. 1997;8:14-52.
20. Flynn BJ, Webster GD. Surgical management of the apical vaginal defect. Curr Opin Urol. 2002;12:353-8.

Advances in Pelvic Repair and Reconstructive Surgeries

CHAPTER 26

Vineet Mishra, Neeta Mishra, Deepa Chaudhary

INTRODUCTION

Female pelvic medicine and reconstructive surgery, while still in its infancy, has undergone a quantum leap over the last decade. Pelvic floor dysfunction is an intricate condition globally affecting urination, defecation, and sexual function. Pelvic organ prolapse (POP), urinary or fecal incontinence, chronic constipation, pelvic pain, and sexual dysfunction are few of inveterate facets of it which dramatically increases with age and menopause.

Pelvic floor is highly assailable to injuries and functional modifications during pregnancy, obesity, and ageing. When identified early, certain nonsurgical therapies, such as pelvic floor muscle physiotherapy, energy source tightening (laser or radiofrequency) can delay apparition of symptoms to some extent but most will require surgery. Pelvic floor reconstructive surgeons have passel of surgical options using either transvaginal or transabdominal (open, laparoscopic or robotic) approach.

Operative approach requires a thorough discernment of pelvic anatomy, requirements of patient, surgical skills of the surgeon. In most patients, the pelvic floor has multiple defects, hence any pelvic reconstructive surgery should take into account all three levels of support and provide comprehensive repair. Thus, a diligent knowledge of the underlying functional status of pelvic organs is paramount for a successful surgical outcome.[1]

FUNCTIONAL ANATOMY OF PELVIC ORGAN PROLAPSE

With the advent of new functional pelvic floor imaging, understanding about the etiology has changed from the old empirical hypothesis based on gross anatomy and physical examination to new mechanistic hypotheses by comparing the structure and function of pelvic floor between living women with and without prolapse using magnetic resonance imaging (MRI), ultrasound and functional pelvic floor testing.

Interactions between the levator ani muscle and pelvic connective tissues is the main stay of pelvic organ support. Puboviscveral portion (PVM) cross-sectional area (CSA) thickness is measured in the injury zone by ultrasound and MRI. MRI examination of the levator in women with and without prolapse have demonstrated that vaginal delivery related injury to the PVM where more than 50% of the muscle is missing causes pelvic organ prolapse in 55% of women as opposed to only 16% of women with intact support. Differential pressure produced on the vaginal wall due to muscle failure causes uneven traction on the fascia and musculature leading to prolapse **(Figs. 1A to C).**[2]

EMERGING FUNCTIONAL ROLE OF FEMALE COSMETIC GENITAL SURGERY

Female cosmetic genital surgery (FCGS) refers to a treatments that address the vulval or vaginal appearance. The surgical techniques used in FCGS have been used for

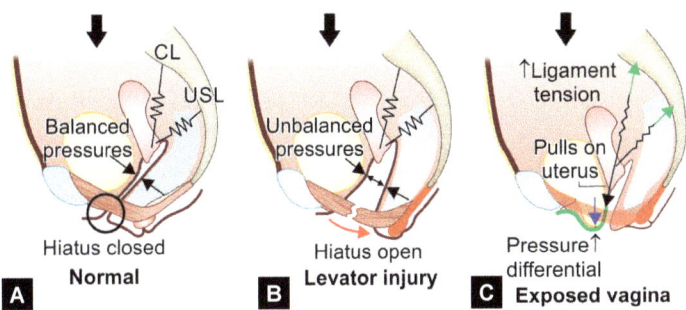

Figs. 1A to C: Diagrammatic representation of interactions between levator ani muscle, anterior vaginal wall prolapse, and cardinal/uterosacral ligament suspension. With normal levator function (A), the vaginal walls are in apposition, and anterior and posterior pressures are balanced. Levator damage (B) results in hiatal opening, and the vagina becomes exposed to a pressure differential between abdominal and atmospheric pressures. This pressure differential (C) creates a traction force on the cardinal ligament (CL) and uterosacral ligament (USL).
Source: Modified from ©DeLancey, 2012.

noncosmetic reasons but their indication for cosmetic and sexual functional reasons is what is garnering attention.

The surgeries performed as part of FCGS have been covered in detail on the Chapter on Cosmetic Gynecology.

Perineum, vulva and vagina of female undergoes anatomical and structural changes during childbirth and with age causing weakness and stretching of tissue resulting in vaginal laxity affecting sensation and sexual function.[3] Prolapse is considered as more severe form of vaginal relaxation. This "wide vagina" as depicted by **Figure 1** is the first preventable stage of POP studies has shown when repaired, it improves sexual function.

Most women with complain of vaginal relaxation will also have anterior/posterior vaginal wall prolapse or cervical decent which should be repaired simultaneously. The two most commonly performed surgeries to address vaginal laxity are Perineoplasty and Vaginoplasty which are modifications of colpoperineorrhaphy but the cosmetic appearance of the introitus and perineal body are also taken into account. Care is taken to avoid tension on the levators as it causes intense perineal pain on penetration due to lateral banding of vagina.

Goal of these surgeries is not limited to aesthetics but also functionality. Sexual function usually improves due to introital tightening, elevated perineum with reconstruction of the perineal body and correcting the posterior compartment defects. Reconstruction of the downward angle of the vagina directs penile pressure against the clitoral complex, pushing it against the pubic bone with coital thrust, presumably helping with clitoral orgasm. Aesthetic surgery of the vulva and vagina is community rather than university or academically driven. It can be medically necessary therapy in one who looks upon self-perceived genital "disfigurement" or "sensation of a wide vagina" as a sexual or body image dysfunction, or as a cosmetic dissatisfaction issue, subject to elective revision. So, the division between cosmetic and functional procedures has become somewhat indistinct combining both of them will improve the sexual quality of life as well as prevent progression of prolapse.[4,5]

SURGERY FOR PELVIC ORGAN PROLAPSE

Anatomic classification of pelvic surgery is based on compartment affected, i.e., anterior, posterior and/or apical. Any of these compartment defects can be dealt by transvaginal or abdominal approach, open or minimally invasive.

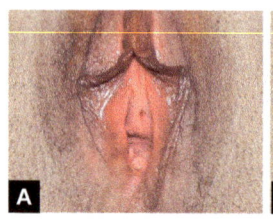 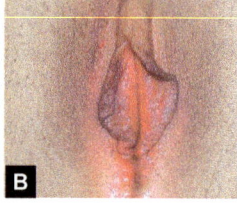

Figs. 2A and B: (A) Preoperative perineoplasty; (B) Postoperative perineoplasty.

Four important clinical parameters will direct the surgical planning:
1. Leading edge of the prolapse 1 cm inside or any distance outside the hymen requires a surgical correction.
2. Each compartment should be evaluated independently using a speculum to identify the origin of prolapse.
3. Understanding the most dependent part of the vaginal apex plays an important role. A cotton swab can be used to measure total vaginal length (TVL) and POP-Q point C (cervix or cuff during Valsalva). A difference of >2 cm between TVL and point C is an indicator of the necessity for apical suspension.
4. Presence or absence of cervix or uterus has critical implications for surgical planning, prolapse is frequently "up-staged" in the operating room due to anesthesia.[6] Newer modalities such as functional MRI are providing a new perspective regarding the relative contribution of the structural components of pelvic organs to prolapse.

There is no universal rule for surgical approach. This needs to be individualized according to patient's need and surgeon's skill. Focus of pelvic reconstructive surgery is now uterine preservation and apical suspension. Apical prolapse refers to prolapse of the uterus, cervix or post-hysterectomy vaginal cuff. This is frequently seen in prolapse which extends beyond the hymen. Therefore, restoration of apical support is paramount during repair of advanced pelvic organ prolapse, failure of which leads to recurrence. Hysterectomy is not mandatory for treatment of pelvic organ prolapse but correction and reconstruction of apex should be performed.[6]

Hysteropexy

Uterine preservation is requested by women for a variety of reasons: Sense of identity, maintenance of fertility, concern on impact of sexual function, and risk involved in hysterectomy. Correct selection of candidates for the procedure is imperative for pelvic surgeons. Patients at greater risk for gynecological cancers and cervical elongation are not ideal candidates for uterine preservation. Obesity is a relative contraindication.

There is reduction in operating time, blood loss, and risk of mesh exposure in uterine preserving surgeries compared with similar surgical routes with concomitant hysterectomy and do not significantly change short-term prolapse outcome.

Hysteropexy procedures can be separated on the basis of vaginal and abdominal approaches and with or without the use of mesh. These procedures are now increasingly being performed by the laparoscopic and robotic techniques. But robust studies comparing efficacy of various hysteropexy procedures are still lacking.[7,8]

In sacrospinous hysteropexy (SSHP), the cervix or utero sacral ligament complex is transfixed to the sacrospinous ligament using permanent or delayed absorbable suture.

There Sascha et al. (2019) in their multicenter randomized control trial ($n = 204$) compared the sacrospinous hysteropexy versus vaginal hysterectomy with utero sacral ligament suspension in uterine prolapse of stage 2 or more by and had shown that uterine preservation is more effective than vaginal hysterectomy with uterosacral ligament suspension, and the risk for retreatment of recurrent prolapse or malignancy is low in a five-year follow-up. So, surgical correction of uterine prolapse is not hysterectomy and women should be given the opportunity to choose uterus preservation.[9]

Abdominal sacrohysteropexy is considered the gold standard procedure. Recent laparoscopic approach has improved the vaginal length and C point of POPQ.[9,10] The challenges with sacrocolpopexy lie with dissection at sacral promontory and extensive endosuturing involved in the minimally invasive approach.

Two newer techniques which conserve uterus include the following.

Uterus-preserving Laparoscopic Lateral Suspension with Mesh for Pelvic Organ Prolapse

Laparoscopic lateral suspension (LLS) with mesh for pelvic organ prolapse aims to treat anterior and apical compartment POP **(Fig. 3)**. The uterus-preserving approach of LLS appears to result in better anatomic outcome for the anterior compartment, better subjective outcome, and greater patient satisfaction.[11,12]

Technique:
- *Anesthesia*: General
- *Position*: Trendelenburg
- *Ports*: Central 10 mm umbilical camera port and three 5 mm working ports in the inguinal regions and suprapubically.
- The vesicovaginal space is dissected until the endopelvic fascia is reached. Deep dissection enables concomitant correction of cystocele.
- This is followed by dissection of the rectovaginal space toward the anorectal and perineal junction. This is facilitated by vaginal manipulation.

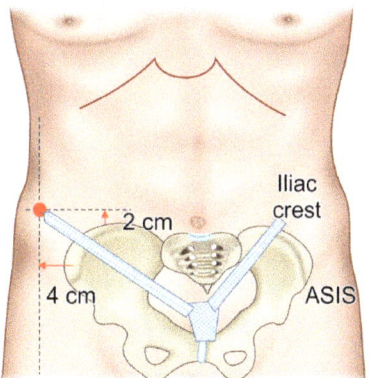

Fig. 3: Placement of mesh in lateral suspension.

- A T-shaped mesh with central rectangular part (~4 × 6 cm) and two long lateral side arms is fashioned and is introduced in the peritoneal cavity. The rectangular part is fixed to the anterior vaginal fascia.
- The skin is incised 2 cm above the iliac crest and 4 cm posterior to the anterior superior iliac spine on either side and a laparoscopic grasping forceps is introduced through this new incision where it stops short of perforating the peritoneum. The mesh is pulled out through the tunnel created and the peritoneum is closed over the mesh.

Pectineal Ligament Hysteropexy or Pectopexy

A new modification of apical suspension is pectineal ligament hysteropexy (PAH) first described by Bannerjee and Noe in 2011. It avoids the risk of vascular injury and sacral disk complications that can be encountered at the promontory by suspending two mesh arms to the lateral iliopectineal ligaments instead of sacral promontory. The RCT performed by Noe et al. in 2015 comparing pectopexy to LSC did not show statistically significant rate of recurrence but however there was a significantly lower rate of defecatory dysfunction in the pectopexy group.

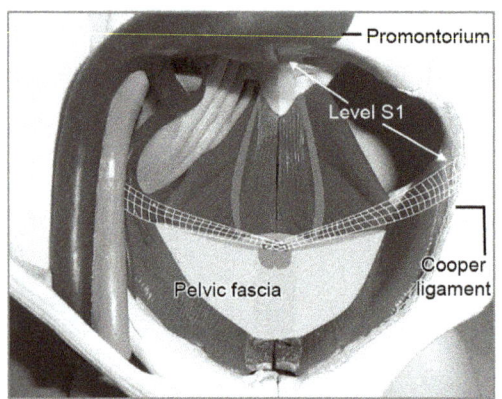

Fig. 4: Bilateral fixation at the iliopectineal ligament and the cervical stump. Fixation level: Sacral vertebra 1.

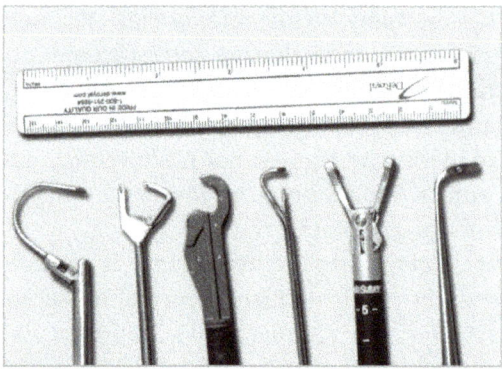

Fig. 5: From left to right, Miya hook, Arthrotek suture punch, Capio device, i stitch, Endostitch, Deschamp aneurysm needle.

Similar results were published by Biler et al. in 2018 who compared PLH to ASC (**Fig. 4**).[13]

RECONSTRUCTION OF APEX IS CRUCIAL FEATURE IN PELVIC RECONSTRUCTIVE SURGERY

Vaginal Sacrospinous Fixation—Use of Special Devices

Sacrospinous fixation is a standard assessed, cost-effective surgical procedure since long and has a definite place in modern pelvic reconstructive surgery. It provides good long-term outcomes, both objectively and subjectively with comparable complication rates to sacrocolpopexy.[14]

Only enigma is vascular anatomy around sacrospinous ligament, which is highly variable and carries risk of hemorrhage during procedure. Suture placement two finger breadths medial to the spine does not guarantee safety and require expertise. Risk of hemorrhage has led to invention of new compact devices which impress and enfold but does not penetrate the ligament. Suture carrying sharp penetrating component should traverse the shortest distance at the shallowest depth allowing adequate bite. These criteria are satisfied by the Caspari, Capio and less so by Endostitch. The Deschamp and Miya devices may be a good compromise for the developing world where cost is important (**Fig. 5**).[15]

Abdominal Sacrocolpopexy: Minimally Invasive Sacrocolpopexy

Abdominal sacrocolpopexy (ASC) is considered the "gold standard" procedure for apical prolapse due to its supremacy in anatomic durability over native tissue vaginal repairs.

Minimally invasive sacrocolpopexy (MISC), either a standard laparoscopic (LSC) or robotic-assisted approach (RSC) has largely replaced ASC advantages being the shorter recovery time, better visualization of tissues for suture intensive procedures, reduction in complication rate and reduced pain. Recent modifications such as nerve-sparing techniques of dissection at the sacral promontory, use of the iliopectineal ligaments and natural orifice vaginal sacrocolpopexy are promising.

Six years (2010–16) database of the American College of Surgeons' National Surgical Quality Improvement Program revealed that women who underwent apical prolapse surgery via MISC have similar rates of complication at the first month and duration of hospital stay compared with non mesh vaginal surgeries for apical prolapse.[16]

Paucity of studies evaluating long-term outcomes of minimally invasive apical procedures requires prospective randomized controlled trials so as to understand the relative risk/benefit ratio of mesh-based techniques.[13]

ROLE OF ROBOTICS IN PELVIC FLOOR REPAIR

Robotic-assisted laparoscopy has numerous advantages notably better depth perception due to three-dimensional (3D) vision, better surgical ergonomics, a more natural surgical feel, and a faster learning curve. Various procedures which can be performed using it are abdominal sacrocolpopexy, high uterosacral suspension and burch colposuspension.

Robotic-assisted Abdominal Sacrocolpopexy

Meta-analysis in 2015 comparing LSC to robotic-assisted abdominal sacrocolpopexy (RASC), revealed that despite the widespread performance of RASC, its advantages in terms of complications and anatomical outcomes remain unclear.[17] A more recent 2016 meta-analysis showed that RASC "boost surgical capacities" in terms of its ability but high cost seems to be the main barrier.[18]

Robotic-assisted Uterosacral Ligament Suspension

Robotic-assisted uterosacral ligament suspension is preferred in patients requiring total hysterectomy or desiring a reconstructive procedure free of synthetic materials that requires an endoscopic approach.[19] The clear visualization of the intra-abdominal anatomy, decreases the risk of ureteral compromise with the robotic approach as compared to the vaginal approach. It is suggested that diagnostic cystourethroscopy be performed after this procedure as with any hysterectomy to ensure no bladder or ureteral compromise.[20]

TRANSVAGINAL NATURAL ORIFICE TRANSLUMINAL ENDOSCOPIC SURGERY FOR SACROCOLPOPEXY: A PILOT STUDY OF 26 CASES

New approaches such as single-incision laparoscopic surgery and natural orifice transluminal endoscopic surgery (NOTES) can be useful for the treatment of pelvic disease. Transvaginal natural orifice transluminal endoscopic surgery (vNOTES) employs the same principles as single-incision laparoscopic surgery. The advantages are lack of any abdominal incision with improved visual field and range of motion and better postoperative recovery. Especially for sacrocolpopexy, vNOTES overcomes difficulty in visualizing the middle sacral artery which is a major limiting step with the other approaches. Randomized control trials are needed to better evaluate the long-term efficacy and safety profile of vNOTES sacrocolpopexy **(Figs. 6 and 7)**.[21]

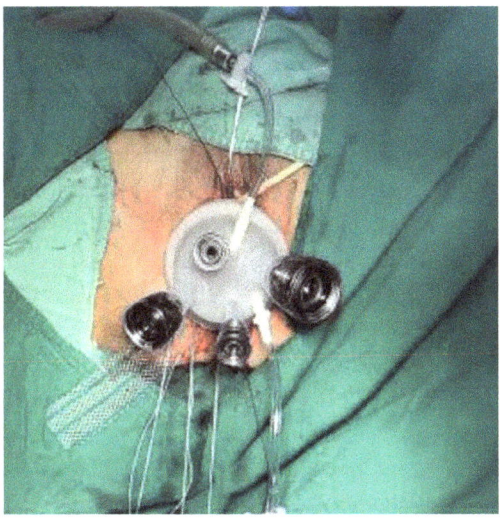

Fig. 6: Placing a port specifically designed for vNOTES.

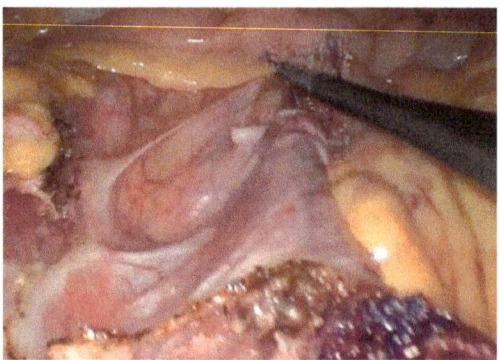

Fig. 7: Completing the retroperitoneal tunnel for the long-arm of the Y-mesh.

NATIVE TISSUE REPAIR VERSUS MESH IN PELVIC RECONSTRUCTIVE SURGERY

Native tissue repair remains a mainstay of prolapse therapy for uncomplicated, primary POP. PROSPECT study (2017)[22] concluded that vaginal repair with mesh or biological graft material did not differ in terms of effectiveness or quality of life but more than one in ten women had a mesh complication. Therefore transvaginal mesh should be used as a second-line procedure, or for patients with a significant grade of prolapse who are at a high risk of recurrence. The patient needs to be made aware of all the risks associated with mesh use. Surgeon experience is a very important prognostic factor for successful outcome.

But however, mesh use in abdominal sacrocolpopexy is safer and has shown to have better outcomes when compared to the vaginal approach. It is prudent to avoid a concomitant total hysterectomy with sacrocolpopexy to limit risk of vaginal erosion.[23]

The US Food and Drug Administration (FDA) released a recommendation regarding safety and effectiveness of transvaginal placement of surgical mesh specifically for pelvic organ prolapse.[19] It created a lot of debate regarding future of mesh in vaginal surgeries. But, as per the FDA, the safety and effectiveness of multi-incision slings is well-established in clinical trials that followed patients for up to 1-year.[24,25] Polypropylene mesh is well established in the field of hernia surgery.[26,27] When the recommended characteristics of mesh for treatment of SUI are adhered to, long term durability, safety, and efficacy up to 17 years has been noted.[28] So MUS are still gold standard for the treatment of stress urinary incontinence.

TISSUE ENGINEERING FOR PELVIC RECONSTRUCTIVE SURGERY

Tissue engineering strategy can be used either alone or as an adjunct to conventional surgery in the treatment of urogynecology diseases. Multiple treatment avenues focusing on cell-based injection therapy for treating stress urinary incontinence have yielded promising results. Few clinical studies recently have described the different types of cells including muscle-derived stem cells, mesenchymal stromal cells or myoblasts and fibroblasts for treatment of patients with SUI, which had shown promising efficacy and safety.[29]

Cell-therapy method for SUI is unsuitable for POP because the vagina is a complex organ with great demands of functionality, strength, and elasticity. Unlike abdominal wall repairs, one significant difference between POP repair with mesh and abdominal hernia repairs is that the pelvic meshes are generally placed adjacent to squamous epithelium rather than muscle. Therefore, the complications such as mesh erosion or shrinkage with associated pelvic pain or pain with intercourse increased after POP repair with mesh. Tissue engineering with three sections: (1) candidate cells, (2) scaffolds, and (3) trophic factors may solve the problem.

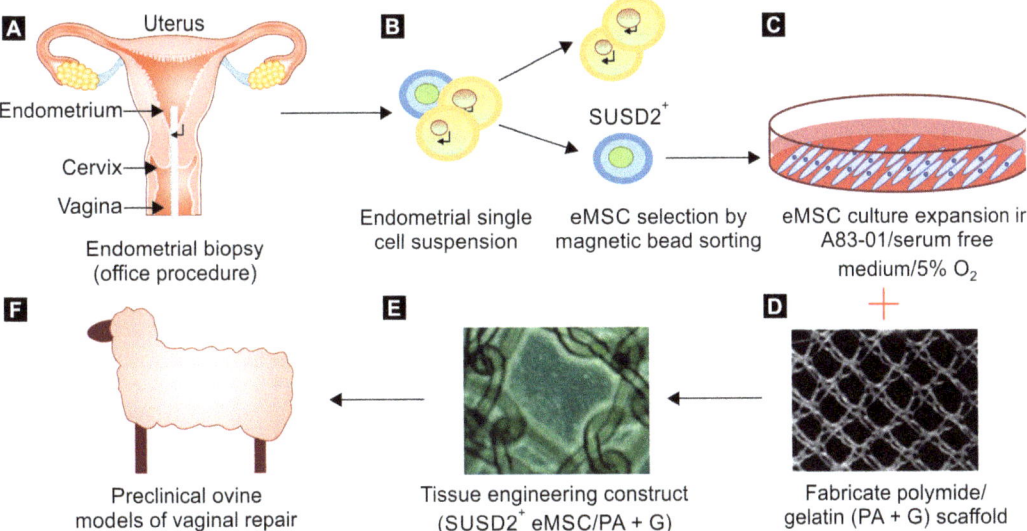

Figs. 8A to F: Solation and application of e-mesenchymal stem cells (eMSC) in pelvic organ prolapse vaginal repair. (A) Simple office-based endometrial biopsies can be used to obtain patients' tissues, which are dissociated, then (B) eMSC selected using SUSD2 magnetic bead sorting, followed by (C) culture expansion in A83-01/serum free medium in 5% O_2 to generate large numbers of undifferentiated SUSD2$^+$ eMSC (90–95%) for (D) seeding onto fabricated scaffolds which will create an (E) eMSC/PA-G tissue engineering construct for implantation into (F) a large animal preclinical model to assess their efficacy in vaginal repair of parous ewes with evidence of pelvic organ prolapse (POP).[29,30]

BIOPRINTING OF ENDOMETRIAL MESENCHYMAL CELLS ON MESH

Endometrial mesenchymal stem/stromal cells (eMSCs) bioprinted mesh can be a potential therapy for pelvic organ prolapse (POP) owing to the excellent regenerative capacity of these cells. Novel blends of electrospun synthetic and natural polymers combined with eMSC shows this approach promotes host cell infiltration and slows biomaterial degradation that has potential to strengthen the vaginal wall during healing in ovine model[30] **(Figs. 8A to F)**.

CONCLUSION

Pelvic reconstructive surgery has to be individualized. Following are the recommendations as per the review of recent studies:
- Functional pelvic floor imaging using MRI or ultrasound will be providing us the additional information regarding cause of pelvic organ prolapse by analyzing the cross-sectional area of pelvic muscles as well as the location of pelvic organs during maximal Valsalva in living women with and without prolapse.
- Vaginal laxity if treated with perineoplasty and vaginoplasty (modification of classical colpoperineorrhaphy) at an early stage will improve sexual satisfaction as well as prevent progression of prolapse.
- Native tissue repair should be first-line treatment for mild first degree POP, unless the surgeon believes that a mesh-augmented repair is indicated.
- An apical defect should always be corrected with or without hysterectomy, abdominal route is an excellent option, especially if the patient is sexually active. Minimal invasive surgery for apical repair is the surgical choice.

- Uterine preservation in cases of uterine prolapse should be thoroughly discussed with the patient.
- Use of transvaginal mesh is controversial, it should be reserved for complex cases at high risk of failure, such as multi-compartment or recurrent prolapse by trained and experienced surgeons.
- Although still emerging, future techniques of tissue engineering such as using cell based injection therapy in SUI and bioprinting of endometrial mesenchymal cells on mesh are promising.

REFERENCES

1. Giannini A, Caretto M, Russo E, Mannella P, Simoncini T. Advances in surgical strategies for prolapse. Climacteric. 2019;22(1):60-4.
2. DeLancey JO. What's new in the functional anatomy of pelvic organ prolapse? Curr Opin Obstet Gynecol. 2016;28(5):420-9.
3. Goodman MP. Female genital cosmetic and plastic surgery: a review. Wormerveer: International Society for Sexual Medicine; 2011.
4. Desai SA, Kroumpouzos G, Sadick N. Vaginal rejuvenation: from scalpel to wands. Int J Womens Dermatol. 2019;5:79-84.
5. Moore RD, Miklos JR, Chinthakanan O. Vaginal reconstruction and rejuvenation surgery: is there data to support improved sexual function? Am J Cosmet Surg. 2012;29(2):97.
6. LeBrun EE. Update on surgical treatments for pelvic organ prolapse. Curr Obstet Gynecol Rep. 2017;6:249-56.
7. Bradley S, Gutman RE, Richter LA. Hysteropexy: an option for the repair of pelvic organ prolapse. Curr Urol Rep. 2018;19(2):15.
8. Gutman RE. Does the uterus need to be removed to correct uterovaginal prolapse? Curr Opin Obstet Gynecol. 2016;28:435-40.
9. Schulten SFM, Detollenaere RJ, Stekelenburg J, IntHout J, Kluivers KB, van Eijndhoven HWF. Sacrospinous hysteropexy versus vaginal hysterectomy with uterosacral ligament suspension in women with uterine prolapse stage 2 or higher: observational follow-up of a multicenter randomized trial. BMJ. 2019;366:l5149.
10. Jefferis H, Jackson SR, Price N. Management of uterine prolapse: is hysterectomy necessary? Obstet Gynecol. 2016;18:17-23.
11. Veit-Rubin N, Dubuisson JB, Lange S, Eperon I, Dubuisson J. Uterus-preserving laparoscopic lateral suspension with mesh for pelvic organ prolapse: a patient-centred outcome report and video of a continuous series of 245 patients. Int Urogynecol J. 2016;27(3):491-3.
12. Veit-Rubin N, Dubuisson J, Constantin F, Lange S, Eperon I, Gomel V, et al. Uterus preservation is superior to hysterectomy when performing laparoscopic lateral suspension with mesh. Int Urogynecol J. 2019;30(4):557-64.
13. Schachar JS, Matthews CA. Updates in minimally invasive approaches to apical pelvic organ prolapse repair. Curr Obstet Gynecol Rep. 2019;8:26-34.
14. Meriwether KV, Antosh DD, Olivera CK, Kim-Fine S, Balk EM, Murphy M, et al. Uterine preservation vs hysterectomy in pelvic organ prolapse surgery: a systematic review with meta-analysis and clinical practice guidelines. Am J Obstet Gynecol. 2018;219(2):129-46.e2.
15. Petri E, Ashok K. Sacrospinous vaginal fixation – current status. Acta Obstetricia et Gynecologica Scandinavica. 2011;90:429-43.
16. Manning JA, Arnold P. A review of six sacrospinous suture devices. Aust N Z J Obstet Gynaecol. 2014;54:558-63.
17. Linder BJ. Minimally invasive sacrocolpopexy versus nonmesh vaginal surgery. Female Pelvic Med Reconst Surg. 2019;25(5):342-6.
18. Pan K, Zhang Y, Wang Y, Wang Y, Xu H. A systematic review and meta-analysis of conventional laparoscopic sacrocolpopexy versus robot-assisted laparoscopic sacrocolpopexy. Int J Gynecol Obstet. 2016;132(3):284-91.
19. Callewaert G, Da Cunha MMCM, Sindhwani N, Sampaolesi M, Albersen M, Deprest J. Laparoscopic versus robotic-assisted sacrocolpopexy for pelvic organ prolapse: systematic review. Gynecol Surg. 2016;13(2):115-23.
20. El-Ghobashy A, Ind T, Persson J, Magrina JF. Textbook of Gynecologic Robotic Surgery. New York: Springer; 2018.
21. Liu J, Kohn J, Fu H, Guan Z, Guan X. Transvaginal natural orifice transluminal endoscopic surgery (vNOTES) for sacrocolpopexy: a pilot study of 26 cases. J Minim Invasive Gynecol. 2019;26(4):748-53.
22. Glazener CM, Breeman S, Elders A, Hemming C, Cooper KG, Freeman RM, et al. Mesh, graft, or standard repair for women having primary transvaginal anterior or posterior compartment prolapse surgery: two parallel-group, multicentre, randomised, controlled trials (PROSPECT). Lancet. 2017;389:381-92.

23. Dällenbach P. To mesh or not to mesh: a review of pelvic organ reconstructive surgery. Int J Womens Health. 2015;7:331-43.
24. FDA (2011). Urogynecologic Surgical Mesh: Update on the Safety and Effectiveness of Vaginal Placement for Pelvic Organ Prolapse. [online] Available from: http://www.fda.gov/downloads/medicaldevices/safety/alertsandnotices/UCM262760.pdf [Last accessed on April, 2021].
25. FDA (2013). Considerations about Surgical Mesh for SUI. [online] Available from: http://www.fda.gov/MedicalDevices/ProductsandMedicalProcedures/ImplantsandProsthetics/UroGynSurgicalMesh/ucm345219.htm [Last accessed on April, 2021].
26. Cobb WS, Kercher KW, Heniford BT. The argument for lightweight polypropylene mesh in hernia repair. Surg Innov. 2005;12(1):63-9.
27. Nilsson CG, Palva K, Aarnio R, Morcos E, Falconer C. Seventeen years' follow-up of the tension-free vaginal tape procedure for female stress urinary incontinence. Int Urogynecol J. 2013;24(8):1265-9.
28. Cox A, Herschorn S, Lee L. Surgical management of female SUI: is there a gold standard? Nat Rev Urol. 2013;10(2):78-89.
29. Gargett CE, Gurung S, Darzi S, Werkmeister JA, Mukherjee S. Tissue engineering approaches for treating pelvic organ prolapse using a novel source of stem/stromal cells and new materials. Curr Opin Urol. 2019;29(4):450-7.
30. Emmerson SJ, Gargett CE. Endometrial mesenchymal stem cells as a cell based therapy for pelvic organ prolapse. World J Stem Cells. 2016;8(5):202-15.

CHAPTER 27

Robotics in Urogynecology

Mohan Keshavamurthy

INTRODUCTION

Robot is a mechanical device incorporated with a computer. The Surgeon controls all the actions of the robotic arms in real time, what is called the "Master-Slave system".

Robot-assisted procedures utilizing the da Vinci system (Intuitive Surgical Inc., California, USA) have been transformative in gynecology especially in patients with complex anatomy.

The da Vinci system was conceptualized originally for remote treatment of war victims in real time. However, it received an impetus for practical application with United States Food and Drug Administration (US FDA) approving it in 2001 for human laparoscopic intervention. There has been a rapid expansion in gynecological robotic surgery subsequent to the first procedure done in 2005. Nearly 30% of all robotic surgeries done on an annual basis belong to this category at present **(Fig. 1)**.

THE PARTS OF DA VINCI ROBOTIC SYSTEM

The da Vinci robotic system is the most commonly employed robotic system across the world for robotic surgeries. It consists of three parts: (1) Surgeon console, (2) Vision cart, and (3) Patient cart **(Figs. 2 and 3)**.

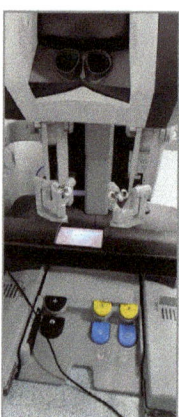

Fig. 2: The da Vinci surgical system: Surgeon console.

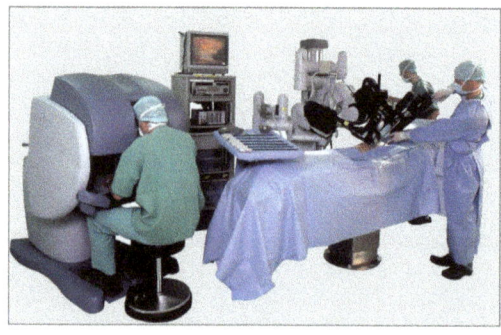

Fig. 1: The da Vinci robotic system.

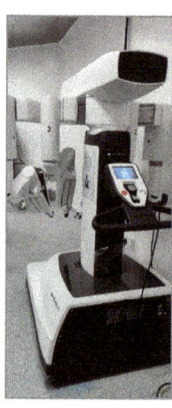

Fig. 3: The da Vinci surgical system: Patient cart.

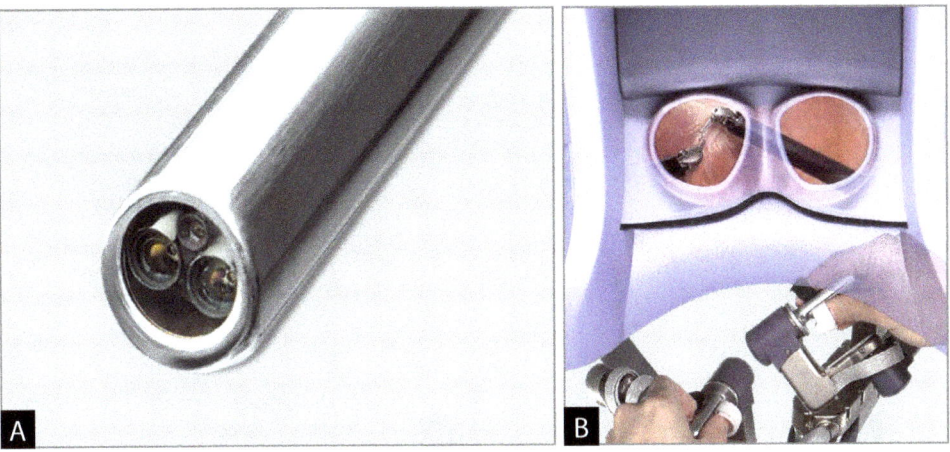

Figs. 4A and B: Double lens laparoscope (3D, high definition); (B) Binocular view (10× magnification).

The surgeon at the console has full control of the camera, instruments and the energy source utilizing ergonomically designed hand controls and foot pedals.

Initially, pneumoperitoneum needs to be established and ports have to be inserted. Thereafter the support team "docks" the robotic system as per the requisite position of the patient needed for surgery and the instruments are inserted via the ports. The assistant positioned besides the patient supports with the retraction, suction and wherever necessary, uterine manipulation.

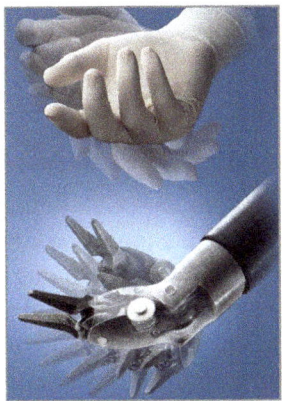

Fig. 5: EndoWrist® Instruments provide enhanced dexterity, precision and control.

Components of da Vinci Robotic Surgical System that Enhance Human Vision and Beyond

The important components of da Vinci Robotic Surgical system that enhance human vision are shown in **Figures 4A and B**.

Components of da Vinci Robotic Surgical System that Enhance Human Hand Dexterity and Beyond

The important components of da Vinci Robotic Surgical system that enhance human hand dexterity are shown in **Figure 5**.
- Filtering of hand tremors
- Scaling down movements 1–5×
- 180° articulation, 540° rotation
- EndoWrist® instruments have 7 degrees of freedom

Patient Positioning

Robot-assisted gynecological surgeries require a steep Trendelenburg position. To prevent postoperative neuralgias, the patient position needs to be secured with shoulder pads, bean bags and gel pads.

Care should be taken to ensure the knee flexion is less than 60° so that neuropathies are avoided. This can be achieved by the use of Yellofin® stirrups. If uterine manipulators

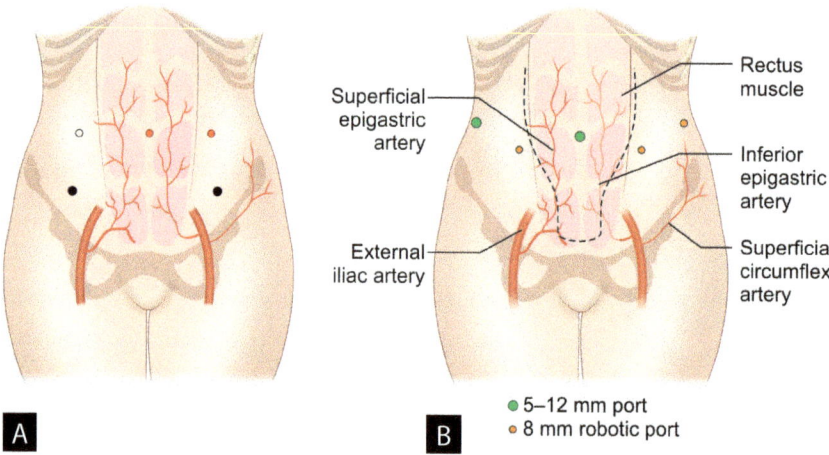

Figs. 6A and B: (A) Four ports are used in the laparoscopic approach to sacrocolpopexy; (B) Five ports were used in the robotic approach to sacrocolpopexy placed in a shallow "W" formation.

are required, they need to be inserted prior to robot docking.

Port Insertion and Trocar placement

The port positioning will depend on the number of arms planning to be used.

If three arms are planning on being used, then four ports are needed: one for the camera, two for the robotic instruments and one assistant port. The camera port size is generally 12 mm while the robotic ports are 8 mm.

An inter port distance of *8 cm distance* is a prerequisite to prevent clashing of the robotic arms. The ports need to be placed vertically and attention needs to be paid to the thick black band on the robotic arm which has to be placed at the level of the parietal peritoneum to prevent slipping and also avoids excessive stretching and consequently, postoperative pain.

The camera port placement, such as in laparoscopy, is crucial to ensure adequate panoramic vision. For a hysterectomy, the camera port is positioned approximately 8–10 cm away from the uterine fundus. For sacrocolpopexy, depending on the presence or absence of the uterus, the camera port is usually placed at or above the umbilicus. The right and left instrument ports are placed 2–3 cm below and 8–10 cm lateral to the camera port. The assistant port can be placed 2–3 cm above and 8–10 cm lateral to the camera port as shown in the **Figures 6A and B.**

DOCKING OF THE ROBOT

This can be of two kinds: (1) *Straight dock* where the Robotic platform is positioned between the patient's legs; or (2) *Side docked* where the patient cart is at right angles to the axis of the patient. The advantage of side dock is more space for the assistant at the vaginal end to perform uterine manipulation.

COMMON INDICATIONS FOR ROBOTIC SURGERY IN GYNECOLOGY

- Robotic-assisted vaginal hysterectomy (RAVH)
- Robot enabled radical hysterectomy with pelvic node lymphadenectomy
- Robotic myomectomy
- Robotic sacral colpopexy
- Robotic vesicovaginal fistula repair (**Fig. 7**)

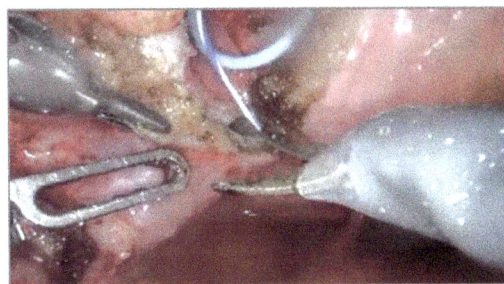

Fig. 7: Robotic vesicovaginal fistula (VVF) repair.

Robotic Gynecological Oncology

Robotic surgery is extremely useful in radical hysterectomy and pelvic node dissection. When sentinel lymph node mapping is required to plan adjuvant therapy, indocyanine green (ICG)-based fluorescence imaging can be used intraoperatively.

There is growing evidence that Robot-assisted procedures are associated with better outcomes in comparison with laparoscopic surgery with regards to complications encountered intraoperatively, need for blood transfusion and duration of hospital stay.

Robotic Hysterectomy for Benign Pathology

Robot-assisted vaginal hysterectomy is an elegant procedure that can be performed in the day care setting. Laparoscopic hysterectomy has proven advantages over open hysterectomy such as less blood loss, shorter stay in hospital, fewer wound infections, and quicker return to normal activity. However, the longer learning curve especially with suturing with laparoscopy resulting in longer operating times has limited the adoption of this technique. Robotic surgery should be able to overcome these hurdles and lead to an exponential increase in the minimally invasive approach.

Robotic Myomectomy

Robotic myomectomy with morcellation for specimen retrieval is an effective technique especially in large multiple myomas. It can be combined with a hysteroscopic myomectomy in case of a submucosal myoma.

Robotic Sacrocolpopexy

Pelvic organ prolapse requiring surgical correction affects about 10% of the female population in their lifetime. It can either be post-hysterectomy vault prolapse or prolapse with an intact uterus requiring a hysteropexy especially in those who intend to preserve fertility.

Robotic surgery offers an excellent solution with significantly reduced blood loss, postoperative pain and much better visualization of the deep pelvic anatomy which will enhance success rates of any urogynecological procedure. It is of particular benefit in patients with severe postoperative adhesions following previous surgeries.

Multiple systematic reviews have established that Robotic-assisted sacrocolpopexy has a shorter learning curve as evidenced by shorter operating time with increasing number of surgeries performed.

TRAINING IN ROBOTIC SURGERY

The learning curve with Robotic surgery is shorter as compared with laparoscopy. This is the direct result of superior ergonomics of the robotic platform. Assisting with a minimum of 50 cases of robotic surgery should suffice to overcome the learning curve.

Credentialing for individual surgeons has no national guidelines. The "DOME" in the United States is the first standardized protocol for initial certification and recertification for robotic surgeons.

Intuitive surgical Inc. has a recommended pathway for institutions to develop a comprehensive training program. The initial phase of training is by simulation on a virtual reality skill simulator. Subsequently, training can be done on animal and cadaveric models. Dual console training can facilitate training between trainer and trainee. Finally, live surgery under a proctor allows direct supervision and learning the finer nuances of robotics.

ADVANTAGES OF ROBOTIC SURGERY

- Excellent camera stability
- Enhanced anatomical accuracy
- Enhanced range of movement
- Elimination of hand tremor
- Elimination of Fulcrum effect
- Efficient Surgeon ergonomics
- Scalable movements
- Enhanced depth perception
- Potential for micro-anastomoses
- Reduced hospital stays
- Reduced postoperative pain
- Reduced wound site infections
- Enhanced cosmesis
- Potential for telesurgery

DISADVANTAGES OF ROBOTIC SURGERY

- Expensive (purchase/upgrade/maintenance)
- Steep learning curve
- Limited training opportunities
- Long setup time
- Heavy, space occupying equipment
- Lack of force and tactile feedback
- Significant risk of mechanical malfunction/failure
- Risks associated with port placement
- Compromised patient safety in case of an emergency
- Requires training of the entire OT team
- Not suitable for morbidly obese patients

ALTERNATIVE ROBOTIC SYSTEMS

- Revo-I (Meere Company Inc., Yongin, Republic of Korea)
- Telelap ALF-X® (SOFAR SpA, Milan, Italy)
- Micro Hand S robot
- Flex system® (The Medrobotics, Raynham, USA)
- SPORT® surgical system (Titan Medical, Toronto, Canada)
- Versius system (Cambridge Medical Robotics)

DOME ROBOTIC TRAINING SYSTEM

The Nicholson center has developed an online curriculum and corresponding psychomotor skills testing model called FRS DOME as part of Fundamentals of Robotic Surgery (FRS) certification.

The Dome has been designed by 80 leading robotic surgeons to teach and test essential skills of an aspiring robotic surgeon in a 3D model in the areas of instrument handling, needle control, third arm control, blunt dissection, suturing, knot tying and safe use of energy sources.

These seven core skills have been integrated on a storable, portable and reusable device, the Dome. This consists of a hard dome shell, magnetically attached towers and a fused flesh and fat/soft tissue cover with embedded vessels. The hard shell and towers are reusable hundreds of times and the other components are reusable three times.

This is an excellent tool to standardize robotic training and assess specialty specific.

CHAPTER 28

Female Genital Cosmetic Surgery

Deepa Ganesh

INTRODUCTION

Female genital cosmetic surgery (FGCS) is relatively a new entry in the field of cosmetic-plastic surgery. In Medical literature, the terms *cosmetic vaginal surgery (CVS), aesthetic vaginal surgery (AVS), female cosmetic genital surgery (FCGS), vulvovaginal aesthetic surgery (VVAS), cosmeto-plastic gynecology (CPG) and vaginal rejuvenation* have been used, which encompasses variety of procedures designed to modify appearance of the external genitalia and improve sexual functioning.

Cosmetic procedures on women's faces, skin and breasts for cosmetic reasons have now become widely accepted. Hence, it may not be surprising that they wish to change, reconstruct or rejuvenate their intimate parts.[1]

For years, surgeons have performed surgical procedures altering the genital size, appearance and function such as anterior/posterior colporrhaphy, perineorrhaphy, labial size alteration, surgical procedures which aimed to repair genitals after obstetrical delivery, pediatric labial hypertrophy and in transgender persons. Honore and O'Hara[2] in 1978, Hodgekinson and Hait[3] in 1984 and Chavis, LaFeria and Niccolini[4] in 1989 were the pioneers in discussing cosmetic gynecological procedures.

In recent years, there has been increasing popularity of FGCS procedures especially vaginal rejuvenation in western countries, to both health care providers and women. Survey by the American Society of Plastic Surgeons (ASPS) in 2013 reported over 3,500 vaginal rejuvenation procedures representing a 64% increase from 2011.[5]

The increasing popularity of female genital cosmetic surgeries obtained academic attention worldwide. The American College of Obstetricians and Gynecologists (ACOG) published a committee opinion paper on FGCS in 2007, stating that these FGCS and vaginal rejuvenation are not medically indicated procedures considering insufficient data supporting their efficacy and safety and its potential complications such as infections, scarring, dyspareunia and altered sensation.[6]

The Royal College of Obstetricians and Gynaecologists (RCOG) and the Royal Australian and New Zealand College of Obstetricians and Gynaecologists (RANZCOG) took the same stand[7,8] and in 2013, the Society of Obstetricians and Gynaecologists of Canada (SOGC) published its policy statement to guide their members and the women requesting FGCS, advocating appropriate training in cosmetic gynecology.[9]

The critics of FGCS also tried to draw analogs to female genital mutilation surgery. According to World Health Organization (WHO), female genital mutilation includes all procedures involving partial or complete removal of the external female genitalia or other injury to the female genital organs for nonmedical reasons.[10] Since it is a thin line between female genital mutilation and FGCS, confusion exists at times. Gynecologist and plastic surgeons should be aware of potential damages being caused while performing these FGCS procedures and in the future it may be classified as "mutilation".[11]

ANATOMY AND FUNCTION OF VULVA AND VAGINA

The female external genitalia is formed from anterior to posterior, by mons pubis, labia majora, labia minora, vulvar vestibule, external urethral meatus, hymen and the perineum. There are a multitude of anatomical variations of the external genitalia which should be explained to the patient. As part of the hormonal changes from puberty to menopause, the external genitalia undergo various changes ranging from prominent labia majora after puberty to changes with childbirth and again post menopause undergo atrophic changes with loss of elasticity. Sexual function is complex and multifactorial apart from anatomy. The vagina will be able to dilate during the normal female sexual response, and this can be impacted adversely by both physiological processes such as childbirth, menopause, and iatrogenic causes such as surgery, cancer treatments, and radiation.

SURGICAL COSMETIC PROCEDURES

Cosmetic surgery on the female external genitalia and vagina are designed to "subjectively" match appearance as per patient's expectations, reduce discomfort, and/or potentially provide functional and psychological improvement in sexual stimulation and satisfaction. The most commonly performed procedures are labiaplasty, labia majora reduction/augmentation, clitoral hood reduction, vaginal rejuvenation (which includes colpoperineoplasty, perineoplasty and vaginoplasty), hymenoplasty, G-spot augmentation and mons pubis reduction.

Labiaplasty (Fig. 1)

Labiaplasty or reduction of labia minora size is the most frequently performed FGCS procedure designed to improve the subjective appearance of the external female genitalia.

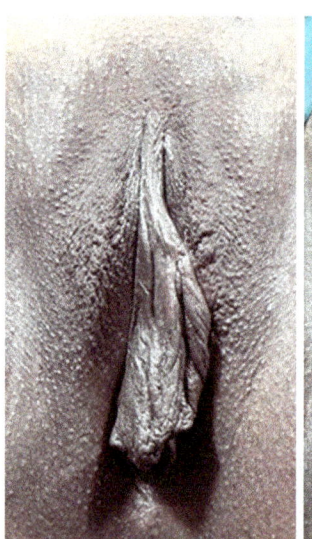 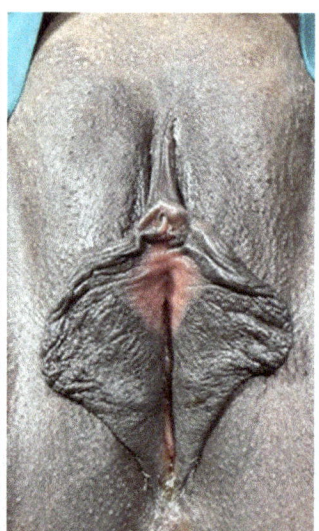 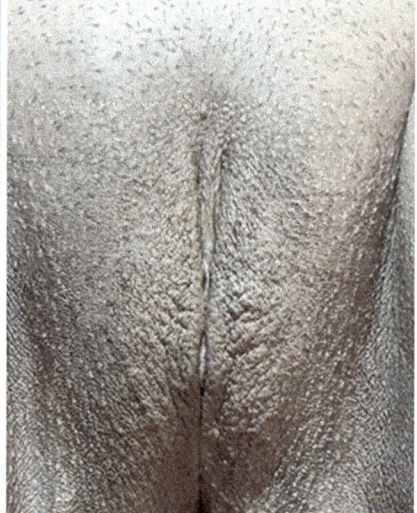

Fig.1: Labiaplasty: Linear edge resection using Laser.

According to textbooks, nine female anatomical types of labia exist, but the perception of normal labia seems to be influenced by culture, media perception and sexual partners. Perception of ideal female external genitalia differs from country to country. In some African countries, elongated labia minora are considered attractive and a sign of modesty, whereas in Japan butterfly shaped labia is most preferred.[12]

Hodgkinson was one of the first to publish a description of the aesthetic vaginal labiaplasty in 1983.[3] Alter subsequently presented innovations to the procedure in 1998 and 2005 and later, modifications of the labiaplasty techniques were described by Rouzier, Choi, Munhoz, Maas and Giraldo.[13-15] There have been eleven surgical techniques of labiaplasty described in the literature so far but no single gold-standard technique exists as each has its unique advantages and disadvantages.[12] Different surgical techniques include edge/linear resection, wedge resection, composite reduction labiaplasty, de-epithelization technique, W-plasty, custom flask, laser labiaplasty and other less utilized techniques. The main goals of labiaplasty is to reduce the hypertrophic labia minora to maintain a minimum labial length of 1 cm, preserve the neurovascular supply, optimal color/texture should match the labial edge with minimal invasiveness. The most widely performed techniques are linear resection and wedge resection techniques.

The *linear edge resection*, one of the first described techniques in literature in 1983 is also known as amputation technique. The labia minora is linearly resected using scalpel, electrosurgical needle or laser and the cut edges are repaired with fine absorbable sutures. In this technique, the preservation of the natural contour is not possible as the main request is to remove the irregular dark edges. Risks may include excess tissue resection and persistent protrusion of clitoral hood. Overall this technique has low complication rate and favorable aesthetic outcomes.[16]

Wedge resection technique was described by Gary Alter, where a V-shaped wedge of labial tissue is excised.[13] The superior edge of the V begins inferior to the clitoral hood fold and the inferior edge of V above the posterior commissure. To prevent dog ears, wedge resection with lateral extension- "hockey stick" curvature is done. The cut edges are sutured with 4-0 or 5-0 absorbable subcutaneous "anchoring" sutures and skin with interrupted sutures. When there is a redundant hood, excess clitoral hood resection can be done at same time by modifying the "V" to "Y" incision. Advantages of V-wedge resection technique include preservation of natural looking edge and prevention of over resection. Disadvantages are postoperative pain, high risk of wound dehiscence, sinus/fistula formation, and clitoral hood excess.[17] To prevent scar contraction, Giraldo et al. performed a 90° Z-plasty where via a "Z"-shaped incision, central wedge of labia is excised.[18]

Inferior wedge resection with superior pedicle flap rotation: This is another modified wedge resection technique where the inferior labial portion is amputated and the superior portion of the labium is brought down as a pedicle flap and anchored to the denuded inferior edge.

Multiple studies of labiaplasties reveal all techniques can give superior results in experienced hands and with a judicious approach.

Clitoral Hood Reduction (Fig. 2)

Clitoral hood reduction, also known as clitoral unhooding or hoodectomy is mostly

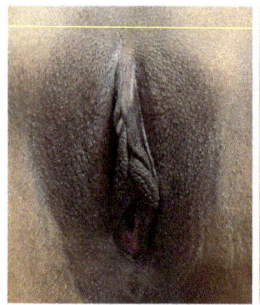
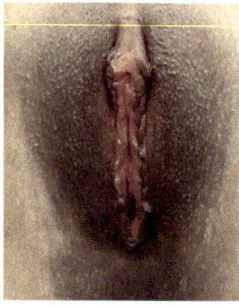

Fig. 2: Clitoral hood reduction combined with labiaplasty using laser.

done concomitantly with reduction of labia minora size. The clitoral hood or prepuce, covers and surrounds the clitoris, which in the female is the highly sensitive and arousing erectile tissue. Often along with enlarged labia minora, this tissue or hood can become enlarged and can negatively impact sexual pleasure. Labia minora flows down from one or more epithelial folds which make up the central, medial and lateral folds of "clitoral hood" and these hood folds often cause tissue protrusion which bothers the patient. Hood size reductions without labial reduction are only occasionally performed solo.[19]

If clitoral hood is not addressed during labiaplasty, it can cause a secondary clitoral hood hypertrophy where revision surgery is often needed. Isolated clitoral hood deformities are rarely observed in cases of congenital anomalies such as pseudohermaphroditism combined with clitoral hypertrophy and labial fusion.[20]

Clitoral hood reduction, is often combined in most of modern techniques for labiaplasty in a single operative session. In case of vertical redundancy, vertical incision is made and if horizontal excess (which is less common), inverted V-shaped incision is used. An H-shaped incision is used when the redundancy is along both the axes.

Vaginal Rejuvenation

Vaginal rejuvenation was first described and marketed by Dr David Matlock as laser vaginal rejuvenation. In FGCS, it is considered as an "umbrella term" comprising a range of elective vaginal tightening surgical procedures designed to tighten the vaginal canal, provide pelvic floor support and increase vaginal wall friction and functional tone to improve sexual and orgasmic pleasure.[21-23] Vaginal rejuvenation includes colpoperineoplasty, perineoplasty and/or vaginoplasty.

Perineoplasty (PP) includes surgical reconstruction of the vulvar vestibule, vaginal introitus, perineum and perineal body, where redundant and scarred tissues are excised along with posterior compartment defect. Then the superficial transverse perinei are approximated in the midline in layers. Reapproximation of the perineum is carefully done in anatomic manner.

Vaginoplasty (VP) is defined as general tightening procedures involving the vaginal canal. Usually this refers to posterior colporrhaphy, limited to the distal half of the vagina and modified to reapproximate the vaginal walls tightly to reconstruct the posterior vaginal wall in a layered fashion. It may or may not involve anterior colporrhaphy and/or excision of elliptical strips of lateral forniceal mucosa to provide superficial mucosal and fascial approximation. The surgical techniques are done with traditional scalpels, needle electrodes, scissors or by using energy sources such as laser or radiofrequency electrodes. Different energy sources have claimed reduced scarring, morbidity and better surgical outcomes in vaginal caliber as well as sensation.

Colpoperineoplasty (CP), first described by Jack Pardo from Chile is a recent addition

Female Genital Cosmetic Surgery 213

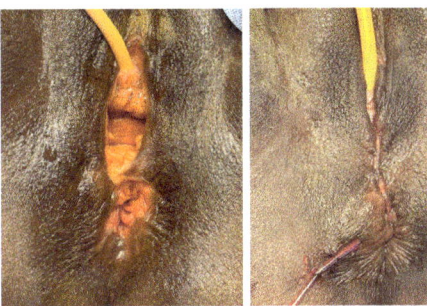

Fig. 3: Colpoperineoplasty: Vaginoplasty (VP) and perineoplasty (PP).

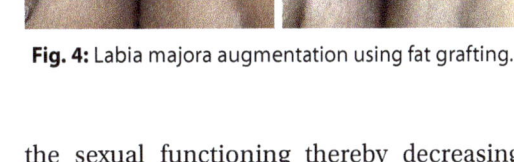

Fig. 4: Labia majora augmentation using fat grafting.

to the nomenclature meant to encompass both VP and PP **(Fig. 3)**.[24]

Labia Majora Reduction

Labia majora reduction also called as labia majoraplasty is a surgical procedure done in women purely for cosmetic reasons as per the patient's expectations.[25,26] Labia majora reduction is done by vertical elliptical excision of labial dermis with or without the underlying adipose tissue with Colles' fascia using the traditional scalpel, needle electrode or the touch laser fiber and radiofrequency energy which are elegant, easy to use and gives better aesthetic outcomes. Closure is usually done in two layers via subcutaneous imbricating sutures and subcuticular skin sutures utilizing 3-0 to 5-0 preferably monofilament. If there is atrophy of fatty tissue, then a small amount of fat transfer is done by liposuction from another area of the body.

Labia Majora Augmentation (Fig. 4)

Female genitalia, such as other body parts, are affected by the normal ageing process. With the decrease in fat, hyaluronic acid and collagen there is volume loss, rhytids development, and an increased minora to majora ratio, where the labia minora become prominent.[25] These age-related changes affect the sexual functioning thereby decreasing sexual self-esteem, resulting in psychosocial impairment.[26]

Labia majora augmentation, a relatively new technique was first described by Felicio in 2007 where the enhancement of deficient labia is done using autologous fat grafting.[27] Fat is harvested from the lower abdomen with 2 mm cobra cannula and 20 cc syringe and it is decanted with normal saline and rinsed until the solution below the fat is clear with no blood. Total injected fat volume ranges from 18 to 120 mL per session. Fat can be injected at multiple sites, on the mons pubis, the anterior, lateral labia and the posterior labia majora. The fat injection is done in three layers: deep, medium and superficial in the subcutaneous tissue to increase the fat survival.[28] Before the placement of the fat tissue, 2 cc platelet rich plasma (PRP) can also be added from top to bottom of the labia majora.

Hyaluronic acid can also be used to augment labia majora subcutaneously. The concentration of the hyaluronic acid used is 19-20 mg/mL and the total volume injected ranges from 2 to 6 mL per session.[29] The injection technique is important to ensure smooth outcome. After the initial injection, retouching can be done after 2-4 months whereas in fat, lipofilling can only be done after 4–6 months.

Mons Pubis Reduction

The mons pubis, also known as mons veneris may vary in size from woman to woman. Pregnancy, weight gain, menopause and hormonal changes with age can cause prominence of the mons pubis and labia majora to uneven fat deposits and skin laxity.[30-32] These can cause issues with sexual intercourse, ill hygiene and discomfort wearing pants and swimsuits thereby affecting self-esteem. Monsplasty or mons pubis reduction surgery either by fat liposuction or open excision along with suspension techniques, i.e., pubic skin lift gives good results.[33] This is commonly performed with abdominoplasty but may be carried out as an isolated procedure. The importance of presurgical counseling to ensure realistic expectation by the patient cannot be overemphasized enough.[34]

Hymenoplasty (Fig. 5)

Hymenoplasty is a surgical repair/reconstruction procedure of the hymenal ring done via approximation sutures, to minimize the size of the introitus and produce temporary introital tightening and bleeding with subsequent intercourse. Usually sought by women of a certain cultural background, where an intact hymen is considered as a sign of virginity.

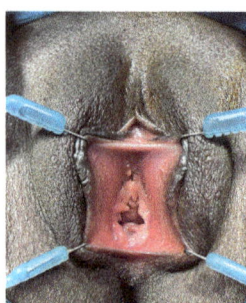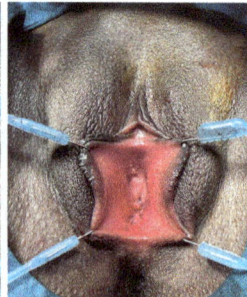

Fig. 5: Hymenoplasty.

NONSURGICAL COSMETIC VULVOVAGINAL PROCEDURES

As demand for cosmetic gynecology procedures increases, patients prefer nonsurgical outpatient procedures with no anesthesia, no admission and quicker recovery time. Energy-based devices such as lasers and radiofrequency are used for treatment of redundant labia majora and vaginal laxity. Fractional laser and chemical peels are used for vulvar hyperpigmentation. These energy-based devices induce new collagen and elastin fiber synthesis with neovascularization thereby tightening the vaginal canal and improving the quality of vaginal wall tissue.

Other nonsurgical popular procedures are G-spot augmentation invented by David Matlock (USA), using collagen fillers to temporarily augment the G-spot to enhance the sexual gratification in women and O-shot by Charles Runnels (USA), using PRP for vulvovaginal rejuvenation and orgasmic female sexual dysfunction.

IDEAL PATIENT CRITERIA FOR SURGERY

- Well informed patients, who understand their alternatives.
- Patients who understand the results which are proposed to them.
- It can be safely performed any time after sexual maturity (minimum patient age of 18 years).

CONTRAINDICATIONS FOR SURGERY

- Active gynecological disease, such as infection or malignancy
- Heavy smokers with poorly controlled comorbid medical illnesses such as diabetes and hypertension
- Patients with "body dysmorphic disorder", psychosis or anxiety disorder
- Patients who have unreasonable expectations based on media images

CONCLUSION

The demand for *female genital cosmetic surgery* has increased over the last decade, in adults as well as in young adolescent girls. Cosmesis, improving sexual function and increasing self-esteem are the reasons women request alterations of their vulvas and vaginas. The growth of FGCS is driven by the media and patients, but the original architects are the gynecological surgeons, but some gynecologists fail to grasp the intimate relationship between a woman's perception of her genitalia and her self-esteem and the psychobiological need for sexual gratification. The cosmetic vaginal surgeon's intent is to alleviate psychological and physical pain caused by perceived unattractive and poorly functioning genitalia. Since the pelvic floor, perineum, and vulva are the rightful domains of the gynecologists, their contributions are very important.

A complete medical, sexual, and gynecological history is mandatory and the absence of any major sexual or psychological dysfunction should be ascertained. Counseling should be a priority for women requesting FGCS. Women should be made aware that by cosmetically or physically altering their external genitalia does not mean that they are developmentally or structurally "abnormal." When an adolescent girl requests FGCS, these procedures should be offered only after complete maturity including genital maturity.

The genital cosmetic surgeon should be properly trained in these procedures and have sufficient training in sexual medicine to withhold these procedures from women with sexual dysfunction, mental impairment or body dysmorphic disorder. It is important that training guidelines for practitioners be established and that long-term outcome, psychosexual and safety data be published.

REFERENCES

1. Goodman MP. Female genital plastic and cosmetic surgery. Oxford: Wiley Publication; 2016. pp. 3-8.
2. Honore LH, O'Hara KE. Benign enlargement of the labia minora: report of two cases. Eur J Obstet Gynaecol Reprod Biol. 1978;8:61-4.
3. Hodgekinson DJ, Hait G. Aesthetic vaginal Labiaplasty. Plast Reconstr Surg. 1984;74(3):414-6.
4. Chavis WM, LaFeria JJ, Niccolini R. Plastic repair of elongated, hypertrophic labia minora. A case report. J Reprod Med. 1989;34:373-45.
5. American Society of Plastic Surgeons (2005) 2006 statistics. [online] Available at: https://www.plasticsurgery.org/documents/News/Statistics/2005/cosmetic-procedures-women-2005 [Last accessed on April, 2021].
6. Committee on Gynecologic Practice. American College of Obstetricians and Gynecologists ACOG Committee Opinion No. 378: vaginal "rejuvenation" and cosmetic vaginal procedures. Obstet Gynecol. 2007;110(3):737-8.
7. Royal College of Obstetricians and Gynaecologist. Ethical considerations in relation to female genital cosmetic surgery (FGCS). London: RCOG Ethics Committee; 2013.
8. The Royal Australian and New Zealand College of Obstetricians and Gynaecologists. RANZCOG College Statement: C-Gyn 24. Vaginal "Rejuvenation" and Cosmetic Vaginal Procedures. RANZCOG College: Melbourne; 2008.
9. Committee Clinical Practice Gynaecology, Ethics Committee, and Executive Council of the Society of Obstetricians and Gynaecologists of Canada Female genital cosmetic surgery. J Obstet Gynaecol Can. 2013;35(12):e1-e5.
10. World Health Organization. Female genital mutilation. Fact sheet no. 241. Geneva: WHO; 2012.
11. Scholten E. Female genital cosmetic surgery—the future. J Plast Reconstr Aesthet Surg. 2009;62(3):290-1.
12. Özer M, Mortimore I, Jansma E, Mullender MG. Labiaplasty: motivation, techniques, and ethics. Nat Rev Urol. 2018;15:175-89.
13. Alter GJ. A new technique for aesthetic labia minora reduction. Ann Plast Surg. 1998;40(3):287-90.
14. Munhoz AM, Filassi JR, Ricci MD, Aldrighi C, Correia LD, Aldrighi JM, et al. Aesthetic labia minora reduction with inferior wedge resection and superior pedicle flap reconstruction. Plast Reconstr Surg. 2006;118:1237-47.

15. Rouzier R, Louis-Sylvestre C, Paniel BJ, Haddad B. Hypertrophy of labia minora: experience with 163 reductions. Am J Obstet Gynecol. 2000;182:35-40.
16. Jeong-Ho S, Jun-Woo J, Yoon-Ho J. Clinical effectiveness of labia minora reduction surgery. J Cosmet Med. 2017;1(1):52-6.
17. Goodman MP. Female genital plastic and cosmetic surgery. Oxford: Wiley Publication; 2016. pp. 53-4.
18. Giraldo F, González C, de Haro F. Central wedge nymphectomy with a 90-degree Z-plasty for aesthetic reduction of the labia minora. Plast Reconstr Surg. 2004;113:1820-5.
19. Philip H. Zeplin. Clitoral Hood Reduction. Aesthet Surg J. 2016;36(7):NP231.
20. Liu L, Fan J, Gan C. Staged reconstruction of the labia minora and reduction clitoroplasty for female pseudohermaphroditism. Aesthetic Plast Surg. 2010;34(5):652-6.
21. Kent D, Pelosi MA. Vaginal rejuvenation: an in-depth look at the history and technical procedure. Am J Cosmetic Surg. 2012;29(2):89.
22. Moore RD, Miklos JR. Vaginal reconstruction and rejuvenation surgery: is there data to support improved sexual function? Am J Cosmet Surg. 2012;29(2):97.
23. Goodman MP. Female Genital Plastic and Cosmetic surgery. Oxford: Wiley Publication; 2016. pp. 29-30.
24. Pardo JS, Solà VD, Ricci PA, Guiloff EF, Freundlich OK. Colpoperineoplasty in women with a sensation of a wide vagina. Acta Obstet Gynecol Scand. 2006;85:1125-7.
25. Goodman MP, Placik OJ, Benson RH, Miklos JR, Moore RD, Jason RA, et al. A large multicenter outcome study of female genital plastic surgery. J Sex Med. 2010;7:565-77.
26. Goodman MP, Placik OJ, Matlock DL, et al. Evaluation of body image and sexual satisfaction in women undergoing female genital plastic/cosmetic surgery. Aesthet Surg J. 2016;36(9):1048-57.
27. de Alencar Felicio Y. Labial surgery. Aesthet Surg J. 2007;27(3):322-8.
28. Salgado CJ Tang JC Desrosiers AE 3rd. Use of dermal fat graft for augmentation of the labia majora. J Plast Reconstr Aesthet Surg. 2012;65(2):267-70.
29. Fasola E, Gazzola R. Labia majora augmentation with hyaluronic acid filler: technique and results. Aesthet Surg J. 2016;36(10):1155-63.
30. Alter GJ. Mangement of the mons pubis and labia majora in the massive weight loss patient. Aesth surg J. 2009;29:432-42.
31. Bloom JM, Van Kouwenberg E, Davenport M, Koltz PF, Shaw RB Jr, Gusenoff JA. Aesthetic and functional satisfaction after monsplasty in the massive weight loss population. Aesthet Surg J. 2012;32(7):877-85.
32. El-Khatib HA. Mons pubis ptosis: classification and strategy for treatment. Aesthet Plast Surg. 2011;35(1):24-30.
33. Michaels VJ, Friedman, Coon D, Rubin JP. Mons rejuvenation in the massive weight loss patient using superficial system suspension. Plast Reconstr Surg. 2010;126(1):45e-46e.
34. Goodman MP. Female Genital Plastic and Cosmetic Surgery. Oxford: Wiley Publication; 2016. p. 74.

29 Her Unspoken Problems

Narendra Malhotra, Molina Patel, Neharika Malhotra, Jaideep Malhotra, Manpreet Sharma, Shemi Bansal

INTRODUCTION

In every phase of a woman's life, the feelings and experiences that a woman holds about herself and her symptoms, largely varies with social, cultural, emotional, and personal biological aspects. Not all of the changes that a woman perceives are reflected in the mirror or spoken frankly about. These "unspoken problems" are often overlooked, rather not even given a thought about.

Fluctuations in sex hormones, trauma from childbirth, ignorance toward macro- and micronutrient supplementation, lack of adequate rest, physically and mentally strenuous lifestyle, and genetics are the few factors which make women vulnerable to alterations in genital anatomy and functionality with age. All this cumulates to—her unspoken problems **(Fig. 1)**.

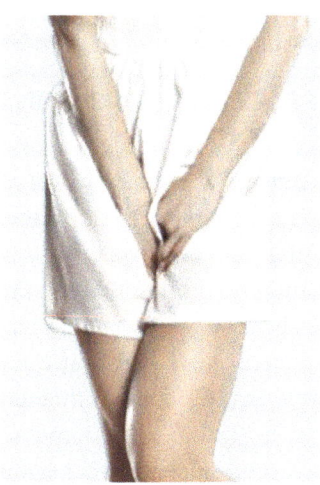

Fig. 1: A woman with "her unspoken problems".

ETIOLOGY OF AGEING ON THE FEMALE GENITALIA

The most significant change is the biological ageing of connective tissue. Matrix component also undergoes postsynthetic modifications and proteolytic degradations. Oxidative stress and environmental factors further increase the matrix metalloproteins (MMPs), which lead to degradation of collagen, elastin fibers and proteoglycans.

With age, advanced glycation end-products (AGEs) accumulate and modify the cross linking of collagen fibrils, making the tissues stiff with impaired flexibility, and compromised function.

There is an atrophy of the following:

Vulva: It appears pale, dry, and dry with reduction of adipose tissue of the labia majora. The prepuce and clitoris also decrease in size. The introitus is narrow and friable.

Vagina: The changes in the vagina are relatively more profound. The vaginal walls show loss of rugosity, tenderness, and patchy edema. The vaginal mucosal changes lead to decreased vascularity and dryness, lower glycogen, higher pH and recurrent vaginal infections. Laxity of the vaginal walls may lead to prolapse uterus/rectocele and/or cystocele in turn leading to urinary or rectal problems.

GENITOURINARY SYNDROME OF MENOPAUSE

Genitourinary syndrome of menopause (GSM) is a new term that describes various signs and symptoms associated with decrease in estrogen production during menopause including:

- *Genital symptoms,* such as vaginal dryness, burning, irritation, pricking sensation
- *Sexual symptoms,* such as lack of lubrication, discomfort during intercourse, impaired sexual function, postcoital lacerations
- *Urinary symptoms,* such as urgency, frequency, stress urinary incontinence, burning, dribbling, recurrent UTI.

The term GSM has been coined by The Board of Directors of the International Society for the Study of Women's Sexual Health (ISSWSH) and the Board of the North American Menopause Society (NAMS) in 2014, and it deals with the unspoken anatomical and functional genitourinary issues faced by the ageing woman.

Approximately 50% of postmenopausal and perimenopausal women develop GSM caused by estrogen deficiency. The vasomotor symptoms resolve as time elapses but the genitourinary symptoms often worsen if not addressed.[1] Although these symptoms are not life-threatening, they are progressive and negatively impact the woman's self-esteem and intimacy with their partners.[2]

Despite the valuable information about the prevalence of GSM, very little evidence is available to describe its impact on well-being and function.

The GENISSE study was a multicentric, cross-sectional, descriptive, observational study that involved 430 postmenopausal women who consulted a gynecologist in Spain for any reason between September and October 2015. It found the prevalence of GSM to be approximately 70%. At the time of diagnosis, only 40% of women reported a prior history of vulvovaginal atrophy (VVA) or GSM. Furthermore, GSM was undetected in 60% of cases, being diagnosed when visiting the gynecologist for a routine visit.[3]

The recently published Clarifying Vaginal Atrophy's Impact on Sex and Relationships (CLOSER) study found that vaginal discomfort had a direct, negative impact on the intimacy of both partners (women: 58%; men: 78%) and resulted in a loss of libido (64% and 52%, respectively). Overall, 38% of women and 39% of their male partners reported that vaginal symptoms had a worse-than-expected impact on their intimate relationships.[4]

In the REal Women's VIews of Treatment Options for Menopausal Vaginal ChangEs (REVIVE) survey, women reported that their vaginal symptoms negatively affected enjoyment of sexual activity (59%), sleep (24%), and overall enjoyment of life (23%).[5]

Furthermore, GSM may also occur in other hypoestrogenic states including hypothalamic amenorrhea, surgical menopause, use of gonadotropin-releasing hormone (GnRH) agonists, or because of cancer treatments such as chemotherapy, pelvic radiation, or endocrine therapy.[6] This patient demographic is usually a relatively younger age group in whom the quality of life is greatly compromised. Addressing GSM in them has become an increasingly important issue.

LATEST PROCEDURES IN VAGINAL REJUVENATION

Recently new, noninvasive, energy-based systems are a welcome development for the many women wary of surgery due to the risk, expense, and downtime involved **(Table 1)**. These devices have opened up a new market for nonsurgical vulvovaginal correction procedures. But before we discuss these devices, as clinical aestheticians, we must follow a few criteria for patient selection, which are as follows:

TABLE 1: Spectrum of procedures in aesthetic gynecology.

Functional	Anatomical	
	Surgical	Nonsurgical
• Vaginal rejuvenation • Vaginal tightening • Enhancement of sexual gratification • Stress urinary incontinence • Lichen sclerosis • Vulvodynia	• Female genital cosmetic surgery (FGCS) • Perineoplasty • Himenoplasty • Labiaplasty • Pubis liposuction • Clitoral hood reduction • Labia majora filling • Genital wart removal • Combination of surgeries	• Perineal whitening • Perineal chemical peels • Perineal skin resurfacing • Episeotomy scar lightening • Perineal skin anti-wrinkle treatment

Today we have Lasers and Designer Laser Vaginoplasty® (DLV®), a procedure in the USA. The Laser Vaginal Rejuvenation Institute of America (LVRIA) claims that only physicians trained at LVRIA are certified to perform DLV®. DLV® is a group of procedures which repair, enhance and beautify the external genitalia of the female. These procedures are known as labiaplasty, perineoplasty, and hymenoplasty.

Many other vulval and vaginal procedures are now possible. Lasers introduced by FemiLift Alma can now treat many of "her unspoken problems".

- After delivery vaginal realignment
- Vaginal toning and lubrication
- Perimenopausal vaginal dryness and dyspareunia
- Urine leak (Stress urinary incontinence)
- Mild prolapse (First and second degree)
- Sexual enhancement therapy
- Aesthetic vulval rejuvenation and whitening

It is a simple, short, noninvasive procedure which gives high success rates.

PRETREATMENT EVALUATION

- Written and informed consent
- Detailed counseling about the treatment modality, its cost, long-term and short-term effect and side effects
- Elaborate history and patient interaction
- Full medical, pelvic and obstetrics report
- Detailed pelvic examination to examine the cervix, vaginal, uterus and adnexa
- Evaluation of vaginal laxity
- Evaluate any cystocele/rectocele and grade according to POP-Q classification
- Vaginal health index (VHI) questionnaire
- Detailed pelvic ultrasound
- PAP smear
- Pregnancy test
- Cough test

CONTRAINDICATIONS

- Active HPV/HSV
- VIN findings
- Acute vaginitis
- Genital malignancy
- Uncontrolled vaginal bleeding
- Pregnancy
- Recent vaginal injury/bleeding
- Patients on menstrual periods
- Patients with body dysmorphic syndrome
- Patients with unrealistic expectations

FRACTIONAL CO_2 LASER

The Pixel CO_2 fractional laser and its principle for vaginal treatment are shown in **Figures 2A and B**.

Effective Mechanism

The mechanism of action of lasers goes through three phases: the first 48–72 hours is where the thermal damage causes shrinkage of collagen followed by proliferation of new collagen fibers over the next 30 days.

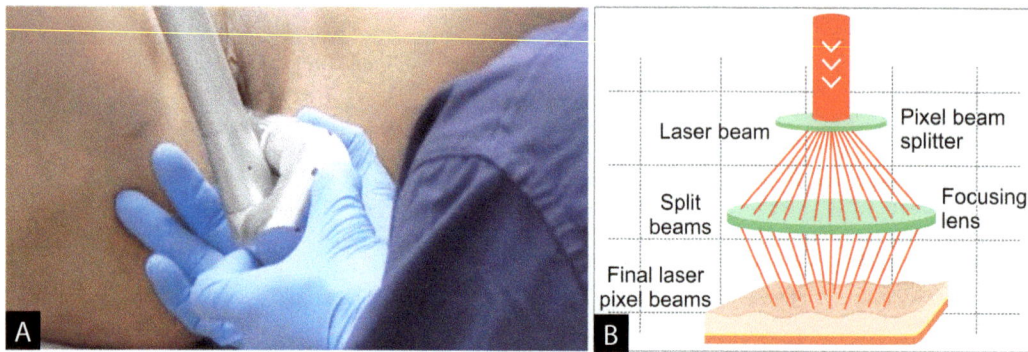

Figs. 2A and B: The Pixel CO_2 fractional laser treatment and its principle.

The collagen fibers mature and new elastic fibers form in the last 3–6 months of remodeling.

Protocol: 3–4 sittings @ 4–5 passes per sitting; 4 weeks apart.

Note: The treatment protocol must be customized according to the case.

THE ER:YAG LASER

Wavelength: 2,940 nm

Principle: Nonablative heating + superficial thermal damage to the vaginal mucosa

Effective mechanism: Erbium is highly absorbed in the water content of the vaginal mucosa itself, hence the thermal injury it creates is much lower than CO_2 fractional laser, which means lower collagen stimulation **(Fig. 3)**.

It has a "smooth" mode technology which delivers pulsatile energy to the vaginal mucosal tissue in 100 milliseconds resulting in nonablative heating.

Protocol: 3–4 sittings 4 weeks apart.

Note: The treatment protocol must be customized according to the case.

Post-treatment Advice

- No sexual activity for at least 2–3 days
- Intravaginal hyaluronic acid for 7 days
- Adequate hydration

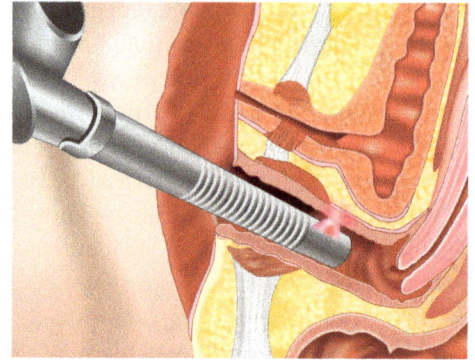

Fig. 3: Erbium:YAG laser 360° scanning scope.

- Take oral vitamin C supplements for the next 4–6 months
- Kegel exercises
- There might be slight blood stained discharge in about 45% of the patients in the early 3–5 days
- Reassurance

RADIOFREQUENCY-BASED DEVICES

Radiofrequency-based device is shown in **Figure 4** (Thermi Aesthetics RF device).

Effective Mechanism: Focused electromagnetic waves generate heat upon meeting tissue impedance.

Advantages over Lasers

- No downtime
- Greater ablative depth + three-dimensional and targeted thermal effect

- Less painful
- More effective for labial and introital skin rejuvenation and/or pigmentation
- Depth of penetration: 3-5 mm
- Safe for all skin types

Protocol: 3-4 sittings 4 weeks apart. Average treatment duration is 15-30 min per sitting.

Clinical endpoint: Targeted tissue temperature of 40-45°C for approximately 3-4 minutes per zone (or longer, depending on tissue tolerance). The next step is to target the mucosal surface of the introitus from the hymenal ring and advancing inwards up to 4-9 cm.

Note: The treatment protocol must be customized according to the case.

HIGH-INTENSITY FOCUSED ULTRASOUND

The principle of high-intensity focused ultrasound (HIFU) is described in **Figure 5**.

Action occurs in two phases: Initial lift and delayed sustained lift (in which effect lasts up to a year).

Protocol: 3-4 sittings 4 weeks apart.

Note: The treatment protocol must be customized according to the case.

ADVANTAGES OF LASERS/RADIOFREQUENCY

- Depth of penetration: 4-4.5 mm
- A thermal effect of 60° is generated in the coagulation zone in the form of dots without damaging the mucosal surface.
- Lifting and tightening effect is seen on the relaxing zone
- Noninvasive
- No bleeding
- No trauma

THE CONTROVERSY ABOUT ENERGY-BASED DEVICES

The use of energy-based devices for vaginal rejuvenation, a practice that sparked a recent safety communication from the US Food and Drug Administration (FDA), was implicated in nearly four dozen adverse event reports

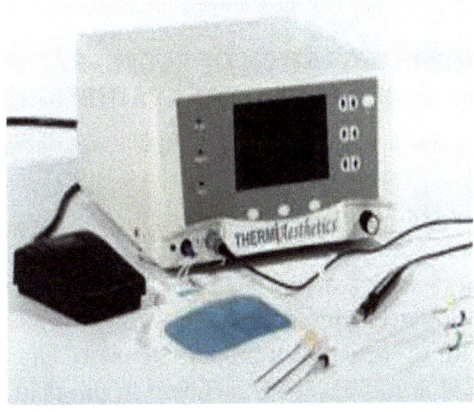

Fig. 4: Thermi aesthetics RF device.

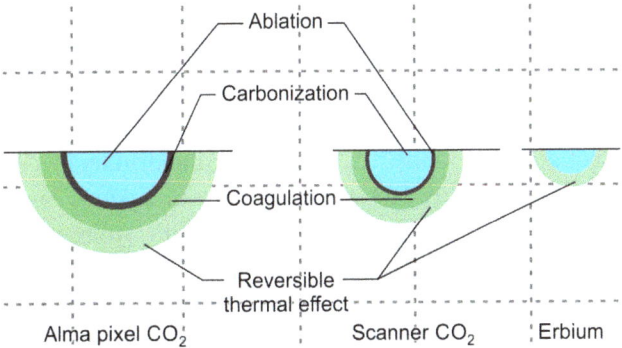

Fig. 5: Principle of high-intensity focused ultrasound.

TABLE 2: Comparison of energy-based devices in aesthetic gynecology.

(a) Laser (Light amplification by the stimulated emission of radiation) Diode laser Er:YAG laser carbon dioxide (CO_2)	Working principle: • Angiogenesis • Microvascularization • Tissue oxygenation • Tissue lubrication • Tissue sensitivity

(b) Radiofrequency-based devices

Monopolar	Bipolar	Multipolar

(c) HIFU (High-intensity focused ultrasound)

Guided waves	Shear waves

found in the agency's medical device adverse event reporting database **(Table 2)**.

The 45 unique event reports, submitted to the FDA during October 2015–January 2019, described 46 patients in total, of whom 33 reported long-term effects including pain, numbness, and burning. They included 31 that were reported by the patients, eight reported by the manufacturer; four reported by the distributor, and two not specified.

These findings highlight the need for randomized control trials to evaluate the safety and efficacy of the energy based devices that have been marketed and used for so-called vaginal rejuvenation procedures. In July 2018, the FDA issued a *safety communication* that the safety and effectiveness of energy-based devices has not been established for procedures described as "vaginal rejuvenation".

In a November 2018 update, the FDA had contacted some device manufacturers to express concerns that the devices were being marketed inappropriately and the manufacturers they had contacted so far "responded with adequate corrections."

Pain was the most commonly adverse event, accounting for 19 reports in the FDA analysis, while 11 patients reported numbness or burning.

Among the laser- and energy-based devices specifically described in the 39 patient-report injuries, the MonaLisa Touch® had the highest number of adverse event reports.

In light of these findings, the authors advised clinicians to ask patients about their reasons for seeking vaginal rejuvenation procedures, and that it must be undertaken in absolutely needed indications only.

THE INTEGRATION OF REGENERATIVE MEDICINE IN VAGINAL AESTHETICS

There are three components essential for tissue regeneration:
1. Cells
2. Growth factors
3. Scaffold

Platelet-rich plasma (PRP) provides two out of three components (growth factors and scaffold) and is included in the field of regenerative medicine.

Vaginal rejuvenation using PRP is a recent innovation in the field of sexual medicine. Here, the patient's own platelets are used to increase sensitivity and improve sexual health. It can also be used in women who suffer from urinary incontinence.

The procedure involves injecting the PRP into the suburethral region for urinary problems or into the clitoris and upper vaginal wall for enhanced vaginal hydration leading to sexual enhancement. This acts by release of growth factors which promote collagen and elastin production thus causing tissue hypertrophy.

The treatment effect is noticed immediately by women who have urinary incontinence but after 3-6 weeks for sexual health issues. The efficacy of the injection lasts for up to a year and is dependent on various lifestyle factors. They usually require a single top up sitting after a year.

What are the Benefits of PRP for Vaginal Rejuvenation?

- Renew sexual intimacy
- Improved functionality of vagina
- Increase libido
- No more painful intercourse
- No more leaking of urine

CONCLUSION

With the increasing life expectancy, it is projected that women spend one-third of their life in the postmenopausal phase, necessitating substantial amount of care for her.

The field of Aesthetic and Regenerative Gynecology is a fresh and emerging field specifically addressing "Her Unspoken Problems".

The need for more multicenter and transnational studies must be emphasized, in order to get more evidence and confidence regarding the various energy-based treatment modalities.

REFERENCES

1. Sturdee DW, Panay N. Recommendations for the management of postmenopausal vaginal atrophy. Climacteric. 2010;13:509-22.
2. Nappi RE, Kokot-Kierepa M. Vaginal health: insights, views and attitudes (VIVA)—results from an international survey. Climacteric. 2012;15:36-44.
3. Moral E, Delgado JL, Carmona F, Caballero B, Guillán C, González PM, et al. Genitourinary syndrome of menopause. Prevalence and quality of life in Spanish postmenopausal women. The GENISSE study. Climacteric. 2018;21:167-73.
4. Nappi RE, Kingsberg S, Maamari R, Simon J. The CLOSER (CLarifying Vaginal Atrophy's Impact On SEx and Relationships) survey: implications of vaginal discomfort in postmenopausal women and in male partners. J Sex Med. 2013;10:2232-41.
5. Kingsberg SA, Wysocki S, Magnus L, Krychman ML. Vulvar and vaginal atrophy in postmenopausal women: findings from the REVIVE (REal Women's VIews of Treatment Options for Menopausal Vaginal ChangEs) survey. J Sex Med. 2013;10:1790-9.
6. The North American Menopause Society. Management of symptomatic vulvovaginal atrophy: 2013 position statement of the North American Menopause Society. Menopause. 2013;20:888-902.

Index

Page numbers followed by *b* refer to box, *f* refer to figure, *fc* refer to flowchart, and *t* refer to table

A

Abdomen 35, 118
    examination 29
    ultrasound of 102
Abdominal apical suspension
        procedures 185
Abdominal leak point pressure 49
Abdominal procedure 185
    concomitant 73
Abdominal uterosacral ligament
        suspension 182, 185, 189
Acupuncture 59
Adhesions 129
Adnexal mass 153
Aesthetic gynecology 222*t*
Aesthetic vaginal surgery 209
Albumin, serum 21
Albuminuria 22
Ambulatory urodynamics
        monitoring 43, 50, 51
American Association for Surgery of
        Trauma 122
American College of Obstetricians and
        Gynecologists 162, 209
American Society of Plastic
        Surgeons 209
American Urological Association
        30, 80, 108
Analgesia, regional 136
Anesthesia 60, 62, 108, 186, 189, 197
    general 68
    local 68
    regional 68
Angiogenesis 222
Angiotensin converting enzyme
        inhibitors 55
Anterior mesh placement 187
Anterior sacrospinous suspension
        technique 168
Anterior vaginal wall
    closure of 76*f*
    cyst of 153
    dissection of 187
    prolapse 151, 151*f*, 152, 195*f*
Antibiotic prophylaxis 108
Anticholinergic 85
    agents 58
Anticipatory pelvic floor
        contractions 59

Anti-incontinence sling surgeries 112
Antimicrobial prophylaxis 99, 108*t*
Apex, reconstruction of 198
Apical suspension
        procedures 156*f*, 165
Arcus tendineus fascia
        pelvis 6, 10*f*, 167
Augment apical suspension 165, 172
Augmentation cystoplasty 86
Autologous fascial sling 72, 77, 78*f*, 80
Autologous retropubic midurethral
        sling 79
Autologous transobturator
        midurethral sling 79

B

Bacteria 21
    promote colonization of 97
Baden-Walker halfway scoring
        system 152
Behavioral therapies 58, 82
Bifid
    collecting system 36
    ureter 36
Bilateral iliococcygeus fascia
        suspension 169, 169*f*
Bile salts 22
Bilirubin 22
Birth injury 150
Bladder 26, 51, 68, 113, 140
    autoaugmentation of 86
    catheterization 117
    compliance 27
    contractions 82
    diary 82
    diverticula 112
    emptying requires 42
    examination of 111
    function 27, 82
    hypocontractility 47*f*
    injury 111, 117, 119, 129, 130, 132*f*
        location of 130*t*
        prevention of 132
        recognition of 130
        repair of 131
        risk factors for 129, 129*b*
        timing of 130, 130*t*
    innervation 42*f*
    lesions 112

    neck 111
    neoplasm 98
    neurogenic 38*f*
    outlet obstruction 93*f*
    overactive 84*f*, 92, 138
    perforation 79
    pillars 18
    sensation 27
    stones 98
    training 59, 82
    visualization of 107
    wall
        ipsilateral side of 126
        irregular thickening of 31*f*
        thickness 38
Bleeding 113
    complications 187
Blood 22
    examination of 20, 21, 24
    sugar 57
    urea nitrogen 154
Board of North American
        Menopause Society 218
Boari flap 126, 126*f*
Body, perineal 153
Bony pelvis 5*f*
Botulinum toxin 85
    injection of 96
    intravesical 85
Breisky-Navratil retractors 167
Broad ligament fibroids 115
Burch colposuspension 6, 62
Burch sutures, placement of 63*f*

C

Calcium 23
Candidal infections 55
Cardiac failure, congestive 55
Cardinal ligament 18
Casts 21
Catheter 44
    externalized 108
    types of 45*f*
Cell 222
    therapy method 200
Cellulitis 55
Central nervous system 55, 85
Cervical
    cytology 153
    fibroids 115

Index

stroma 18
stump 198f
Cervix, congenital elongation of 153
Cesarean delivery 129
  previous 129
Cesarean section 129, 136
Chemical
  analysis 20, 22t
  peels, perineal 219
Chest X-ray 154
Chloride 23
Chronic obstructive pulmonary
    disease 55, 185
Ciprofloxacin 99, 108
Clean intermittent
    catheterization 73, 136
  self-catheterization 84, 94, 95f
Clitoral hood 212
  reduction 211, 212, 212f, 219
Coccygeus-sacrospinous ligament
    complex 166
Colpocleisis 158f, 159f
  total 158
Colpoperineoplasty 212, 213f
Colpoperineorrhaphy,
    posterior 157, 178
Colpopexy, sacrospinous 156f
Colporrhaphy
  anterior 155, 157, 157f
  posterior 155, 157f
Combination therapy 85
Comorbidity, history of 28
Complete blood count 154
Complete urethral obstruction 107
Complex neuropathic bladder
    dysfunction 146
Compression 34
Computed tomography scan 35, 93
Connective tissue 18
Conservative treatment 144
Constipation 98
Continuous antibiotic
    prophylaxis 99
Cooper's ligament 5, 6, 18
Corticosteroid 108
Cosmetic vaginal surgery 209
Cosmeto-plastic gynecology 209
Cotton swab test 57
Cough
  chronic 55
  test 219
Crawford fascial stripper 78
Crystals 21
Cystitis 136
  acute 137
  complicated 99

recurrent 31f
  uncomplicated 99
Cystocele 40
  formation 9f
Cystogram 31f
Cystometry 43, 48
Cystoplasty 86
Cystoscope
  flexible 109, 110
  sheath 109, 109f
  types of 109
Cystoscopic-guided ureteric
    catheterization 116f
Cystoscopy 29, 58, 61, 76f, 93, 98,
    107, 108, 111, 112, 118f,
    119, 120f, 123, 188, 190
  basics of 107
  use of 112
Cystotomy 107, 131b
  intentional 118
Cystourethroscope, flexible 111f
da Vinci robotic system 204, 204f
  components of 205
  parts of 204

D

Darifenacin 58, 85
Deep perineal reflexes 153
Deep tendon reflexes 56
Depression 55
Detrusor
  instability, stress-induced 57
  myomectomy, partial 86
  pressure 48, 49
Diabetes mellitus 28, 55
Diarrhea 98
Dietary modifications 59
Diode laser 222
Distal ureteral calculus 102f
Distant coexistent infection 108
Diverticulum
  acquired 39
  congenital 39
  formation 146
Dorsal lithotomy position 68
Double collecting system 36
Double lens laparoscope 205f
Double ureter 36
Double-kink sign 103f
Duplex kidney 36
Dye testing 29
Dyspareunia 69, 146, 157, 219
Dysuria 98
  symptoms of 137

E

Electrical stimulation 59, 86
Electrocardiography 154
Electrolytes, serum 22
Electromyography 43, 49, 93, 94
Emergency delivery 129
E-mesenchymal stem cells 201f
Endocrine therapy 218
Endometrial mesenchymal stem 201
Endopelvic fascia, hammock of 12
Episeotomy scar lightening 219
Episode, acute 99
Epithelial cells 21
Erbium:YAG laser 220
  360° scanning scope 220f
  carbon dioxide 222
Escherichia coli 39, 98, 99
Estrogen 58
Excretory system, duplication of 36f
Extended-spectrum
    beta-lactamase 137
Extracorporeal magnetic resonance
    therapy 59

F

Fascia lata 77, 78, 78f, 79
  pubovaginal sling 62
  suburethral sling 62
Fascial repair, anterior 177
Fat 18
Fecal incontinence 98
Fecaluria 98
Female cosmetic genital surgery
    194, 209, 215, 219
  emerging functional role of 194
Feminizing genital reconstructions
    surgery 141
Fesoterodine 58
Fever 131
Fibrin glue, use of 146
Fibrinogen 21
Fibroid 153
Fistula 40, 140
  classification systems 143
  iatrogenic 140
  postpartum 40
  urogenital 140f
Flank pain 98
Fluoroscopy 43
Foley bulb
  appearance of 131
  visualization of 118
Foley catheter 68, 74, 76, 77
  intraperitoneal 118f

Index

Fowler's syndrome 94f, 96
Fractional CO_2 laser 219
Fractures 55
Fulcrum effect, elimination of 208

G

Genital hiatus 153
Genital malignancy 219
Genital prolapse 150
Genital symptoms 218
Genital wart removal 219
Genitalia, female 210, 213, 217
Genitourinary fistula
   identification of 140
   management of 140
Globulin, serum 21
Glomerular filtration rate 24, 101
   measurement of 24
Glucose 22
Goh's classification system 144
Gonadotropin-releasing hormone
   agonists 218
Granulomas 146
Growth factors 222

H

Hand tremor, elimination of 208
Hematuria 98, 118, 131
Hemoglobin 22
Hemorrhage 68
Hiatus urogenitalis 153
High-intensity focused ultrasound 221, 222
   principle of 221, 221f
High-uterosacral ligament
   suspension 165, 175
Himenoplasty 219
Hormone replacement therapy 28, 95, 154
Horseshoe kidney 36f
Hyaluronic acid 213
Hydrodissection 167f
Hydronephrosis 102f
   gestational 101
Hydroureteronephrosis 37, 37f
Hymen 210
Hymenoplasty 214, 214f
Hypercalcemia 23
Hyperchloremia 23
Hyperkalemia 23
Hypernatremia 23
   euvolemic 23
   hypervolemic 23
   hypovolemic 23

Hyperphosphatemia 23
Hypersensitivity 26
Hypocalcemia 23
Hypochloremia 23
Hypokalemia 23
Hypomagnesemia 23
Hyponatremia 23
   hypervolemic 23
   hypovolemic 23
Hypophosphatemia 23
Hysterectomy 160, 190
   abdominal 123f
   laparoscopic 207
   robotic 207
Hysteropexy 196
   procedures 196
   sacrospinous 196

I

Ileal ureter 127f
Ileum, arcuate rim of 17
Ileus 131
Iliac artery, internal 18
Iliococcygeus fascia 170
Iliopectineal ligament 5f, 198f
   fixation 192f
Inadvertent cystotomy, urological
   assessment of 131fc
Incision 186, 189
Incontinence 40, 98
   types of 27t
Indocyanine green 207
Indwelling catheter drainage 144
Infections 112
   persistent 99
Infertility 146
Injury
   iatrogenic 1
   mechanism of 114, 122
   perineal 136
   prevention of 119
   site of 114
International Consultation on
   Incontinence Committee 138
International Continence Society 53, 67, 135
   classification 27t
   Female Lower Urinary Tract
   Symptoms 88
International Federation of
   Gynaecology and
   Obstetrics with
   International Society of
   Obstetric Fistula
   Surgeon 144

International Prostate Symptom
   Score 89, 89t
International Society for Study of
   Women's Sexual Health 218
Intestine 140
Intravenous indigo carmine 122
Intravesical pressure 48
Intrinsic sphincter deficiency 53, 54, 72
Invasive urodynamic 44
   evaluation, indications of 47

J

Joel-Cohen and Misgav-Ladach
   methods 130

K

Kegel's exercises 58
Kelleher questionnaire 55
Kelly's stitch 157
Ketone bodies 22
Kidney 20
   autotransplanted 127f
   normal sonographic appearance
   of 34f

L

Labia
   central wedge of 211
   majora 210, 213, 213f
   majoraplasty 213
   minora 210, 212, 213
Labiaplasty 210, 210f, 219
Labor 129, 130
Laceration, perineal 153
Laparoscopic electrosurgical
   complications 116
Laparoscopic procedure 165, 185
Laparoscopic uterosacral ligament
   suspension 182
Laparoscopy 117f, 118f
Lasers, advantages of 221
Le Fort's colpocleisis 158
   Goodall-power modification of 158
Le Fort's modifications 154
Le Fort's operation 154
Levator
   ani muscle 6f, 18, 195f
   complex 54f
   detachment 7
   muscles 153
Lichen sclerosis 219
Light amplification by stimulated
   emission of radiation 222

Index

Light source 109
Lignocaine gel, local application of 108
Linear edge resection 211
Lower ureteric injury 123*f*
Lower urinary tract 26, 28*t*
　afferent pathways of 11
　symptoms 26, 47, 88, 98, 146
Lumbar sympathetic nerves 10
Lynch syndrome 161

M

Mackenrodt's complex 171*f*, 172*f*
Mackenrodt's ligament 171, 172
Magnesium 23
Magnetic resonance imaging 31, 33, 35, 93, 102, 103, 194
Malignancy 39
Manchester operation 154
Marshall and Boney's test 57
Master-Slave system 204
Matrix metalloproteins 217
Maximum urethral closure pressure 50, 50*f*
McCall culdoplasty 158, 165, 170, 170*f*, 171, 172
　modified 171
　technique of 171
McCall procedure 172
McCall sutures 171
　external 171
　internal 171
McGuire's technique 72
Meatal stenosis 47*f*
Medical therapy 82
Medicolegal issues 92
Menopause, genitourinary syndrome of 217
Menstrual periods 219
Mesh 156*f*
　erosion 188
　placement 187, 188
Methylene blue dye 122
Metzenbaum scissors 68
Michigan four-wall technique 168
Microvascularization 222
Micturition, dynamics of 42
Midurethral complex deficiency 72
Midurethral sling 60, 73
　placement, types of 60*f*
Minimally invasive sacrocolpopexy 189, 198
Mirabegron 85
Mixed urinary incontinence 63, 72

Mons pubis 210, 214
　reduction 214
Mons veneris 214
Movement, enhanced range of 208
Multipara, risk factors in 150
Muscles forming pelvic floor 6
Myelodysplasia 72
Myomectomy, Robotic 206, 207

N

Native tissue repair 200
Natural orifice transluminal endoscopic surgery 199
Nephrogram 34
Nephrographic phase 5*f*, 35
Nephrolithotomy, percutaneous 105
Nephrostomy, percutaneous 124, 124*f*
Neurogenic incontinence 72
Neurogenic lower urinary tract symptoms 51
Neurological disorders 43, 92
Neuromodulation 95
Nifedipine 104
Nitrite 22
Nocturia 98
Non-antimicrobial prophylaxis 99
Non-contrast computed tomography 35, 102
Noninvasive tests 43
Noninvasive urodynamics 45
Nonsteroidal anti-inflammatory drugs 103
Nonsurgical cosmetic vulvovaginal procedures 214
Normal sonographic appearance 33, 34*f*
Normal uroflowmetry
　curve 46, 46*f*
　graph 91*f*
Nulliparous prolapse 150

O

Obesity 55, 115
Obliterative procedures 158, 159*f*
Obliterative surgery 158
Obstetric fistula 138, 140, 143
Obstructive lower urinary tract symptoms 88
　causes of 88*t*
Obturator internus 18
　fascia 6, 6*f*
One-hour pad test 29*b*
Onuf's nucleus 11
Operative injuries 138
Oral contraceptive pills 28

Ovarian cysts 115
Overflow incontinence 88
Oxybutynin 58

P

Packed cell volume 25
Pad tests 29
Pain management 103
Para-aminohippuric acid 25
Paracervix 15, 18
Parametrium 15, 18
Pararectal space 15, 18
Paraurethral bulking agents 63
Paravaginal defect 10*f*
Paravesical spaces 15, 17, 18*f*
Patch slings 62
Pectineal ligament
　anatomy of 192*f*
　hysteropexy 197
Pectopexy 185, 191, 197
Pelvic fascia 8
Pelvic floor 5, 135
　dysfunction 6, 194
　examination 56
　exercises 82
　map 152*f*
　muscle training 58, 59, 84, 138
　repair 199
　supporting pelvic organs 59*f*
Pelvic hypogastric plexus, formation of 11*f*
Pelvic mass 118
Pelvic medicine, female 30, 194
Pelvic nerves, importance of 10
Pelvic node lymphadenectomy 206
Pelvic organ 32*f*
　prolapse 55, 150, 152, 154, 155*t*, 165, 175, 176*f*, 185, 194, 197, 201
　　after surgery, recurrence of 163
　　burden 150
　　etiology of 150
　　examination of 153*b*
　　functional anatomy of 194
　　management of 154
　　pessary treatment of 154, 154*b*
　　prophylaxis of 154
　　quantification system 150, 153
　　risk factors for 150, 150*b*
　　surgery 195
　　symptoms of 150, 151*b*
　　types of 151, 151*b*
　　vaginal repair 201*f*
Pelvic reconstructive surgery 198, 200, 201
　tissue engineering for 200

Index

Pelvic repair 194
Pelvic retroperitoneum 14
Pelvic ureter 1, 15, 18, 19f
  course of 1, 1f
  crossing uterine artery 2f
Pelvic viscera 15f
Pelvic walls 18
Pelvis 35, 181f
  female 15
  ultrasound of 102
Perineal skin
  anti-wrinkle treatment 219
  resurfacing 219
Perineal whitening 219
Perineoplasty 212, 213f, 219
  postoperative 196f
  preoperative 196f
Perineorrhaphy 155
Perineum, sensation of 56
Peripheral nervous system 10
Peritoneal cavity 131
Peritoneal closure 188
Peritoneal incision 186
Peritonitis 131
Pessary 156f
Pfannenstiel method 130
Pharmacotherapy 95
Phosphates 23
Plasma clearance 24
Plasma proteins, estimation of 21
Platelet rich plasma 213, 222
Plexuses, importance of 10
Pneumaturia 98, 118
Polyp 153
Polypropylene suture 78
Poor urinary stream 88
Port placement 189
Postcoital prophylaxis 99
Posterior abdominal wall, muscles
  of 16f
Posterior vaginal wall 10f, 151, 172f
  deflection 167f
  dissection of 187
  prolapse 151f, 152, 157
Post-hysterectomy vault prolapse
  165
Postvoid residual urine 30, 43, 46
Potassium 23
Pregnancy 219
  test 219
Pressure 48
  abdominal 48
  flow study 43, 49

Prolapse 40
  anterior 161
  apical 152f
  posterior 161
Prolene sutures, retrieval of 76f
Prophylaxis management 99
Protein 22
  total 21
Proteinuria 22
Psoas hitch 126
Pubic bone 7f
Pubis liposuction 219
Pubocervical fascia 8, 8f, 9f, 17,
  177, 177f
  detachment of 9f, 10f
Puborectalis 7f
  detachment 7f
  unilateral 7f
  sling 6f
Pubourethral ligament supporting
  proximal urethra 54f
Pubovaginal sling 62, 72, 80
  surgery 64
Push and spread technique 74
Pyelogram 34
Pyelography, intravenous 36f, 116
Pyelonephritis 137, 146
Pyeloureterography, retrograde 123,
  123f

R

Radiation 141
Radical hysterectomy, Robot
  enabled 206
Radiofrequency 220-222
Randomized controlled trial 146
Reconstructive surgery 158, 160, 194
Rectal catheter 45
Rectal prolapse 153
Rectocele 40
Rectovaginal fascia 8f, 9, 10f, 177,
  177f
Rectovaginal fistula 140f
Rectovaginal septum 14, 16, 17f
Rectum 140
Rectus fascia
  pubovaginal sling 62
  suburethral sling 62
Rectus sheath
  closure of 77f
  defattening of 73f
Red blood cells 21

Regenerative medicine, integration
  of 222
Renal autotransplantation 127
Renal blood flow 24, 25
  calculation of 25
  measurement of 25
Renal disease 24
Renal function
  assessment of 20
  tests 20, 22, 24t
Renal plasma flow 24, 25
  measurement of 25
Retention
  acute 88
  risk factors for 135
Retroperitoneum 14, 14f, 15f
Retropubic sling placement 61f
Retropubic space dissection 75f
  initial steps of 75f
Retropubic space of Retzius 15, 17,
  17f, 74
Rigid cystoscope 109, 111
  parts of 109
Robotic gynecological oncology 207
Robotic procedure 165, 185
Robotic surgery 206, 207
  advantages of 208
  disadvantages of 208
  fundamentals of 208
Robotic systems, alternative 208
Robotic vesicovaginal fistula repair
  206, 207f
Royal College of Obstetricians and
  Gynaecologists 135, 209

S

Sacral
  agenesis 72
  colpopexy 156f
  neuromodulation 86
  parasympathetic
    nerves 10
    pathway 10
  suture
    placement of 187
    site, selection of 186
Sacrocolpopexy 160, 165, 185, 185f,
  189, 199, 206f
  abdominal 154, 155, 160, 178,
    185, 198
  laparoscopic 156f, 160b
  robotic 199, 206, 207
Sacrohysteropexy, abdominal 197

Sacrospinous fixation 155, 198
Sacrospinous ligament 5f, 167f
    anatomy of 166f
    suspension 165, 166, 168f, 178
Sacrum 18
    structure of 16f
Serotonin norepinephrine reuptake inhibitor 58
Sexual dysfunction 55, 146
Sexual enhancement therapy 219
Sexual gratification, enhancement of 219
Shirodkar's operation 154
Shock wave lithotripsy 105
Sims' speculum 153
Single ureter 36
Skene's gland abscess 98
Skin 140
    irritation 55
Sling, tension-free fixation of 77f
Sodium 23
    fluorescein 120f
Solifenacin 58, 85
Somatic efferent pathway 11
Somatic pudendal nerves 10
Sonography 37
Space of Retzius 18, 68
Speculum examination 153
Sphincter 51
Spinal cord
    injury 72
    issues 55
Squamous cell carcinoma 40
Stamey needle 77, 78f
Stress urinary incontinence 6, 11, 28, 51, 53, 54, 67, 72, 146, 157, 219
    causes of 137
    management of 53, 67
    prevalence of 137
    primary 70
    surgery for 92
Stromal cells 201
Suburethral sling surgery 141
Sulfamethoxazole 108
Superficial perineal reflexes 153
Superior pedicle flap rotation 211
Suprapubic bruising 118
Surgery 122
    combination of 219
    contraindications for 214
    previous abdominal 129
    principle of 144
    route of 145
    timing of 145
Surgical cosmetic procedures 210
Surgical therapy 86
Surgical treatment 95, 144
Sutures, placement of 177f, 190
Synthetic mesh erosion 73

T

Tamsulosin 104
Telescope 109, 110
    lenses 110t
Tension-free vaginal tape 60, 67, 70, 72
Thoracolumbar sympathetic pathways 10
Three swab test 141, 142f
Tibial nerve stimulation, posterior 86
Tissue
    flaps 146
    lubrication 222
    oxygenation 222
    sensitivity 222
Tolterodine 58, 85
Transabdominal procedures 165
Transobturator tape 62
    procedure 70
    sling 61
Transobturator tension-free vaginal tape 71
Transureteroureterostomy 126, 126f
Transvaginal high uterosacral ligament suspension procedures, outcome of 179t
Transvaginal mesh
    placement 165
    use of 202
Transvaginal natural orifice transluminal endoscopic surgery 199
Transvaginal procedures 160
Trauma 141
    psychological 146
Trimethoprim 108
Trocar placement 206
Trospium 58, 85
Tubo-ovarian mass 115
Tumor 153
Typical 3-day frequency volume chart 90t

U

Ultrasonography 30, 92, 154
    transabdominal 102f
Umbilical folds, lateral 17
Upper genitourinary tract 33
Upper tract
    imaging 98
    instrumentation 108
Urea clearance test 25
Ureter 114
    anatomy of 181f
    duplex 4
    identification of 181
    inserts
        heterotopic 37
        orthotropic 37
    malformations of 4
Ureteral defect 131b
Ureteral injury 107, 112, 115, 180
Ureteral orifice, normal fish mouth opening of 118f
Ureteral reimplantation technique 125f
Ureteric blood supply, surgical significance of 2, 3, 3f
Ureteric fistula, management of 147
Ureteric injury 122, 124f, 138, 141
    incidence of 140
    management of 122
    risk of 140
Ureteric obstruction 146
    management of 178
Ureteric patency, evaluation of 177
Ureteric stenting 124
Ureterocalycostomy 127, 127f
Ureterocele 40
Ureteroneocystostomy 125, 126f
Ureteropelvic junction 102f
Ureteroscopy 103
Ureteroureterostomy 124, 124f
Ureterovesical junction 102f, 103f
Urethra 68, 113
    examination of 111
    visualization of 107
Urethral dilatation 95
Urethral diverticulum 39, 39f, 98, 141, 153
    complications of 39
Urethral function 27
Urethral hypermobility 53, 72
Urethral lumen 39f
Urethral meatus, external 210

Index

Urethral obstruction 92
Urethral occlusive devices 60
Urethral pressure 48, 50
   profile 43, 50
   recording, types of 50
Urethral procedure, concomitant 73
Urethral sphincter
   external 12f
   incompetence 146
Urethral stricture 47f
Urethropelvic angle, measurement
   of 38f
Urethrotomy 95
Urethrovaginal fistula 140f, 141
   management of 147
Urethrovesical junction 62, 111
Urge incontinence 51, 82, 138
Urinalysis 20
Urinary bladder 42, 117f
   dome of 118f
   injuries 129
Urinary calculi, symptomatic 101
Urinary distress inventory 55
Urinary diversion 86
Urinary fistula 98, 140
   initial management pathway of
      145fc
Urinary incontinence 27, 28fc, 36f,
   53, 153
   postpartum 137
   recurrence of 146
   types of 53
Urinary infection
   postpartum 136
   treatment of 155
Urinary issues, postpartum 135
Urinary retention 70, 135
   acute 68
   chronic 135, 153
   postpartum 135
Urinary stasis 88
Urinary stone
   disease 101
   formation 101t
Urinary symptoms 218
Urinary tract 1
   anatomic anomalies of 108
   calculi 101
   infection 55, 88, 107, 146
      active 107
      chronic 55
      complicated 98
      recurrent 30, 97
      risk factors for 97
   injury 107, 114, 147
   involvement 107
   trauma 138
Urine
   analysis 29, 57, 98
   chemical analysis of 22t
   composition of 20
   culture 98
   drainage 118
   examination of 20, 24
   extravasation 131
   leak 219
   microscopic examination of 21t
   obstructed flow of 46f
   physical examination of 21t
   reduce flow of 97
   solid components of 20f
Urobag 131
Urobilinogen 22
Urodynamic
   basics of 42
   contraindications for 43
   prerequisites for 43
   study 30, 58, 80, 92, 94
      clinical applications of 51
Uroflowmetry 43, 45, 90
   abnormal patterns of 46
   machine 43, 44f
   parameters 46f
   patterns 91f
   test 90
Urogenital reconstruction 30
Urogram, intravenous 34t
Urogynecology 5, 10, 33
   robotics in 204
Urolithiasis 55
   diagnosis of 102
   management of 104fc
Uropharmacology 82
Urosepsis 146
Uterine
   descent 151
   incision, Misgav-Ladach
      technique of 130
   preservation 160, 196, 202
   prolapse 160
Uterosacral complex 172f
Uterosacral ligament 8, 155, 158,
   171, 175, 176, 177f, 180,
   189, 190
   anatomy of 190f
   colposuspension 165
   fixation 191f
   suspension 156f, 172, 178, 195f
      robotic-assisted 199
   visualization of 176
Uteroscacral complex 171f
Uterovesical fistula 141, 147
Uterus 115, 197
   preservation of 161
   size of 153

V

Vagina 140, 217
   anatomy of 210
   anterior compartment of 8
   function of 210
   improved functionality of 223
   posterior compartment of 9
Vaginal aesthetics 222
Vaginal apex 177f
Vaginal apical suspension
      procedures 165
Vaginal atrophy 218
Vaginal bleeding 219
   uncontrolled 219
Vaginal cones 59
Vaginal discharge 98
Vaginal dryness, perimenopausal
   219
Vaginal epithelial penetration 188
Vaginal hysterectomy
   laparoscopic-assisted 115
   robotic-assisted 206, 207
Vaginal injury 219
Vaginal length, total 196
Vaginal mesh 172
Vaginal peritoneal closure 188
Vaginal prolapse
   anterior 175
   repair 157
Vaginal rejuvenation 209, 212, 219,
   222, 223
   latest procedures in 218
Vaginal repair
   anterior 155
   posterior 155
Vaginal sacrospinous fixation 198
Vaginal stenosis 146
Vaginal support, Delancey's three
      levels of 185t
Vaginal swab, high 154
Vaginal tightening 219
Vaginal toning 219
Vaginal transperitoneal HUSLS 176
Vaginal uterosacral ligament
      suspension 190
Vaginal wall 195f
   suburethral sling 62

Vaginitis 154, 219
Vaginoplasty 195, 212, 213f
Valsalva maneuver 38
Vault prolapse 152f, 176f
   classification of 152
   prevention of 163
Vesicoureteric junction 38f
Vesicouterine fistula 140f
Vesicovaginal dissection 17f
Vesicovaginal fistula 112, 112f, 140f
Vesicovaginal septum 15, 17
Video cystourethrography 91
Video urodynamics 43, 50
Visceral ligaments 14, 16f
Visceral pelvic fascia 14
Visible detrusor muscle
   laceration 131
Visual urethral dilatation 107
Voiding
   cystourethrogram 30, 31f, 39f, 93
   dysfunction 79, 92
      postoperative 80
   pressure-flow study of 49
Vulva 153, 217
   anatomy of 210
   function of 210
Vulval cyst 153
Vulvar vestibule 210
Vulvodynia 219
Vulvovaginal aesthetic surgery 209
Vulvovaginal atrophy 218

W

Waaldijk's classification system 143
Ward Mayo's hysterectomy 154
Wavelength 220
Wedge resection technique 211
Weigert-Meyer
   law 4
   rule 37
Weight loss 59, 82
White blood cells 21
Wound infection 69, 146

Z

Z- shaped incision 211

EU GSPR Authorised Reprsentative
Logos Europe, 9 rue Nicolas Poussin
1700, La Rochelle, France
Phone: +33 (0) 6 67 93 73 78
E-mail: contact@logoseurope.eu

www.ingramcontent.com/pod-product-compliance
Ingram Content Group UK Ltd.
Pitfield, Milton Keynes, MK11 3LW, UK
UKHW051138270226

468476UK00003B/28